Body, Society, and Nation

HARVARD EAST ASIAN MONOGRAPHS 414

Body, Society, and Nation

*The Creation of Public Health and Urban Culture
in Shanghai*

Chieko Nakajima

Published by the Harvard University Asia Center
Distributed by Harvard University Press
Cambridge (Massachusetts) and London 2018

The Harvard University Asia Center publishes a monograph series and, in coordination with the Fairbank Center for Chinese Studies, the Korea Institute, the Reischauer Institute of Japanese Studies, and other facilities and institutes, administers research projects designed to further scholarly understanding of China, Japan, Vietnam, Korea, and other Asian countries. The Center also sponsors projects addressing multidisciplinary and regional issues in Asia.

Library of Congress Cataloging-in-Publication Data

Names: Nakajima, Chieko, author.
Title: Body, society, and nation : the creation of public health and urban culture in Shanghai / Chieko Nakajima.
Other titles: Harvard East Asian monographs ; 414.
Description: Cambridge, Massachusetts : Published by the Harvard University Asia Center, 2018. | Series: Harvard East Asian monographs ; 414 | Includes bibliographical references and index.
Identifiers: LCCN 2017060558 | ISBN 9780674987173 (hardcover : alk. paper)
Subjects: LCSH: Public health—China—Shanghai—History. | Medical policy—China—Shanghai—History. | Health attitudes—China—Shanghai—History. | Health behavior—China—Shanghai—History. | Shanghai (China)—Civilization—Foreign influences.
Classification: LCC RA528.S48 N35 2018 | DDC 362.10951/132—dc23
LC record available at https://lccn.loc.gov/2017060558

Index by the author

♾ Printed on acid-free paper

Last figure below indicates year of this printing
27 26 25 24 23 22 21 20 19 18

For my parents

Contents

Tables and Figures

Tables

Figures

Acknowledgments

Writing a book is challenging and, at times, even grueling. But it is also a great pleasure. It is exciting, fascinating, and gratifying. Throughout the long and winding road of research and writing, I encountered many friends and teachers who helped and supported me in various ways.

In Japan, the late Nakajima Mineo first kindled my interest in American scholarship on China and East Asia. His advice opened my eyes and inspired me to embark on my journey to China, Taiwan, and the United States.

At the University of Michigan, I was privileged to have a wonderful group of professors. Ann Arbor will always be a very special place for me. The vigorous and creative environment of Ann Arbor and the collective expertise of the Michigan faculty encouraged me to freely explore and develop an interdisciplinary approach to Chinese studies. Foremost, I would like to express my sincere gratitude to my advisor, Ernest Young, for his continuous support, patience, and enthusiasm. His keen insight helped me expand and refine an idea into a theme, a theme into a dissertation, and a dissertation into a book. In addition to his encouragement, the late Albert Feuerwerker, Yi-tsi Mei Feuerwerker, the late Paul Forage, Noriko Kamachi, Martin Pernick, and Leslie Pincus, all provided me invaluable academic input.

In Shanghai, Zhao Nianguo and other devoted staff at the Shanghai Academy of Social Sciences extended me warm hospitality and made all the necessary arrangements for my initial visit to the city. Lu Ming, Luo

Suwen, Ma Jun, and many other scholars generously shared not only their knowledge about Shanghai but also practical skills for conducting research there.

In Taipei, Keng Li-chun, Jane Liau, and other staff of the Center for Chinese Studies of National Central Library were wonderful hosts. They were most welcoming and congenial and made my time in Taipei really productive, enjoyable, and unforgettable. Chen Den-wu, Sean Hsiang-lin Lei, and Lien Ling-ling kindly invited me to their institutions and facilitated my ability to discuss my project with their colleagues and students. I profited immensely from their intellectual stimulation.

I was fortunate to have been able to present parts of this research at various venues, including at several meetings of the Association for Asian Studies, at National Taiwan Normal University, at Academia Sinica, and at the Center for Chinese Studies. I was truly grateful for and enormously benefitted from questions and comments from the audience, panelists, and discussants. Earlier versions of chapters 3 and 4 were published in *Twentieth-Century China* 34, no. 1 (2008): 42–72, and *Twentieth-Century China* 37, no. 3 (2012): 250–74. Portions of them are reproduced with permission from the Johns Hopkins University Press. James Carter, Christopher Reed, and anonymous reviewers for the journal offered criticisms and suggestions, which helped sharpen my thinking. I am also grateful to three anonymous readers for the Harvard University Asia Center. Their constructive and insightful comments helped significantly improve the quality of the manuscript and strengthen my arguments.

I had the distinctive honor of receiving guidance and help from remarkable individuals. I owe a tremendous debt to intellectual and moral support from Paul Ropp and Karen Turner. Their constant advice and encouragement greatly enriched my scholarship and helped me literally "survive." I am also profoundly indebted to Mark Elliott, who inspired me with his inquisitive and critical mind, and to Sophia Lee, who read part of the manuscript and gave me thoughtful feedback. Hsiu-ling Kuo shared her knowledge of history and sense of humor. Special thanks go to Deborah Kisatsky. Without her unflagging support, this book might not have been completed. I am also grateful to Bob Graham for helping me with the publication process of this book and to Cynthia Col for painstakingly editing the manuscript.

My research depended on assistance from dedicated and knowledgeable staff and librarians of several archives and libraries: the Shanghai Municipal Archives, the Shanghai Municipal Library, the Harvard-Yenching Library, the Widener Library of Harvard, Harlan Hatcher Graduate Library of Michigan, Taubman Health Sciences Library of Michigan, the National Diet Library of Japan, the National Central Library of Taiwan, and Academia Historica. It was also made possible by the financial support of the University of Michigan, the Fulbright-Hays Doctoral Dissertation Research Abroad Fellowship, and the Research Grant for Foreign Scholars in Chinese Studies of the Center for Chinese Studies.

Peter Sandusky always made my life interesting and adventurous. My deepest appreciation goes to my parents. Sadly they did not live to see the completion of this book, but they steadily supported me for many years even though they lived on the other side of the earth and seldom saw me.

Abbreviations

CCWEC	Central China Water and Electric Company
CIDH	Chinese Infectious Disease Hospital
CMB	China Medical Board
CMJ	*Chinese Medical Journal*
DSCG	Dispatch from the Shanghai Consulate General to the Ministry of Foreign Affairs
EPC	Epidemic Prevention Committee
FMC	French Municipal Council
GDP	Gross Domestic Product
GK	Gaimushō kiroku
GZHB	*Gezhi huibian*
JCHB	*Jiating changshi huibian*
LMS	London Missionary Society
NHA	National Health Administration
PEPC	Provisional Epidemic Prevention Committee
PHB	public health bureau
PHCC	Patriotic Hygiene Campaign Committee
PHD	Public Health Department
PRC	People's Republic of China
PT	preparation team

PUB   Public Utilities Bureau
PUMC   Peking Union Medical College
RC   residents' committee
SARS   Severe Acute Respiratory Syndrome
SCMS   Shanghai Chinese Medical School
SEH   Shanghai Emergency Hospital
SMA   Shanghai Municipal Archives
SMC   Shanghai Municipal Council
SPH   Shanghai Public Hospital
SSGY   *Shanghai shizheng gaiyao*
SWZ   *Shanghai weishengzhi*
WC   waterworks company
WEC   water and electric company
WG   *Weisheng gongbao*
WHO   World Health Organization
WY   *Weisheng yuekan*

INTRODUCTION

In this book I offer a story of the various ideas, practices, and systems related to health and body in late nineteenth- and early twentieth-century Shanghai. The pursuit of good health loomed large in Chinese political, social, and economic life. Yet, "good health" did not refer simply to the physical well-being of individuals. It had a range of associations—it was a goal of charitable activities, an integral part of Chinese nation-building, a notable outcome of Western medical science, a marker of modern civilization, and a commercial catchphrase. Although the question of how to maintain and improve corporeal health was a private matter, it also raised social issues and invoked national concerns. In this study, through a discussion of these various implications and meanings about body and health, I address the complexity and plurality of China's unfolding modernity.

Over the course of the late nineteenth and early twentieth centuries, with the advent of Western powers, notions about personal hygiene and the private body gradually expanded and came to be linked to and incorporated into broader concepts of public health, national power, and racial strength in China. In her pathbreaking work, Ruth Rogaski examines the Chinese term *weisheng* to illuminate this process and contends that *weisheng*, which originally meant "personal regimen," transformed into public health and hygienic modernity.[1] This transformation was not

1. Rogaski, *Hygienic Modernity*.

unilinear or straightforward. It was further complicated by indigenous medical ideas, preexisting institutions, various social groups, and local cultures and customs.[2] China's hygienic modernity took various forms to adapt to the Chinese environment. In this study I explore many ways the various strata of Shanghai society—from administrators and medical doctors to merchants and consumers—experienced and understood multiple meanings of health and body within their everyday lives. I trace the institutions they established, the rules and regulations they implemented, the practices they brought to the city, and the kinds of merchandise they sold—all as part of an effort to promote their health, seeking to understand how local practices and customs fashioned and constrained public health and, in turn, how hygienic modernity helped shape and develop local cultures and influenced people's behavior and mentalities. Global public health and Shanghai's local culture mutually accommodated and interacted. Together, they facilitated and structured new ideas, practices, and institutions related to health and hygiene.

Shanghai is an ideal setting for this inquiry. From the nineteenth century, with two foreign concessions within its borders, people in Shanghai lived under the shadow and pressure of foreign powers; Westerners introduced new medical institutions, theories, and practices to the city. In spite of this, the Chinese maintained their own jurisdiction and opened their own public health administrations. A tradition of medical philanthropy and a vibrant medical market thrived in the city, long before the arrival of the West, and survived into the 1940s.[3] Western powers created concessions and took advantage of China economically, but they did not impose complete control over China. This lack of a formal colonial structure allowed the Chinese to maintain a flexible and open attitude toward the West. They skillfully adopted a number of Western ideas, systems, and products and appropriated them for their own purposes. Under such circumstances, Shanghai Chinese devised and implemented strategies and methods to protect their physical well-being. The city served as a flexible scaffold and a fertile ground on which they operated medical-care facilities and undertook public health activities.

---

2. Leung and Furth, eds., *Health and Hygiene*; Lei Hsiang-lin, "Weisheng weihe bu shi baowei shengming?"

3. Leung, "Organized Medicine"; Kohama, *Kindai Shanghai no kōkyōsei to kokka*.

Scholars of modern China have made Shanghai probably the best-studied of all Chinese cities. As a treaty port, Shanghai experienced extensive direct contact with the West and Japan. Western arts, literature, and cinema flourished there. Shanghai was an important locus of China's economic and industrial development. It was also the birthplace of the Chinese Communist Party and home to labor activism and higher education. Because of its significance and the abundance of available sources, Shanghai has been a popular research site since the 1990s, and Shanghai studies are well established as a legitimate subfield of Chinese studies. Shanghai studies cover a range of topics, from the city's law enforcement to gangsters, bankers, capitalists, beggars, rickshaw pullers, and prostitutes; scholars have studied Shanghai's campus life, alleyways, cabarets, films, publishing houses, and corpses and graves.[4]

Clearly the variety of topics addressed by scholarly literature about Shanghai is quite robust; yet, to date, Kerrie MacPherson's *A Wilderness of Marshes: The Origins of Public Health in Shanghai, 1843–1893* is the only work in English that exclusively concerns the public health of the city.[5] MacPherson discusses primarily the construction of the medical and sanitary infrastructure in the International Settlement during the nineteenth century, focusing on how Western settlers transformed the "City of Reeds" into a "habitable and salubrious" place from scratch and what they brought into the city from elsewhere. By contrast, my study focuses on the twentieth century, Chinese Shanghai is central, and the majority of the actors are Chinese. During the first four decades of the twentieth century, different groups of Chinese people sought out institutions, therapies, and commodities to stay well and to create a healthy city; in doing so, they capitalized on preexisting as well as Western-driven systems, ideas, and practices available in the city. By analyzing the visions and voices of these Shanghai Chinese, I bring into focus how Shanghai

4. Wakeman, *Policing Shanghai*; Wakeman, *Shanghai Badlands*; Martin, *Shanghai Green Gang*; Bergère, *Golden Age*; Hanchao Lu, *Beyond the Neon Light*; Hanchao Lu, "Becoming Urban"; Hershatter, *Dangerous Pleasures*; Henriot, *Prostitution and Sexuality*; Yeh, *Alienated Academy*; Bracken, *Shanghai Alleyway House*; Field, *Shanghai's Dancing World*; Yingjin Zhang, ed., *Cinema and Urban Culture*; Zhen Zhang, *Amorous History*; Reed, *Gutenberg in Shanghai*; Henriot, "'Invisible Deaths, Silent Deaths'"; Henriot, "Colonial Space of Death."

5. MacPherson, *Wilderness of Marshes*.

Chinese understood hygienic modernity and translated it into mundane behavior and practices within the contexts of the city's urban milieu and the culture of which they were part. Unlike the European settlers of the mid-nineteenth century discussed in MacPherson's work, I do not see Chinese Shanghai as a "dull and unprepossessing spot"[6] that was the "most unlikely place" to develop public health. Rather, borrowing Elizabeth Perry's words, I argue that Shanghai was not a tabula rasa on which Westerners and Western-educated elites could freely draw their schemes and directives, nor were Shanghai Chinese passive and malleable recipients of "scientific knowledge" or "medical orders" delivered to them by outside forces. The city had its own life, and Shanghai culture was not static or monolithic. People in Shanghai had an ability to capitalize on official and popular modes of communication, to devise strategies for mass mobilization, and to appropriate Western medical knowledge.

In studying Shanghai history, culture can be a particularly useful analytical framework. In this regard, Elizabeth Perry's study on labor activism in Shanghai is particularly noteworthy. Perry shifted the focus from workers' class consciousness and party ideology to their workplace culture and their own tradition of collective actions. She convincingly argues that Shanghai workers had their own culture and repertoire of protest, and such culture strengthened and radicalized labor activism.[7] Bryna Goodman, Jeffrey Wasserstrom, and Sherman Cochran, among others, have elaborated on and added nuance to the concept of culture.[8] My study is informed by these studies and this work fully acknowledges the flexible and creative nature of Shanghai's urban culture. By "culture," these scholars do not mean static sociopsychological patterns or fixed and self-contained frameworks. Rather they see culture as encompassing, diverse, and fluid sets of values, customs, dispositions, and norms that shaped attitudes toward life and death, structured the forms of social interactions and communication, and provided underlying

6. Ibid., 15.
7. Perry, *Shanghai on Strike*.
8. Goodman, *Native Place, City, and Nation*; Wasserstrom, *Student Protests*; Cochran, ed., *Inventing Nanjing Road*; Cochran, *Big Business in China*; Lee, *Shanghai Modern*; Cochran, *Encountering Chinese Networks*; Cochran, *Chinese Medicine Men*; Perry, *Anyuan*.

logic to collective actions. They do not sharply distinguish between elite/high culture and popular/low culture or Western culture and traditional culture. These cultural realms often overlapped and coexisted in Shanghai, and the city offered a wide range of readily available cultural resources and assets, both high and low. Culture was also changeable and porous. The Chinese could localize Western culture and incorporate selected aspects into Chinese traditions. They could also mimic styles and techniques of official ceremonies and rituals and re-create them as popular culture.

These points are relevant to this study. In this book I address the emergence and development of new health-care institutions (chapter 1), public health administration (chapter 2), mass programs (chapter 3), and hygiene products (chapter 4) and illustrate how they evolved from and were influenced by Shanghai's urban culture and distinctive local contexts. New institutions and ideas about body and health were not autonomously transformative; they were responsive and applied to social and political arrangements of the local society, and they became part of the city's urban culture. Shanghai's administrators, medical elites, and merchants strategically and liberally drew on some of the city's cultural assets to communicate with the general populace of the city. They creatively deployed indigenous values and norms, such as patriotism, philanthropy, national unity, Confucian morality, and medical knowledge, to implement their agenda on health and hygiene; they also took full advantage of the city's cultural resources to make them intelligible and available to local people. People in Shanghai were surrounded by a variety of medical-care facilities, and they were exposed to information and admonitions on health delivered by various publicity methods. Depending on their financial means and personal preferences, they enjoyed a certain degree of freedom and flexibility in choosing what to do to stay well; in doing so, they freely crossed the borders between Western and Chinese medicine. When they became sick, they visited general hospitals and had their bodies x-rayed. They also saw Chinese-style physicians and had their pulses examined. When they found a doctor's diagnosis inaccurate or a prescription ineffective, they simply refused to comply and sought alternatives. They listened to radio programs on germ theory, attended public lectures on the harms of spitting, and, as they perused magazines, they read advertisements for mosquito coils. Altogether Shanghai people with different backgrounds experienced hygienic modernity in their own ways and participated in the creation of public health.

Diverse approaches to health and hygiene were juxtaposed in Shanghai. They were integrated into mundane practices and quotidian activities and generated popular consciousness about the body, Shanghai society, and the Chinese nation among the city's people. Hospitals, food shops, injection booths, city streets, and bathhouses all became sites where ordinary citizens encountered public health initiatives and claimed their hygienic citizenship. Disparate-but-still-related agents, events, and institutions contributed to the process of building a sanitary city and creating the ideals of a healthy population, and this process transformed many features of Shanghai's medical culture and public life. For people in Shanghai, efforts to protect themselves from germs, dirt, and pests and to build a strong China were part of everyday life. These stories of Shanghai suggest complex and multiple ways in which concerns for their physical well-being shaped people's relations to medical workers, to the city authorities, to their neighborhood communities, to foreign imperialists, and to each other.

Figures 0.1, 0.2, and 0.3 exemplify some important implications of the idea of health and body. All were printed and circulated in Shanghai in the 1920s and 1930s. The first (fig. 0.1) appeared in a book published by the YMCA in 1928 to promote the citywide hygiene campaigns, which are the subject of chapter 3. Pictured is a young man in sportswear who is sweeping rubbish. Street sweeping was one of the major programs of the municipal hygiene campaigns that aimed at mobilizing the entire population of the city. The texts make a clear connection between healthy bodies and a strong nation, and describe diseases as analogous to national disorders. The illustration and the attached texts present a healthy body, sweeping as a virtuous activity, a strong nation, and germ theory side by side.

Unlike figure 0.1, figures 0.2 and 0.3 are commercial promotions that appeared in the pictorial, *Liangyou*.[9] These two suggest that consumers

9. On *Liangyou* and its advertisements, see Lee, "Cultural Construction," 44–53; Pickowicz, Shen, and Zhang, eds., *Liangyou, Kaleidoscopic Modernity*.

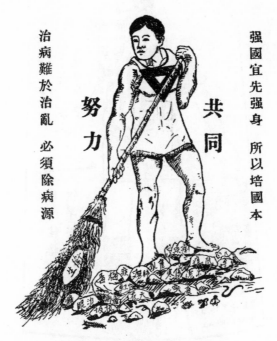

康而壽俾

FIGURE 0.1 Street sweeping. Lou, *Weisheng yundong*, 8. The triangle across the man's chest is a YMCA logo, and the broom he is holding is marked *weisheng*. The four characters surrounding him read, "Let us make an effort together"; the line above him, "Health and longevity"; the vertical line at right, "To make a strong nation, we must first make a strong body so that we can cultivate the national foundation"; and the vertical line at left, "Treating diseases is as difficult as controlling national disorders; we have to eliminate pathogens." Each piece of rubbish is labeled with a word such as *laji* (trash) or *bujie* (filth), as well as the name of an infectious disease, such as tuberculosis, cholera, dysentery, trachoma, smallpox, scarlet fever, typhoid, plague, malaria, or syphilis.

can make themselves fit and healthy by purchasing their products. Figure 0.2 is an advertisement for Quaker Oatmeal. Quaker Oatmeal adopted various Chinese people, including men, women, couples, youth, babies, and convalescents, as the subjects of their commercial advertisements; athletic men were one of their favorite models. Like figure 0.1, figure 0.2 shows a young man in sportswear, but, rather than cleaning,

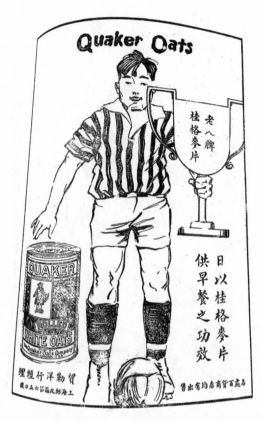

FIGURE 0.2 Quaker Oatmeal. *Liangyou* 18 (August 1927), 36. Pictured is a man holding a trophy that reads "Quaker Oatmeal"; the caption at the lower-right declares, "Eating Quaker Oats everyday makes for a successful breakfast."

he is dribbling a soccer ball.[10] In this ad, the man shows off his fitness while promoting the nutritional value of the American product. Whereas the man in figure 0.1 is making efforts with others (*gongtong nuli*) to sweep streets and strengthen the nation, the man in figure 0.2 is athletic. He is more concerned about keeping himself in a good shape through diet, nourishment, and exercise than cleaning the environment and removing germs.

10. On athletics and physical exercise in Republican China, Morris, *Marrow of the Nation*.

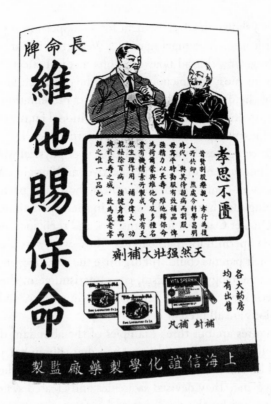

FIGURE O.3 Vita Spermin. *Liangyou* 142 (May 1939), inside front cover. The left top horizontal line reads "Longevity Brand" (*changming pai*), and the vertical line reads "Vita Spermin" (Weita cibaoming; literally "life-saving vitamin supplement"). The right line in the box reads "Filial piety should never be a deficit." The text cites a traditional Chinese story about a filial son who cuts a piece of flesh from his thigh to cure his sick parents, and continues, "Nowadays science is flourishing. Give your parents this effective tonic when they are feeling fine; it will give them energy and help them gain longevity—so much better than cutting off a piece of your thigh when they are sick!" According to the ad, Vita Spermin contains hormones, vitamins, and other precious and refined elements (*jingsu*); exerts a natural physiological effect; greatly helps increase vitality; prevents many illnesses and strengthens the body; is a scientific product that vitalizes old people; and can be taken as a tablet (*buwan*) or ampoule (*buzhen*).

Figure 0.3 shows an advertisement for Vita Spermin, a Chinese supplement.[11] It features a younger man in a Western suit and an older man in a Chinese gown. This ad boasts various medical effects for this supplement, but its most conspicuous point is the parent-child relationship, emphasizing the duty of a filial son. With its presentation of Western medical terminology serving the ideal of traditional family ethics, the ad exemplifies the mixing of Chinese and Western values.[12]

These three figures depict certain aspects of physical well-being and healthy life, but present different perspectives and insights. Yet, they are not necessarily in conflict with each other. Those who participated in a street-sweeping march might play sports in their spare time. Those who purchased Quaker Oatmeal for themselves and their spouses might also purchase Vita Spermin for their parents. Those who were always respectful toward their parents could still organize the city's hygiene campaigns and study bacteriology. Patriotism, consumerism, germ theory, athleticism, Western food, collective actions, faith in science, and traditional family relations are all present here.

These figures are but three examples of the abundant depictions of physical well-being in Republican Shanghai. Shanghai people were surrounded by various images of and information about health, medicine, and hygiene. They devised strategies and created systems and institutions, evoked by these images and information, to protect their bodies and city from sickness and filth. An in-depth analysis of these presentations and agencies and a critical examination of the motivations, politics, and desires behind them bring to light the multiple ways in which the Shanghai Chinese experienced social and cultural changes in the city and nation and understood the interplay of local and colonial powers. In this book, I address three lines of academic inquiry: Western medicine in a non-Western context; Republican China; and colonialism in Shanghai.

11.   Vita Spermin is a product of Xinyi (Trust and Friendship) Chemical Pharmaceutical Manufacture. Xinyi was originally established by a German in Shanghai. Later Bao Guochang purchased the company. See *Xiandai shiyejia*, 127.

12.   Sherman Cochran's study has demonstrated that Chinese pharmaceutical companies shrewdly drew on print media and produced a considerable body of commercial ads for their Chinese-made Western drugs. See Cochran, "Marketing Medicine"; Cochran, *Chinese Medicine Men*.

Western Medicine and Science in China

Implicitly or explicitly, each of the above illustrations makes reference to something foreign—foreign threats, Western medical terminology, and Western food are particularly conspicuous. Without a doubt, foreign presence played a significant role in modern Chinese history in general and in the history of Shanghai in particular. From the late Qing through the Republican era, China faced unrelenting foreign pressure; and, since the mid-nineteenth century, the city of Shanghai experienced particularly extensive and intensive foreign influence. Westerners forced Shanghai to open as a port for international trade as the result of the Opium War (1839–42), and Great Britain, the United States, and France created concessions to carve out territory within the city borders. Eventually the British and American concessions merged to form the International Settlement.[13] During the Second Sino-Japanese War (1937–45), Japanese military forces occupied Shanghai. Overall, Western and Japanese imperialists arrived in Shanghai with violence and demanded extraterritoriality for more than a hundred years. At the same time, they also introduced new ideas, systems, and customs to the city. Most relevant to this discussion, Westerners brought Western biomedicine and medical technology, public health administration, and hygiene practices, and they helped shape Chinese perceptions and understanding of the body and health. In sum, Western medicine set forth a model of hygienic modernity. Yet, it was not a simple process. The practitioners, advocates, and critics of Western medicine, and their beliefs, visions, and experiences, all contributed to the formation and transformation of public health in Shanghai.

Founded and developed in Western Europe, the practices of biomedicine and bacteriology spread throughout the world during the twentieth century. Medicine was always a significant component of imperialism, and Western medicine facilitated Western expansion and invasion.[14] Various non-Western medical ideas and practices still survived, but once Western medicine was introduced, they were often marginalized and

13. For a history of foreign concessions in Shanghai, see appendix 1.

14. Bashford, *Imperial Hygiene*; Bu, Stapleton, and Yip, eds., *Science, Public Health, and the State*.

treated as merely "traditional" or "old" forms of medicine. In examining medical history in non-Western societies, conventional scholarship often views the West either as a "benevolent modernizer" that eradicated endemics, eliminated pathogens, and created new public health systems in local societies or as an "oppressive imperialist" that destroyed ecological balance, brought about new diseases, and scrutinized and controlled the bodies of the colonized. Assuming that indigenous populations had completely different notions about health and medicine from the West, these scholars describe local responses to the West in terms of "acceptance" or "resistance."[15] These views have their merits, and they certainly describe some aspects of the Chinese experience.

However, since the 1990s, studies on colonial medicine have presented a much more complex picture. Historians of colonial medicine have pointed out that "acceptance" and "resistance" are not necessarily antithetical to each other. Although indigenous elites and intellectuals in colonies resisted the imposition of Western medicine, they also perceived it as a benefit and adopted it to enhance their own prestige.[16] They also "blended" Western-driven bacteriology with preexisting miasmic theories.[17] Other scholars further develop this line of inquiry and question the existence of clear boundaries separating medical practices in metropoles, colonial medicine, and local therapies. Moreover, Western medicine itself consisted of multiple contesting theories. Scholars contend that biomedicine was not universal or transcendent; it was a local medicine of Western Europe in the nineteenth and twentieth centuries.[18] By "provincializing" Western medicine and juxtaposing Western and non-Western medicine without privileging either of them, scholars seek to understand how the colonizers and the colonized observed and discovered the character of their own medicine and medical practices and also that of others.

China was not a formal colony in the same way that India and Hong Kong were British colonies. However, many points made by historians

---

15. For *review* and critique of the present literature, see, for example, Rogaski, *Hygienic Modernity*, 4–10; Cunningham and Andrews, "Introduction."

16. Arnold, *Colonizing the Body*.

17. Sutphen, "Not What, But Where."

18. Cunningham and Andrews, eds., *Western Medicine as Contested Knowledge*; Sutphen and Andrews, eds., *Medicine and Colonial Identity*; Michael Shiyung Liu, *Prescribing Colonization*.

of colonial medicine might well elucidate the ways in which the Chinese manipulated and reformulated the concepts of "Western medicine" and "Western drugs." Even after the introduction of global public health and biomedicine, Chinese medical vocabulary coexisted with Western terms, and Chinese traditional explanations and understanding of infectious diseases played a significant role in developing strategies to defend communities from contagion.[19] Also, in commercial promotion, "Western drugs" (*xiyao*) indicated a variety of products, including imported drugs, Chinese-made drugs, nutrition supplements, plasters, and tonics.[20] Moreover, Western medical personnel in China's treaty ports generally had only limited power or authority to engage in preventive medicine. They had little interest in undertaking sanitation or medical work that might provoke local resistance or riots.[21] In sum, Western medicine had multiple dimensions and was not a single, dominate force. Cooperation with, coercion of, and resistance to Western-defined public health all took place in China.[22]

I also shed light on the ways in which various people in Shanghai skillfully appropriated Western medical ideas and systems for their own use. Although they emulated and followed Western models, they did not simply copy from them; rather, they challenged, contested, and reinterpreted them. By doing so, they invented methods and practices similar to, but different from, Western examples and served Shanghai's local needs.[23] China's hygienic modernity did not emerge in a vacuum, nor was it directly transplanted from the West; it was shaped by local conditions and became part of Chinese ways of life. Yet it was also a means through which China could globalize and surpass the West. The central focus here is the processes by which various Shanghai Chinese observed and understood Western medical science in their own terms; acting on this understanding, they developed and elaborated strategies to protect and improve individual, municipal, and national health and hygiene. They were engaged in behavioral and corporeal reforms based on Western

19.   Andrews, "Tuberculosis and the Assimilation"; Leung, *Leprosy in China*.
20.   Yeh, "Shanghai Modernity," 131.
21.   Bretelle-Establet, "French Medicine," 148.
22.   Rogaski, *Hygienic Modernity*, 7–9.
23.   On the process of this appropriation and reinvention, see de Certeau, *Practice of Everyday Life*, 165–89.

biomedicine to create healthy Chinese citizens who could outperform the West. In doing so, they incorporated Western ideas and systems into political and commercial visions and, in tandem, created new health-related images, institutions, and merchandise for local consumption.

Chinese perceptions of health and body were closely related to Chinese understandings of science and scientism. Science, "one crucially powerful category of knowledge for Chinese intellectuals in the twentieth century,"[24] was a significant element of Western modernity. China had a long history of natural studies since ancient times, but since the late nineteenth century, Chinese intellectuals had also learned modern science as part of Western scholarship.[25] By the early twentieth century, Chinese elites and political leaders came to believe that science was the key to a strong, modern nation and a solution to China's weaknesses and backwardness. In their minds, science was not only an academic discipline or research activity, but also a way of life that could lead Chinese people to a better future and rejuvenate the state.[26] Late Qing reformers believed that Western science and technology could easily coexist with and strengthen Confucian doctrines, but their confidence was severely damaged by their crushing defeat in the First Sino-Japanese War (1894–95) and the Boxer Protocol (1901).[27] In the early twentieth century, Chinese intellectuals challenged Chinese values per se, and along with democracy, "science" became one of the key terms in intellectual discourse that criticized Chinese values and systems. In particular, May Fourth intellectuals embraced "an intense faith in the capacity of 'science' to dismantle 'tradition,' and to achieve its opposite, dubbed 'modernity.'"[28] Many of the Chinese discussed in this study, both elites and non-elites, also embraced and advocated science and scientific attitudes; they strove not only to make their professional practices and medical instruments scientific, but also to align their mundane behavior and commodities meant for regular and everyday use with the latest scientific knowledge.

24.   Helen Schneider, *Keeping the Nation's House*, 12.
25.   Elman, *On Their Own Terms*; Sivin, *Science in Ancient China*; Needham, *Science and Civilisation*.
26.   Kwok, *Scientism in Chinese Thought*; Zuoyue Wang, "Saving China through Science."
27.   Kwok, *Scientism in Chinese Thought*.
28.   Dikötter, *Sex, Culture, and Modernity*, 2.

But what qualified as "science" differed greatly depending on when, how, and by whom the word was used. The "universality" of science could coexist and even reinforce the "particularity" of nationalism;[29] it could be a means to modernize or Westernize China and to preserve Chinese traditional values at once.[30] Scientific knowledge and scientific data are rarely culturally neutral.[31] Through an examination of health and hygiene, I highlight the sociopolitical meanings of "science," paying close attention not only to medical discourses and public policies, but also to science experienced in everyday life. At the same time, I carefully look at Shanghai's sociocultural arrangements, to which medical knowledge and technology were introduced and applied. Shanghai residents came across science by receiving injections, catching flies, cleaning streets, and buying soap. Political actors, medical doctors, and businessmen used science to contest their differing agendas and concerns about how to make the people of Shanghai healthy and clean, how to serve the nation, and how to promote their own interests.

Body, Society, and State in Republican China

This study covers the period from the late nineteenth century through the present time, with a focus on the Republican period, and is situated within a broad scholarly reconsideration of Republican China. During this period it was the state, rather than charitable and religious organizations, that gradually rose to assume the responsibility for the health and hygiene of the general populace and environmental sanitation. I discuss many ways the state came to dominate, discipline, and serve individual bodies and the urban population through biological knowledge and public health administration. I also address how Shanghai people participated in and committed to this process, enhancing our understanding of the synergetic relations between the state and society.

29. Mizuno, *Science for the Empire.*
30. Greene, "GMD Rhetoric."
31. Lam, *Passion for Facts.*

Between the fall of the Qing dynasty and the establishment of the People's Republic of China (PRC) in 1949, China was called a republic. The Republican government was founded in 1912, but it soon lost its ability to control the country after 1916. Chinese politics were dominated by regional warlords until the Nationalist Party (Guomindang) established the Nationalist government in Nanjing in 1928. The Nanjing government incorporated several contradictory elements. It was a "Republican" government that was the product of a nationalist revolution. When it was inaugurated, the government set itself the goal of restoring national order and expelling foreign imperialists. Despite its intentions, the Nanjing government was never able to consolidate its control over the entire territory of China. Local strongmen still had considerable influence over many regions, and after the breakout of the Second Sino-Japanese War in 1937, parts of the country were ruled by various Japanese puppet governments. Because the Nanjing government suffered from its ongoing battles with warlords, Communists, and later Japanese aggression, a large part of the national expenditure went to the military. Coordination within the government was poor, and factionalism and corruption were prevalent. After World War II and a bitter civil war, the Communists defeated the Nationalists and took control of the mainland.

The Republican period is sometimes regarded as merely a transitional time between imperial China and the People's Republic; the Nationalists are dismissed as a failed party. In the last two decades, however, scholars have seriously reconsidered this period. Recent historical studies on the Republican era place less emphasis on 1949 as a dividing line and see great continuity between the Republican and Communist periods.[32] In *Reappraising Republican China,* a pioneering work forwarding this scholarly trend, leading scholars of the period present a comprehensive review of academic debates and issues regarding Republican China.[33] Following their lead, many scholars now recognize the complexities, ambiguities, and potentials of this era.[34] In particular, reflecting on the dynamics of state-society relations is one of the significant academic themes of studies

32. Cohen, "Post-Mao Reforms"; Andrew Nathan, "Some Trends in the Historiography"; Dirlik "Reversals, Ironies, and Hegemonies."
33. Wakeman and Edmonds, eds., *Reappraising Republican China.*
34. For a literature review, see Young, "Introduction"; Dikötter, *Age of Openness.*

on Republican China.[35] In the 1990s, the translation of Jürgen Habermas's work triggered active debates about civil society and the public sphere. Scholars of Republican China have duly noted the emergence of new entrepreneurs and capitalists, professionals, and modern voluntary organizations and pointed out that members of these groups could challenge and bargain with the state.[36] The central question here is whether modern Chinese cities had a public sphere in which city residents enjoyed autonomy outside of state control.[37]

I also place the issues of health and hygiene in Shanghai within the broader sociocultural developments in Republican China. The creation and development of Shanghai's public health system coincided with China's transformation from an imperial dynasty based on the Mandate of Heaven to a Republican state consisting of modern citizens. Chinese elites were convinced that, along with public morality and loyalty to the nation, physical well-being and cleanliness were also indispensable prerequisites to the making of a modern citizen. The Chinese state under different political regimes concurred with them. Being stigmatized by the foreign stereotype of China as a "sick man," the state strove to convert the weak and dirty Chinese body into a healthy and clean one. With this effort, they strove to build a strong nation. When the Nationalists came to power, they viewed public health as a significant part of their state-building program and attempted to build a nationwide public health administrative system based on biomedicine. The Shanghai municipal government also opened a public health bureau to carry out sanitary reforms in the Chinese sector of the city. The bureau provided not only necessary services and assistance to promote welfare but was also involved with inspecting, supervising, controlling, and regulating people's lives and bodies and interfered in business affairs. Implementation of efficient public health policies was a form of political technology and was closely related to the outreach of the state. General optimism about medical science cleared the way for efficient operation of state power

35. Coble, *Shanghai Capitalists*; Bush, *Politics of Cotton Textiles*; Fewsmith, *Party, State, and Local Elite*.

36. Xiaoqun Xu, *Chinese Professionals*; Strand, *Rickshaw Beijing*.

37. Strand, *"Civil Society" and "Public Sphere"*; Bergère, "Civil Society and Urban Change"; Philip Huang, "Public Sphere/Civil Society in China?"; Wakeman, "Civil Society and Public Sphere"; Lean, *Public Passions*.

and helped the expansion of state authority. The coercive dimension of public health came to a fore under the Japanese occupation.

At the same time, however, state expansion did not always take place in a unidirectional, hierarchical manner. Rather, modern state power circulates and becomes disseminated among the general populace through a variety of channels and media.[38] Chinese administrators and medical doctors designed a number of strategies and methods and took advantage of mass media to convey knowledge and information on health and hygiene to the urban masses and to educate them. Moreover, the state was not the only agent involved in public health and the dissemination of medical norms to the public. Social elements such as local philanthropists, religious organizations, businessmen, and consumers all participated in this process as they pursued their varied goals and looked after their particular interests; with their involvement, these groups and individuals at once advocated and promoted their own versions of hygienic modernity, while at the same time they reaffirmed connections among health, hygiene, public welfare, and national strength.

Corporeal health is related to human fundamentals, including birth, pain, and death. Staying well was a common concern of all Shanghai residents; unsurprisingly, a discourse on health became a field in which the state and various social groups contended for the importance of their agenda. Government directives, medical texts, journal articles, and commercial advertisements all produced a vast array of discourses on health and hygiene, and studying such discourses provides a promising venue for gaining a comprehensive view of Shanghai society. In this book I present competing conceptions of the body and health and examine how the state and various segments of Shanghai society understood them in ways that they found meaningful.

Colonialism in Shanghai

In this study I place Shanghai and its particularities at the center of inquiry while remaining conscious of Shanghai's position in a global context, and hope to sharpen our understanding of colonialism in

38. Gluck, *Japan's Modern Myths.*

China. Since the mid-nineteenth century, multiple imperial powers, including Britain, France, Japan, Germany, Russia, Germany, Italy, and Portugal, have encroached on Chinese sovereignty. These powers colonized Hong Kong, Taiwan, and Macao, and created treaty ports and leased territories to take advantage of China. Yet, unlike India, China remained independent. China was never conquered, and the Chinese did not regard themselves as colonial subjects. Scholars and political theorists have used a number of terms to capture distinctive features of modern China.[39] Sun Yat-sen once called China a "hypo-colony." By this he meant that China's international status was worse than that of a formal colony, because China was a colony of many and the Chinese people were everyone's slaves.[40] Ruth Rogaski has called Tianjin a "hyper-colony," in which eight different foreign powers created concessions; each of them offered different models for modernity, and they all competed against each other.[41] "Semi-colony" is probably the most commonly used term. First coined by Lenin, and in spite of its impreciseness, this term has been used to describe pre-1949 China by not only Mao Zedong but also PRC historians. More recently, Shu-mei Shih's study on Chinese modernists analyzes contradictory features of colonialism in China and redefines the term "semi-colony." Shih argues that because their rule was informal and fragmented, imperial powers in China were also exempted from "colonial benevolence." Moreover, fragmentation and multiplicity of colonial arrangements made it difficult for Chinese intellectuals to unite and target a single colonial enemy.[42] James Hevia and Tani Barlow take different approaches. Hevia does not find Chinese experience particularly unique and writes that "we might consider all the entities produced in the age of empires as forms of semi-colonialism."[43] Barlow calls attention to the universalizing power of "colonial modernity" that dominated Europe and colonies.[44] Although these discussions challenge and overlap each other, scholars are increasingly shifting from the formulaic binaries of colonizers versus colonized and aggressors versus exploited to

39. Goodman and Goodman, "Colonialism and China."
40. Sun Yat-sen, "Sanmin zhuyi, minzu zhuyi," 345.
41. Rogaski, *Hygienic Modernity*, 10–18.
42. Shih, *Lure of the Modern*, 32.
43. Hevia, *English Lessons*, 26.
44. Barlow, "Introduction: On 'Colonial Modernity.'"

more multidirectional approaches. The foreign population in China's treaty ports was not monolithic, and foreign powers did compete and cooperate with each other over hegemony.[45] The Chinese also participated in this competition to maximize their profits, and the resistance and accommodation to colonial authorities by Chinese elites and commoners influenced and shaped colonial management. Although the power relations between foreign powers and the Chinese were unequal, some groups of Chinese enjoyed certain freedoms, power, and autonomy and took advantage of extraterritoriality. In James Hevia's words, "Colonization was always a messy process, with diverse parties pulling and pushing in many directions at once."[46]

Several scholars have examined ambivalent self-identities of Chinese elites under such "messy" circumstances. They point out that the absence of a formal colonial structure and the lack of aggressive imposition of Western values enabled Chinese elites to embrace Western-driven modernity without much reservation and resentment. These elites were able to distinguish the image of the West and Japan as liberal modernizers from the image of the West and Japan as aggressive colonizers. They also distanced themselves from the "uneducated" masses and identified themselves with universal values of modernity, science, and progress. Shih calls this process the "strategy of displacement through bifurcation."[47] Though not uncritically, Chinese elites accepted colonial science and colonial modernity; in doing so, they established their authority and prestige vis-à-vis others.[48]

With two foreign concessions within the city, Shanghai was a semicolony in concrete terms; in my study, Shanghai elites also fit this "bifurcation" model. Even though modern biomedicine and public health were brought into Shanghai with violence by imperial powers, Shanghai's medical elites were convinced that Western science would benefit Chinese society and save Chinese lives. They emulated public health systems and policies in the International Settlement and praised the cleanliness and orderliness there. Even those who practiced traditional Chinese medicine

45. For example, in 1930 Shanghai's population consisted of some forty-eight nationals; among these citizens and colonial subjects were Jews, Russians, Indians, and Taiwanese. Bickers and Henriot, "Introduction."

46. Hevia, *English Lessons*, 19.

47. Shih, *Lure of the Modern*, 304.

48. Rogaski, *Hygienic Modernity*, 252; Lam, *Passion for Facts*, 13–14, 117–41.

raised no doubt about the efficacy of science. At the same time, Shanghai's administrators set up laws and rules about hygiene to regulate the behavior of the masses and carried out coercive epidemic control programs directed at the Chinese poor. Shanghai elites saw themselves as champions of Western science and guardians of the masses. They assumed that they were the ones to undertake the "civilizing mission" of commoners and that it was their responsibility to supervise and educate the masses.

However, the "bifurcation" was not always fixed, and boundaries between elites and masses as well as cosmopolitanism and colonialism were often blurry. While advocating the universal value of medical science, Chinese administrators were also sensitive to the presence of imperial powers and the unequal distribution of wealth in the city. They were well aware that the International Settlement had much larger financial resources at its disposal than the Chinese sector; they also knew that such resources significantly contributed to the sanitary facilities in the Settlement. Non-elites were not always under governmental tutelage. Chinese businessmen who had received only an elementary education in science took part in discussions on science and the nation, and they also eagerly participated in the "civilizing mission." In promoting their products, they often championed global science and dismissed its imperialist origin. At the same time, they advocated nationalism and attacked economic imperialism. When necessary, Shanghai Chinese distinguished themselves from Westerners and differentiated their products from foreign brands. In this study I suggest that colonial medicine and hygienic modernity could become part of local culture without undermining Chinese identities or destroying local businesses.

Focusing on local actors in Shanghai, I illustrate how they were engaged in the issues of health and hygiene as well as politics, evangelism, and business simultaneously, and how Shanghai's everyday life and mundane practices reshaped and reframed colonial medicine. As Mary P. Sutphen and Bridie Andrews point out, the study of health and medicine can provide an excellent arena for examining the "hybridity" and "contingencies" of Chinese perceptions of themselves and colonialists.[49] By presenting a "local history" of colonialism, I hope to contribute not only to Shanghai studies but also to studies on colonialism more broadly.

49. Sutphen and Andrews, "Introduction."

An Overview

The research for this study is based primarily on documents housed at the Shanghai Municipal Archives (SMA), as well as on medical journals, popular magazines, and newspapers published in the Republican period. In addition to these Chinese sources, chapter 2 of this study also draws on the materials from the Diplomatic Archives of the Ministry of Foreign Affairs of Japan.

The four chapters of this book are organized thematically rather than strictly chronologically. In each chapter I take up different aspects of Shanghai's urban life and introduce various relevant agents. The focus of chapter 1 is on hospitals (*yiyuan*) and this chapter presents Shanghai's "medical map" as observed and experienced by city residents. Hospitals were significant institutions that defended people's lives from sickness and other misfortunes. The city's hospitals, first opened by Westerners, quickly became part of Shanghai's landscape. In chapter 1, I investigate three different types of nongovernmental hospitals that coexisted in the city: missionary hospitals operated by Westerners, communicable disease hospitals run by local elites and social organizations, and Chinese hospitals operated and supported by those who practiced traditional Chinese medicine. I also look at how preexisting institutions, customs, and ideas in the city provided bases for the opening and development of these hospitals, each with its own goals, strategies, and clientele. Although they were business rivals, these institutions also imitated and influenced one another. Many of these hospitals began as philanthropic institutions to serve the general public, but hospital managers were also aware that well-run hospitals were more likely to earn social prestige and yield profits. All the hospitals adopted "scientific methods" and used "scientific instruments" to practice medicine, yet they also offered various nonmedical social services. In chapter 1, I demonstrate that hospital operation developed by responding to local needs. I also shed light on how philanthropy, business interests, and medical science intertwined in the founding, running, and success of hospitals, and how each of these forces facilitated the growth of medical services.

The focus of chapter 1 was on private health-care providers; the subject of chapter 2 shifts to issues of administration. After a brief discussion of the nationwide public health system, I examine how those who governed the city managed health-related matters to create a clean and healthy city. In Shanghai, the British first opened the Public Health Office (Weishengchu) in 1898 in the International Settlement to take charge of sanitation. The International Settlement served as a model, and the comparison between the "clean" foreign sector and the "dirty" Chinese sector hurt Chinese pride. When the Nationalists arrived in Shanghai, they opened the Shanghai Municipal Public Health Bureau (Weishengju) (PHB). Following the example of the International Settlement, the Shanghai PHB carried out various sanitation and public health programs. However, the Shanghai PHB was not an imposition from the state, nor was it a simple imitation of its Western counterpart. It evolved from indigenous organizations, and its operation was supported and supplemented by local elites. It also represented Chinese interest and challenged the British authorities. Chapter 2 illustrates how state authority, local interests, and Western presence interacted and became mutually engaged as the field of public health evolved in the city. As the PHB expanded its activities, it not only provided necessary services but also began to control people's behavior and intrude into their personal lives. The intrusiveness of the public health administration became particularly explicit during the war. In this chapter I also examine how building on the recent "bottom-up" approach to the occupation, the war and occupation influenced the city's public health programs and prewar notions of national strength and racial hygiene.[50] Finally, I address the issue of collaboration. In all likelihood, those who remained in the city and worked with Japanese occupiers did not believe they were collaborating with Japan. Chinese doctors and public health workers were convinced that they were upholders and conveyers of modern medical science, and that epidemic control work had no national or racial boundaries.

In chapter 3, a narrower focus considers hygiene campaigns (*weisheng yundong*)—a type of mass mobilization program undertaken in Shanghai throughout the twentieth century that aimed at linking medical knowledge, hygiene practices, and political participation. In chapter 3 I look at how an educational program organized by YMCA members and

50. Yeh, ed., *Wartime Shanghai*; Yeh and Henriot, eds., *In the Shadow*; Brook, *Collaboration*.

medical doctors transformed into an official event that promoted national unity, modern civility, and public etiquette among the general populace in the city. Although Westerners introduced some campaign programs, Shanghai Chinese took full advantage of the city's "repertoire of collective actions" and arranged specific methods intended to be suitable for Shanghai people. Drawing on theories of mass movements, I closely examine five major campaign methods: exhibitions and performances, texts and cartoons, lectures and talks, opening ceremonies and street sweeping, and monitoring and policing. An analysis of these methods becomes particularly important in understanding the politics and logic of mass campaigns. The Nationalist government depended heavily on political symbols, rituals, and protocols to claim its legitimacy. It also used various mass media and organized ceremonies and rallies to appeal to and to mobilize the people. Hygiene campaign organizers borrowed such methods and symbols. In chapter 3 I highlight stylistic similarities between hygiene campaigns and other public gatherings and examine how personal bodies and customs became a subject of a political event. I suggest that campaign organizers and their agents did not attempt to exclude or eliminate the "unfit" or "unclean." Instead they affirmed that making a hygienic city was a responsibility that belonged to all Shanghai residents, regardless of social class. They encouraged or coerced everyone to take part in the campaigns and promoted the idea that each and every individual body was a constituent part of the nation. Republican-era hygiene campaigns created a readiness among the population to accept similar mass campaigns in the later Communist period.

In chapter 4 I examine the issues of health and hygiene from the viewpoint of Shanghai's business world. As problems of the nation's health became critical to administrators and intellectuals, Shanghai's industrialists and merchants realized that they could sell health and hygiene. Of the various types of businesses that promoted the healthful effects of their products, I focus on the light chemical industries that manufactured and sold daily-use items like soap, toothpowder and toothpaste, insecticides and mosquito coils, and other personal hygiene items. I highlight the example of Fang Yexian (1893–1940) and Chen Diexian (1879–1940), two successful entrepreneurs of Republican Shanghai. Drawing theoretically from the rich scholarship on China's business history and material culture, I suggest that Chinese manufacturers of this industry played a significant role and were even more successful than the state in localizing and popularizing hygienic modernity among Shanghai residents through their advertising and sales. Most importantly, they actively participated in and took advantage of government-sponsored mass movements. They encouraged consumers to practice hygiene as prescribed by the state and to purchase their commodities as a means to do so.

Finally, in the conclusion I trace the trajectory of public health in post-1949 Shanghai by discussing the history of medical-care institutions and patriotic hygiene campaigns in the People's Republic. When Communists took power, they reorganized hospitals, clinics, and other medical facilities and personnel to conform to socialist ideology and ideals. They also launched patriotic hygiene campaigns to unite people, raise their patriotism and consciousness of sanitation, and urge them to undertake cleaning work. Thanks to these and other measures, the Maoist era brought considerable gain in the field of public health. However, since the beginning of the Reform era, as the state increasingly relinquished its control over and responsibility for the nation's health care, the medical market once again has become privatized and commercialized. Likewise, as the market economy has created economic disparities among the Chinese population and has made new kinds of mass media available, it has become increasingly difficult to unite Chinese people and motivate them to participate in mass movements.

Residents of Shanghai defined "health" in their own variety of ways and strove to transform their society and nation by making their bodies cleaner and healthier. Health was an area in which state authority, local elite and commercial interests, and Western and Chinese medical ideas interacted in a complex manner.

CHAPTER I

Caring for the Sick, Helping the Poor

The Development of Hospitals in Shanghai

In early twentieth-century Shanghai, the preservation of good physical health was a significant concern for the city's general populace. The city's environment was not salubrious. During Shanghai's hot and humid summers, city residents contended with gastrointestinal disorders; in the winter, they often suffered from respiratory diseases. Social and economic pressures and other uncertainties associated with modern urban life caused further anxiety for Shanghai's urbanites about their well-being. Overcrowding, sprawling shantytowns, the inadequate supply of clean water, a shortage of public latrines, and the presence of abandoned corpses on the street all contributed to the breakout of disease.[1] Shanghai residents conformed to traditional Chinese regimens, such as following the Yin and Yang principle, eating and drinking properly, keeping harmony with the cosmos, and avoiding harmful winds, to maintain their health. Still they succumbed to illness, and when they did, they sought treatment from various institutions and individuals in the city.

Long before the arrival of Westerners, Shanghai embraced a vibrant medical-care market. The range of the medical-care providers included hospitals, clinics, pharmacies, drugstores, and various charitable organizations, along with acupuncturists, bonesetters, itinerant drug sellers, and

---

1.   On shantytowns, see Hanchao Lu, "Creating Urban Outcasts"; on the disposal of bodily waste and latrine reforms, see Peng Shanmin, *Gonggong weisheng yu Shanghai dushi wenming*, 257–83; on abandoned corpses, Henriot, "'Invisible Deaths, Silent Deaths.'"

other folk healers. This "market" expanded and diversified significantly during the Republican period. During the 1920s and 1930s, medical development and capitalist competition established a hierarchy among these medical-care providers. General hospitals that employed doctors with medical degrees from Western universities and drugstores with eye-catching window displays on the main streets of the city garnered the greatest prestige. Unlicensed practitioners who primarily served the indigent and vendors and itinerant peddlers who sold simple drugs were at the bottom. These institutions and individuals embraced diverse—even contradictory—ideas about sickness, well-being, and medical treatment and adopted various strategies to attract patients and customers; nevertheless, they were not mutually exclusive. Shanghai residents often engaged in "doctor shopping." Individuals with adequate financial resources could choose from different medical-care services and products.

Hospitals (*yiyuan*) were a distinctive feature of Republican Shanghai's medical culture. Early hospitals were introduced by Westerners, but they had become a familiar institution in the city by the early twentieth century. No single, standardized definition of "hospital" existed at that time, however: it was vaguely understood that hospitals were sites where sick people could receive medical treatment and drugs from professionals, but the term *yiyuan* was applied to a range of institutions and agencies. These included general hospitals that had multiple departments and inpatient facilities, private clinics run by those who practiced traditional Chinese medicine, isolation hospitals that admitted patients with communicable diseases exclusively, specialized hospitals for those with mental illness and other chronic diseases, and charitable clinics that offered free medical services and accommodations for the indigent. Significantly, most of the major hospitals in the city were established and run by nongovernmental initiatives. Not only doctors, but also religious organizations, commercial guilds, pharmaceutical companies, native-place associations, and even a mutual help association of rickshaw pullers all ran "hospitals." In addition, some pharmacies were staffed by Chinese physicians and provided medical consultation and prescriptions.

It is difficult to say just how many "hospitals" were in operation in Republican Shanghai. According to an investigation carried out by the Central Field Health Station, as of 1933, Shanghai had 31 hospitals with a total of 1,967 beds.[2] A list made in 1933 by Pang Jingzhou (1897–1966), a doctor and medical critic in the Republican period, names thirty-one public (*gongli*) hospitals and sixteen "famous" private (*sili*) hospitals.[3] The Chinese Medical Association, a nationwide association of Western-style doctors, provides a range of figures for hospitals in Shanghai in its annual *Chinese Medical Directory* as follows: 38 (1932), 43 (1934), 34 (1937), 54 (1939), 46 (1940), and 53 (1941).[4] Still other sources give different figures. In 1935, the Dōjinkai, a Japanese medical philanthropic organization, lists 282 hospitals in its directory of Shanghai hospitals.[5] According to *Shanghai weishengzhi* (*SWZ*), the city had 108 hospitals with a total of 9,000 beds in 1936.[6] In 1939, Xu Wancheng carried out a more comprehensive survey of more than two hundred hospitals and nine hundred doctors.[7] As of 1934, the Public Health Department of the International Settlement drew up a list of 202 hospitals within the Settlement.[8]

The ambiguous definition of *yiyuan* is one source of the variance in these figures. Even in the 1930s, when the modern definition of "hospital" was emerging in China, the term was applied to a diverse range of organizations. Whereas some lists included only general hospitals with inpatient accommodations, Xu Wancheng's list embraced municipal clinics, specialized clinics, sanatoriums, and dental clinics as well. Likewise, the Dōjinkai's directory comprised personal clinics, charitable clinics, ophthalmologists, and mental health clinics. Lu Ming, a contemporary medical historian, estimates that some two hundred hospitals, large and small, operated in the city in the 1930s.[9] Based on these figures, it is reasonable to estimate that 1930s Shanghai had some 30 to 40 general hospitals and more than 150 smaller medical institutions. These figures

2.   Guomin zhengfu zhujichu tongjiju, ed., *Zhonghua minguo tongji tiyao*, 395.
3.   Pang, *Yiyao niaokan*, 22–24, 34–35.
4.   Chinese Medical Association, ed., *Chinese Medical Directory* 1932, 59–63; 1934, 148–53; 1937, 369–73; 1939, A147–A152; 1940, A155–A160; 1941, A86–A90.
5.   Ono, ed., *Zhonghua minguo yishi zonglan*, 75–83.
6.   *Shanghai weishengzhi* bianzuan weiyuanhui, ed., *Shanghai weishengzhi* (*SWZ*), 84–85.
7.   Xu Wancheng, *Zhanhou Shanghai*.
8.   The list is filed in Shanghai Municipal Archives (SMA) U1-16-548.
9.   Lu Ming of the People's Number Four Hospital, interview by author, May 1999.

do not include smaller operations run by Chinese-style practitioners and other folk healers. Nor can we assume that all these institutions had good reputations. Some were operated by unqualified personnel;[10] some illegally appropriated the names of famous hospitals in their ads and signs;[11] and some had only two or three beds and were in business simply to pursue private gain.[12]

Three types among these institutions are the focus of this chapter, reflecting, in part, the availability of archival sources: missionary hospitals, summer-disease hospitals, and hospitals operated by those who practiced traditional Chinese medicine. More importantly, even though they had different origins and goals, all the hospitals in this chapter were, more or less, successful. They optimized the use of available resources, responded to local needs, and survived the 1940s and the Communist Revolution. Some of them are still flourishing today. And although they were all inaugurated and operated by private initiatives, they were open to the general public and received public funding. This chapter explores the important role that these hospitals played in creating Shanghai's medical culture. The evolution of these hospitals reflects the changing definitions of medicine and illness, the role of religion and charity, and the realities of urban economy and demography.

The complex relations among Western medicine, Chinese medicine, and the Republican state have been well studied, but little attention has been paid to the significant role that hospitals played in China's medical history. Since Western missionaries introduced hospitals to the city in the mid-nineteenth century along with Western medical techniques, hospitals were often regarded as "Western" and "novel." Indeed, some historians have viewed the introduction of missionary hospitals as a tool of Western cultural imperialism.[13] However, a close examination of missionary hospitals in Shanghai reveals that they were not unlike Chinese charitable clinics. When they were first established, missionary hospitals rented Chinese-style buildings and offered free medical services to demonstrate Christian benevolence.[14] Meanwhile, after the turn of the

10. Yuan Fu, "Tingle lutian zhenliaosuo."
11. Pang, *Yiyao niaokan*, 36–37.
12. SMA U1-16-519.
13. Li Jingwei, *Zhongwai yixue jiaoliushi*, 280.
14. Renshaw, *Accommodating the Chinese*.

twentieth century, increasing numbers of Chinese students studied Western biomedicine in China and abroad. These Western-educated Chinese not only worked at missionary hospitals, but also established hospitals of their own. Moreover, in an effort to enhance their professional prestige and compete with Western medicine, practitioners of Chinese medicine opened hospitals as well. Studying the range and nature of these institutions brings into question the simple dichotomies of "Western medicine versus Chinese medicine" and "scientific medicine versus traditional medicine." It also helps clarify the ways in which Shanghai Chinese understood and indigenized Western medicine and medical systems and how they took advantage of Western ideas for their own use within their society.

Hospitals were also a venue in which charity, business, and medical care intersected with one another.[15] Throughout Chinese history, medical care was associated with charity and social welfare; moreover, providing free medical care and drugs had been a significant part of local charity efforts since the Ming-Qing period. A considerable number of benevolent halls (*shantang*) led by local elites remained active until the 1940s, and they engaged in various charitable activities: they provided medical care, drugs, clothing, food, and coffins; they ran vocational schools and provided free education; they also raised orphans and cared for the aged. In all these activities, medical care was considered a form of social welfare—not an arena for science and research. The sick occupied the same category as the poor, aged, and orphaned.[16] Shanghai's local elites and entrepreneurs also operated charitable clinics and hospitals. In the early twentieth century, these preexisting charitable clinics came to emulate the hospital system and hired doctors who practiced Western medicine. At the same time, as doctors established themselves as modern professionals, the hospital became a site in which doctors conducted research and experiments, which required advanced medical facilities and instruments. Hospitals also provided wealthier patients with comfortable environments and better treatment. As hospitals accommodated those who were able and willing to pay, they began seeking profits. Pharma-

---

15. Sinn, *Power and Charity.*
16. Elvin, "Administration of Shanghai"; Rankin, *Elite Activism*, 202–47; Kohama, "Minkokuki Shanghai no toshi shakai to jizen jigyō."

ceutical companies were also involved in hospital management as a way to expand their market.

Hospitals were autonomous institutions in which various actors, including medical doctors, students, Chinese elites, missionaries, and patients, encountered and interacted with each other. A close examination of the goals, functions, and strategies of Shanghai hospitals provides a window onto major trends in professionalization, institutionalization, and commercialization that were transforming Shanghai's medical-care market. These transformations were a part of larger socioeconomic changes concurrently sweeping across Shanghai, but the development of medical sciences and technologies also played a major role in the evolution of health-care-providing institutions. In turn, hospitals and clinics changed popular perceptions of health and medicine and made a visible impact on the city's landscape.

Christianity and Medical Care: Missionary Hospitals

In the 1930s, among some two hundred hospitals of all sizes in the city, missionary hospitals were distinguished by their history, physical scale, and the quality of medical treatment they provided. Most importantly, missionary hospitals were the first institutions to introduce Shanghai residents to Western medical techniques, practices, and facilities. According to Ruan Renze and Gao Zhennong, at least five Catholic hospitals and seven Protestant hospitals existed in pre-1949 Shanghai.[17] Pang Jingzhou gave missionary hospitals high marks. According to Pang's list from 1933, out of thirty-one public hospitals, six were directly operated by Western churches. If a hospital was open to everyone and financed by endowments and annual funds, Pang considered it "public." He noted that foreign public hospitals, including missionary hospitals, commanded stable funding and were generally well managed. On Pang's list, all six church-related hospitals were classified as "large," out of only twelve hospitals in

17. Ruan Renze and Gao Zhennong, eds., *Shanghai zongjiaoshi*, 715–20, 896–913.

this category.[18] The accounts of the Hospitals and Nursing Services Commission of the International Settlement concur with Pang's observation. The commission commented that Renji Hospital and Tongren Hospital, the two major missionary hospitals in the city, were "large and efficient."[19] The Shanghai Municipal Council (SMC) listed five "large" hospitals in the Settlement that received municipal grants in 1938; those five included Renji, Tongren, and Guangren, all of which were missionary hospitals.[20] Altogether, missionary hospitals tended to a significant number of patients.

FROM CHARITABLE CLINICS TO GENERAL
HOSPITALS

Of the missionary hospitals, Renji Hospital (Renji yiyuan), the oldest Western hospital in Shanghai, serves as an excellent example of how a Western institution developed and transformed, accommodating to Shanghai's urban environments and progress in medical science. Both historically and currently, Renji is one of the most popular and successful hospitals in the city. Founded by a British missionary just after the Opium War, it followed the British "voluntary hospital" tradition and served as Shanghai's "charitable enterprise."[21] The British asserted that it was *their* hospital.[22] However, the hospital quickly adapted to Shanghai's popular needs and grew into a large general hospital by the 1930s. When the Communists took over the hospital in 1949, it had a wide range of departments, including internal medicine, surgery, obstetrics and gynecology, pediatrics, otolaryngology, ophthalmology, and dentistry. It also had operation rooms, laboratories, X-ray facilities, ultraviolet ray facili-

18.   According to Pang Jingzhou, of the twelve "large" hospitals in the city, nine were general hospitals that accepted all cases; of these nine general hospitals, four were church-related. The other "large" hospitals included two obstetric hospitals, both of which were tied to churches, and one isolation hospital run by the International Settlement. Altogether these "large" hospitals had 2,317 beds, and six church-related hospitals had 1,154 beds, constituting 49.8 percent of the total. See Pang, *Yiyao niaokan*, 23–25.

19.   SMA U1-16-519.

20.   SMA U1-4-212.

21.   For the early history of Renji Hospital, see MacPherson, *Wilderness of Marshes*, 143–71.

22.   Ibid., 159.

ties, electric therapy facilities, pharmacies, and ambulances; it had three hundred to five hundred beds and employed forty to fifty doctors. Renji Hospital accepted a total of 150,000 to 166,000 outpatients and more than 7,000 inpatients per year.[23] Until 1941, when the Japanese military took over the International Settlement and the hospital became a Dōjinkai hospital, it was sponsored by the London Missionary Society (LMS). All successive presidents of the hospital until 1941 were British, and many of the Chinese doctors associated with the hospital trained at Anglo-American medical institutions. Because of its close ties to the West, some historians regard Renji Hospital as an imperialist institution.[24] During the Maoist era, the hospital was reorganized several times, but maintained its position as a key medical institution in the city. Currently associated with Shanghai Jiaotong University Medical School, it operates its original Western Division (Xiyuan) on Shandong Road and has new branches: an Eastern Division (Dongyuan) in Pudong and a Southern Division (Nanyuan) in Minhang. Research on digestive organs and cardiology carried out at Renji is highly regarded.[25]

Renji Hospital is a leading medical institution today, but it made its start as a small clinic opened by William Lockhart (1811–96), a medical missionary from the LMS. With support from the Medical Missionary Society in China, Lockhart first went to Canton in 1839 to help Peter Parker and other medical missionaries in south China. Between 1839 and 1843, he moved around Canton, Macao, Ningbo, and Zhoushan and opened a small clinic in Dinghai. He eventually arrived in Shanghai in 1843 with a plan to establish a permanent medical institution there.[26] Lockhart rented a Chinese-style house near the South Gate of the Walled City in February 1844. There he opened a clinic with modest facilities to provide free medical care for local residents, called Lockhart Clinic (Luoshi zhengsuo). Its facilities were simple, Lockhart examined outpatients only, yet the clinic proved to be a success. To meet popular

23. These figures vary depending on sources. See SMA B242-1-131-35; SMA B242-1-146; SMA B242-1-351-107; SMA B241-1-377.

24. For example, see SMA B242-1-146, 14.

25. *SWZ*, 91; Xinkangwang, *Zuixin Shanghai jiuyi zhinan*, 12–13. For Renji's official website, see www.renji.com. For Shanghai Jiaotong University Medical School's official website, see http://english.shsmu.edu.cn/default.php.

26. Wang Ermin, *Jindai Shanghai keji xianqu*, 21–22.

demand, Lockhart invited British doctors already practicing in Shanghai to work for his clinic. He also trained Chinese assistants. In October of the same year, he rented a courtyard house outside of the South Gate with financial assistance from the LMS.[27] With high ceilings and rooms of various sizes, this new building was more suitable for use as a hospital. Lockhart brought in twenty beds so that he could admit inpatients. This new operation was named Renji Yiguan (Renji Medical Office) in Chinese.[28] Renji is an abbreviation of *renshu jishi*, which literally means "arts of benevolence helping society," and was also the name of a Chinese charity organization.[29] In both name and appearance, the hospital was not unlike a traditional Chinese charity clinic— clear indication that, though this hospital was a British institution, the British were familiar with China's traditional charity organizations. Renji's goal was not to boast the efficacy or benefits of Western medicine. Rather, Lockhart and his staff hoped to make the hospital look domestic and neighborly, an example of an amalgam of Chinese and British elements.

Bolstered by the hospital's initial success, a decision was made to expand and acquire property for a permanent site. To this end Lockhart raised contributions from British and Chinese merchants in the city and took out a loan of $10,000 from Turner and Son Co. Bank. In 1846 he used these funds to purchase a parcel of land to erect a new building at the intersection of Shandong and Fujian Roads.[30] In the same year, subscribers held their first meeting. At this meeting, they selected directors (*dongshi*) and four trustees (*baochan weiyuan*). The board of directors in charge of the hospital's general operation included both Chinese and British professionals. But all the trustees, who were in charge of property management and fund-raising, were British, and one of them was required to represent the LMS. The LMS was also responsible for inviting a president and some qualified doctors from Great Britain and paying their

---

27. Chen Pei and Fan Guanrong, eds., *Renshu jishi*, 608.
28. Ge Zhuang, *Zongjiao*, 119; Ruan Renze and Gao Zhennong, eds., *Shanghai zongjiaoshi*, 897.
29. In the late twenties, Renji Shantang was a charity organization in Shanghai, but it was not associated with Renji Hospital.
30. Wang Ermin, *Jindai Shanghai keji xianqu*, 24.

salaries.[31] Though the hospital was sponsored by the LMS, it was housed in a Chinese-style building and served the local Chinese population; it therefore came to be known in English as the Chinese Hospital.[32]

The quality of medical treatment provided by this hospital in its early years is difficult to measure. In the mid-nineteenth century, bacteriology had not developed in Europe, and anesthesia and antiseptic were ineffective. Western treatment was not necessarily superior to Chinese medicine at that time.[33] Lockhart himself was a surgeon, but the hospital had no specialization and treated all cases. It performed surgeries, admitted infectious disease patients, and administered smallpox vaccinations.[34] Renji attracted a large number of patients from its opening. Some nineteen thousand patients visited the hospital between February 1844 and the end of 1845, and they came not only from Shanghai but also from Suzhou, Songjiang, and Chongming Island.[35] In 1861, the hospital moved to yet another location on Shandong Road. In Chinese it was now known as Renji Yiyuan and in English as Shandong Road Hospital for the Chinese. The hospital enjoyed considerable popularity among Shanghai's general populace.

Throughout the nineteenth century, conveying religious teaching through free medical care remained the mission of Renji Hospital—its primary function was providing philanthropy rather than scientific medicine. Its operation had a strong religious flavor.[36] According to the hospital's regulations, all inpatients and hospital staff were supposed to assemble in the hall every day at 7:30 in the morning and at noon to read the Bible and say prayers. Outpatients could not obtain a consultation ticket unless they participated in religious activities. Missionaries from

31. Ibid., 31–33; Zhu Mingde and Chen Pei, ed., *Renji yiyuan*; Ruan Renze and Gao Zhennong, eds., *Shanghai zongjiaoshi*, 897; Ge Zhuang, *Zongjiao*, 120; SMA B241-1-377, 63.

32. Ge Zhuang, *Zhongjiao*, 119–20.

33. For an analysis of medical cases treated at early missionary hospitals, see Yan Yiwei and Zhang Daqing, "Jibingpu yu zhiliaoguan."

34. "Lester Chinese Hospital"; Chen Pei and Fan Guanrong, eds., *Renshu jishi*, 10, 33.

35. Ge Zhuang, *Zongjiao*, 120; Ruan Renze and Gao Zhennong, eds., *Shanghai zongjiaoshi*, 897; Wang Ermin, *Jindai Shanghai keji xianqu*, 48; Chen Pei and Fan Guanrong, eds., *Renshu jishi*, 6–8.

36. Wang Ermin, *Jindai Shanghai keji xianqu*, 48–49.

the LMS visited hospital rooms and examination rooms every day to preach the Gospel.[37]

Renji provided nonmedical community services as well. In times of famine, it dispensed free food to the local poor. Even during the Small Sword Uprising (1853–54), its business continued; moreover, as a humanitarian gesture, hospital staff treated the wounded on both sides.[38] In 1852, the hospital opened a soup kitchen (*zhouchang*) for ten weeks to feed the poor; a similar kitchen was opened in 1856.[39] Thus, except for its evangelical Christian and British origins, Renji was not unlike other charitable clinics run by local elites. No records are available to identify the nineteenth-century patients of Renji Hospital. In all likelihood, many belonged to the same socioeconomic class that frequented other charitable clinics. Presumably the simplicity of the hospital's facilities even drew such patients to its doors.

During the Republican period, Renji continued to expand; with some fluctuations, the number of patients visiting Renji also steadily increased. In the 1900s, the total number of outpatients per year ranged from a low of 61,552 (1909) to a high of 98,300 (1902); in the 1910s, 60,889 (1910) and 103,699 (1913); in the 1920s, 80,482 (1927) and 143,517 (1928); and in the 1930s, 133,121 (1930) and 240,910 (1938). The number of inpatients also steadily increased. Before 1898, the total number of inpatient cases per year did not reach 1,000. However, in the 1900s, the number was between 871 (1906) and 1,289 (1916); in the 1910s, between 1,064 (1910) and 2,209 (1916); in the 1920s, between 2,651 (1922) and 3,817 (1928); and in the 1930s, between 2,869 (1930) and 6,770 (1938).[40]

Several factors contributed to Renji's growth. First, its growth reflected the demographic changes in the city. Renji's development coincided with the development of the city itself. As Shanghai opened as a

---

37. Ge Zhuang, *Zongjiao*, 119–20; Wang Ermin, *Jindai Shanghai keji xianqu*, 47–48; MacPherson, *Wilderness of Marshes*, 153–54.

38. Ge Zhuang, *Zongjiao*, 121.

39. Wang Ermin, *Jindai Shanghai keji xianqu*, 49; Ge Zhuang, *Zongjiao*, 121.

40. These figures are based on E. S. Elliston, *Ninety-Five Years: A Hospital*, 34–35, quoted and tabulated in Wang Ermin, *Jindai Shanghai keji xianqu*, 51–52. Also *The Lester Chinese Hospital Annual Report and Statement Accounts* (*Lester Annual Report*) for various years list these figures. In Wang's table, he differentiates the total number of patients or patient days (*binghuan*) and number of cases (*bingli*).

treaty port and became the nation's industrial and commercial center, the city attracted immigrants, and the city's population grew exponentially. Consequently sickness and injuries also increased. Shanghai in the 1930s was different from Shanghai in the 1840s. Even though Shanghai had about two hundred medical institutions in the city, some were small and some were temporary hospitals open only during the summer to admit acute gastrointestinal disease patients. (More discussions on summer hospitals follow.) There was always a shortage of medical facilities.[41] Moreover, in the 1920s and 1930s, not only the urban poor but also Shanghai's *xiaoshimin*, or "petty urbanites," became interested in hospital care.[42] These people expected not just shelter or simple care but advanced medical care and cures from Renji. Renji responded to socioeconomic realities and popular demand.

To carry out its operation, Renji needed financial support. The London Missionary Society sponsored its founding and, in the early years, also paid the rental fees for the hospital premises.[43] However, over the years, the LMS subsidies covered an increasingly smaller portion of the hospital's total financial requirements. To accommodate its expansion, Renji turned to three other sources of revenue: individual subscriptions and donations, grants from the SMC, and patient fees. An examination of these sources suggests that Renji's operation was funded by Western and Chinese as well as public and private money.

For its first source of income, Renji Hospital raised money widely from both the British and Chinese communities in the city. Before the 1870s, regular subscriptions and individual donations were the hospital's only sources of income. Until 1905—when Renji began charging patient fees—these funds represented the major portion of the hospital's revenue. In addition to annual subscriptions, the hospital occasionally received large sums of money from wealthy families. For example, in 1907, a certain Ms. Chu Yo-chee gave 10,000 taels to build a women's ward; in 1911, Dr. Lalcaca's family made a donation to establish the Lalcaca Memorial Ward. The most significant donation came in 1927, when the late Henry

41.   SMA U1-16-519.

42.   *Xiaoshimin* usually refers to middle and lower-middle class urban residents. See Hanchao Lu, *Beyond the Neon Lights*, 61–64.

43.   Chen Pei and Fan Guanrong, eds., *Renshu jishi*, 6–8.

Lester, a British millionaire and architect, left the hospital an endowment of two million taels of silver and real estate. (Since that time, the hospital's English name has been changed to Lester Hospital.) Renji Hospital established a fund with Lester's donation and embarked on a total reconstruction of its premises. After three years of makeshift operation, the construction was completed in 1931. The new building was impressive. A seven-story building made of reinforced concrete, it housed 270 beds. The building was well heated and well ventilated, and adopted the most advanced architectural techniques of the time. All patient rooms faced south to assure that each benefited from the most sunlight. The walls of all surgery rooms were painted green, since green was believed to relieve eye fatigue. Wang Yiting (1867–1938), a well-known Shanghai entrepreneur and philanthropist, wrote the name of the hospital in calligraphy, and it was engraved in the front wall.[44] Whereas the simple, familiar appearance of the original building might have attracted some patients, the new Western-style building seemed almost "arrogant," and may have frightened some patients away.[45] Income from the rentals of the late Lester's properties contributed to the maintenance and running expenses of the hospital.

The hospital's second source of revenue came from subsidies from the SMC. Whereas individual donations varied every year[46] and incomes from estates also fluctuated,[47] annual grants from the SMC were a stable source of hospital revenue. In particular, the Settlement authorities recognized the charitable nature of the hospital and its positive reputation in the Chinese community. They believed that the hospital treated and accommodated a large Chinese population who lived in the Settlement,

---

44.   Ge Zhuang, *Zongjiao*, 120; Ruan Renze and Gao Zhennong, eds., *Shanghai zongjiaoshi*, 899; Chen Pei and Fan Guanrong, eds., *Renshu jishi*, 17–21; Zhu Mingde and Chen Pei, eds., *Renji yiyuan*, 6–7; *Shanghai Evening Post*, November 8, 1933 (filed in SMA U1-16-822).

45.   Pang, *Yiyao niaokan*, 22.

46.   For example, the amount of donations from Chinese sources dropped from $10,259 in 1924 to $8,990 in 1925. The amount in 1934 was $1,138.68, whereas that of 1935 was $2,719.33. A letter from Renji to the SMA, dated on March 19, 1926 (filed in SMA U1-16-823); *Shanghai Times*, April 1, 1936 (filed in SMA U1-16-822).

47.   For example, income from Lester's estates was $169,984 (1934), $121,042 (1935), $98,131 (1936), and $178,000 in 1940. *North China*, May 20, 1937 (filed in SMA U1-4-216); *Lester Annual Report* (1940).

and that it rendered invaluable community service. On these grounds, Renji became a regular recipient of the SMC's grant-in-aid program. Starting in 1870, Renji received 200 taels from the SMC, and the amount steadily increased. It was raised to 600 taels in 1876, 1,000 taels in 1901, 2,000 taels in 1906, 3,000 taels in 1913, 5,000 taels in 1916, 20,000 taels in 1925, 28,000 taels in 1934, and 35,000 taels in 1940.[48] The SMC was always supportive of Renji and made favorable remarks. Settlement authorities indicated that Renji was well managed and agreed that it would be more cost-effective to subsidize Renji than to open and run a separate municipal hospital.[49] Renji was a private institution run by a religious group located in the Settlement, independent from the Chinese state. Yet, it served Chinese people and was subsidized by Chinese taxes collected by the colonial administration. It functioned as if it were a public organization and made up for deficiencies in state or municipal medical service, looking after public and private interests and presenting a venue in which colonial authorities, Shanghai's local society, and a Christian church interacted with one another.

Patient fees provided the hospital with a third source of income. From its foundation in 1844 to 1904, Renji Hospital treated all patients without charge. However, during the tenure of C. J. Davenport (1862–1926) as its president (1904–26), some important changes took place in Renji's operation. As an eminent physician himself, Davenport upgraded the standard of internal medicine at Renji. Most importantly, starting from 1905, the hospital rolled out an itemized scale of charges and began asking some patients to pay fees for examinations, treatments, and accommodations. In 1905, patient fees totaled 1,848 taels; this increased to 3,359 taels the following year—earnings that were greater than the income from regular subscriptions (2,873 taels) and the SMC grant (2,000 taels) of the same year. According to the fee schedule of June 1927, "ordinary outpatients" received treatment and medicine for free, and "first-class outpatients" paid $1 per visit. Inpatients were sorted into three categories in accordance with the particular ward in which they stayed: general ward patients,

48. Rate applications are filed in SMA U1-4-216 and U1-16-823. From 1928 to 1940, the SMC granted 20,000 taels, or $2,800, to the hospital. This amount was raised to $35,000 in 1941.

49. SMA U1-4-212.

private ward patients, and private room patients. Patients in each category were charged $0.30, $1.50, and $3–$4 per day, respectively. The inpatient fees included food, treatment, and medicine. In addition, operation fees and X-ray fees were established, and "private ward patients" were charged more than "ordinary patients."[50] Renji's fee schedule was revised from time to time, and fees came to account for a considerable portion of the hospital revenue. To put this in perspective, when the Chinese Municipal Public Health Bureau was opened in 1927, the revenue from patient fees was 38,894 taels, which accounted for 53 percent of the total income. In 1935, when Renji began operating in the new building, patient fees amounted to 76,764 taels, or 63 percent of the total income.[51]

Charging fees for services marked a significant change in the management of Renji Hospital. The very fact that people were willing to pay for treatment is indicative of the growing popularity of Western-style hospitals and Western medicine. Western medicine had been widely recognized by the 1920s. In addition to Renji, other Western-style hospitals were opened in the city; city residents became familiar with Western medicine, with some preferring Western medical care over traditional medicine. Chinese disinclination for Western medicine was on the wane, and Renji was aware that Western medicine was in "vogue." The hospital's annual report for 1936 pointed out that numerous small dispensaries and clinics had opened recently that took care of simple cases, implying Renji should focus on more complex cases.[52] Renji attracted patients not just because it offered free or inexpensive treatment, but also because of the high quality of its medical care. The presence of paying patients meant that some people in the city were both able and willing to pay more to receive better treatment and accommodations. Clearly, both the socioeconomic status of the patients of Renji Hospital and their expectations had changed. Wu Tiecheng (1883–1953), who served as a mayor of Chinese Shanghai (1932–37), was once a patient at Renji. Such a fact evidences the high social standing of at least some of the patients served by Renji.[53]

50. These scales of charges are filed in SMA U1-16-822.
51. E. S. Elliston, *Ninety-Five Years*, 36–37, quoted and tabulated in Wang Ermin, *Jindai Shanghai keji xianqu*, 41–42.
52. *Lester Annual Report* (1936).
53. *China Press*, May 3, 1937 (filed in SMA U1-16-822).

Renji Hospital management responded by opening different classes of accommodation, with first- and second-class rooms. What had begun as a small clinic for the indigent now offered patients of the middle and even the upper class medical treatment and surgery done by distinguished experts. In short, Renji was no longer a genuine charity institution. It aimed at both attracting wealthy patients to generate more profits and offering free medical care and other services to the poor.

In grant application letters, Renji Hospital always identified itself as a charitable organization and emphasized its community service. The hospital continued to accept free patients and bore their expenses, and it promoted its charitable nature when it requested donations and grants. In fact, a condition of the late Lester's will prevented the hospital from charging the poor.[54] The hospital admitted accident casualties and attempted-suicide cases brought by the police and others, and it covered their expenses; it also cared for those who became ill from malnutrition.[55] According to the *Shanghai Times* of January 1939, over 50 percent of inpatient services were still performed for free. In addition, the hospital provided other social services in the 1930s. For example, hospital staff offered ongoing care to those who had attempted suicide and helped them identify and overcome their problems. They also opened a Women's Auxiliary Department to foster the independence of convalescent female patients.[56] These services were part of Renji's social welfare program, but they contained subtle differences of emphasis from traditional charities. Here, hospital staff served as counselors and social workers. They did not view patients as helpless victims; rather, they promoted the self-help mentality associated with Western ideals. In the early years, Renji was more like a Chinese charity institution. As time progressed, the hospital became more "Westernized" in response to changing Chinese expectations.

Renji Hospital was not unique. The history of Tongren Hospital (Tongren yiyuan, also known as St. Luke's Hospital) followed a similar trajectory.

54. A letter from the hospital to the SMC, dated March 28, 1928 (filed in SMA U1-16-823). Also see SMA U1-4-212.
55. SMA U1-16-822.
56. *Lester Annual Report* (1939).

Tongren was founded by the American Episcopal Church. It merged with Guangren Hospital (Guangren yiyuan, also known as St. Elizabeth Hospital), another hospital sponsored by the Episcopal Church, and became Shanghai Municipal Thoracic Hospital, which specialized in cardiopulmonary medicine.[57]

Like Renji, Tongren Hospital started as a charitable clinic. In 1866, Reverend Elliot Thomson and Wu Hongyu, a Chinese minister, received a donation from unidentified church members. They used the money to rent a house on the north bank of the Suzhou River and opened a small medical establishment to proselytize the local population. At this time, the Episcopal Church did not even have its own medical mission. The church invited Dr. D. J. MacGowan to be a medical adviser to the hospital. Dr. MacGowan was originally sent to China by the Baptist Church in America. After working in Ningbo, Canton, and other cities, he left China in 1859 and later returned. As of 1866, he was practicing privately in Shanghai.[58] In addition to Dr. MacGowan, the church asked several local doctors to provide their services for free.[59] Since the hospital was located in the Hongkou area, local Chinese called it Hongkew (Hongkou) Hospital. Hongkou is in the northern part of the International Settlement, and the local population in this area—comprising primarily factory workers—became the targeted patient base of Hongkew Hospital. Like other missionary hospitals, the one in Hongkou offered free medical care to attract patients and raised donations from the local business community. In 1877, the hospital had nineteen beds and accepted some 130 inpatients and 15,000 to 20,000 outpatients annually.[60] Tongren also prepared Christian tracts and pictures, and it offered Christian teaching to its patients. Chaplains visited patient rooms and gave Christian leaflets and tracts to the literate and picture cards to the illiterate. Doctors and nurses identified responsive patients and alerted the chaplains.[61]

57. *SWZ*, 91.
58. Wong and Wu, *History of Chinese Medicine*, 205, 208, 234, 273; Xu Yihua and Han Xinchang, *Haishang fanwangdu*, 9.
59. Lamberton, *St. John's University*, 17.
60. Ruan Renze and Gao Zhennong, eds., *Shanghai zongjiaoshi*, 901.
61. *68th Annual Report of St. Luke's Hospital for Chinese for the Year Ending December 31, 1934 (Annual Report of St. Luke's)*, 38.

In the 1880s and 1890s, Hongkew Hospital expanded its business and improved the standards of its medical treatment. In 1880, H. W. Boone (1839–1925), the first medical missionary from the Episcopal Church, arrived in Shanghai and became the director of the hospital.[62] With a donation from Li Jiuming, a wealthy Cantonese merchant, the hospital moved to a new location and constructed a new building. When the construction was completed in 1881, the hospital was renamed Tongren.[63] Tongren, which literally means "universal benevolence," was a common name given to China's charitable organizations. Since the hospital had become famous for surgery, around 1878–80 an obscure Shanghai resident composed the following *zhuzhici*—Shanghai popular verse—about Tongren:

> Tongren Hospital helps many people.
> In the hospital, sores and wounds meet the eyes on every side,
> Patients call out asking what to do.
> Their healing all depends on those who use scalpels.
> Indeed, Hua Tuo lives on in the West.[64]

We do not have a way to measure the actual quality of the operations, nor do we have success or recovery rates from Tongren. Likely, most of the operations in the 1870s and 1880s involved the simple removal of tumors or the extraction of teeth. Yet the author of this verse was impressed by the dedication of hospital staff and the techniques of those who used scalpels. Although Tongren was an American hospital, the author equated Western doctors with Hua Tuo, a legendary Chinese surgeon who was believed to have been active in the second century BCE. In the sense that miraculous cures could be attributed to surgery, this author did not draw a clear line between Western and Chinese doctors.

Like Renji, Tongren developed and expanded its business. As of 1893, Tongren Hospital was staffed with pharmacists and doctors in various

62. Guo Dewen, "Mingyi de yaolan," 335; Xu Yihua and Han Xinchang, *Haishang fanwangdu*, 14.

63. Ruan Renze and Gao Zhennong, eds., *Zongjiaoshi*, 901.

64. Gu Bingquan, ed., *Shanghai yangchang zhuzhici*, 52. This verse originally appeared in *Chun Shengpu zhuzhici* (Verse on Shanghai's Spring), which was compiled around 1878–80.

specialties, including internal medicine, surgery, gynecology, ophthalmology, and dentistry.[65] By the medical standards of late nineteenth-century China, or even compared with the West, the comprehensiveness and diversity of the faculty at Tongren were remarkable.[66] In the early twentieth century, Tongren further upgraded its buildings and facilities. In 1901, it added new wards, including X-ray rooms, consultation rooms, emergency rooms, and other facilities.[67] The hospital observed a growing interest in medical cases, as opposed to surgery, among Chinese patients. As of 1934, the hospital employed nine surgeons, three physicians, two ophthalmologists, and a dentist, in addition to four resident interns and seven assistant interns.[68]

Tongren also relied on SMC grants and patient fees for its finance. Along with Renji, Tongren became one of the largest hospitals in the city and a major recipient of the SMC's annual grants. Commissioners of public health and police both supported Tongren's grant applications on the grounds that Tongren accepted a considerable number of free patients and police cases and thus served the public.

Though it began as a charitable institution, over the course of the twentieth century, as part of its efforts to secure its finances, Tongren, too, opened first- and second-class rooms and began charging patients fees. The amount of revenue collected from inpatients in these rooms gradually increased. Income from this source accounted for 11.9 percent of the total revenue in 1904, 46.9 percent in 1910, 59.8 percent in 1934, and 74 percent in 1936.[69] The total amount of patient fees also increased every year. It was $57,879.62 in 1929, $71,635.81 in 1930, $79,748.63 in 1931, $73,779.21 in 1932, $91,806.29 in 1933, and $98,906.17 in 1934.[70]

65.   Ruan Renze and Gao Zhennong, eds., *Shanghai zongjiaoshi*, 902; Ge Zhuang, *Zongjiao*, 127; Lu Ming, "Shanghai jindai xiyi yiyuan gaishu," 23.

66.   In the West in the early nineteenth century, most practitioners were generalists, and specialists were regarded as "marginal" or even "quacks." Whereas medicine in German-speaking nations was becoming increasingly ramified, specializations were established only in the 1880s in Anglo-American hospitals. See Rosenberg, *Care of Strangers*, 169–73.

67.   Ruan Renze and Gao Zhennong, eds., *Shanghai zongjiaoshi*, 902–3.

68.   *Annual Report of St. Luke's*, 1–3.

69.   Ruan Renze and Gao Zhennong, eds., *Shanghai zongjiaoshi*, 903–4; *Annual Report of St. Luke's*, 22.

70.   *Annual Report of St. Luke's*, 18.

But Tongren never completely abandoned its charitable mission. The hospital offered higher-class rooms and also had wards to accommodate the poor. It also accepted a considerable number of police cases, and in the 1930s, the hospital still provided free care for refugees and beggars.[71] After the war against Japan broke out, Tongren opened its second hospital in December 1937. This hospital had 250 beds and provided full outpatient services; it also operated bathhouses for refugees and their children.[72] Throughout the hospital's history, the patients of Tongren were diversified and stratified, and the hospital provided different types of rooms to accommodate the needs of the broad range of patients that it served. By doing so, it engaged in charity and business simultaneously.[73]

SCIENCE AND EDUCATION

Renji and Tongren were Shanghai's two major missionary hospitals; in the twentieth century, they became engaged in two new services: scientific research and medical education. The development of these hospitals roughly coincided with the development of medical technology in Europe. In the mid- to late nineteenth century, European medical scientists made several important breakthroughs: the effective use of anesthesia, development of bacteriology, and the invention of X-ray and radiation technology. Modern anesthesiology started in the 1840s, and physicians began using narcotic drugs—including ether and chloroform—to anesthetize patients during surgery. In the 1870s and 1880s, Louis Pasteur (1822–95) inaugurated modern bacteriology, and Robert Koch (1843–1910) further advanced microbiology by identifying and isolating specific bacteria. Pasteur, Koch, and their students developed new concepts of germs,

71. Ruan Renze and Gao Zhennong, eds., *Shanghai zongjiaoshi*, 901–5; Lamberton, *St. John's University*, 155–56.

72. "Memorandum of the Members of Health and Finance Committee"; Xu Yihua and Han Xinchang, *Haishang fanwangdu*, 48–49.

73. There is an obvious parallel between the trajectory of missionary hospitals in China and hospitals in the United States. Though they developed in a different sociocultural setting, by the early twentieth century, American hospitals had also evolved from being "receptacles" for the poor and those who had no families to places that provided advanced medical care by experts. Yet, American hospitals have always been a "hybrid" of business and charity. Rosenberg, *Care of Strangers*; Stevens, *In Sickness and in Wealth*.

vaccines, immunity, and sterilization. In the 1890s, Wilhelm Konrad Roentgen (1845–1923) and others discovered X-ray radiation. By the 1910s, it was common practice among medical personnel to use X-ray technology to produce radiographic images of the body and internal organs. Both Renji and Tongren were quick to respond to these developments and adopted new techniques for diagnosis and treatment. As Chinese interests in internal medicine grew, Renji and Tongren attached more importance not only to surgical skills but also to scientific medicine.[74] Both hospitals were promoted as sites in which well-qualified medical professionals conducted advanced research and carried out state-of-the-art examinations using modern technologies.[75] A comment made by a participant at Renji's annual subscriber's meeting in 1934 is illustrative: twenty-six years ago, the hospital was packed with crowds of patients; doctors provided diagnoses and prescriptions "at an amazing rate"; and the outpatient clinic was "rough-and-ready." But, everything was different now. Doctors carry out an "intricate investigation" for each case and pay more attention not only to how to treat and cure patients, but also to what is causing the symptoms.[76] This summary of a comment evinces that the hospital's emphasis had shifted from quantity to quality and from therapy to pathological study.

Renji's scientific development was in part supported by the Henry Lester Research Institute. The Lester Institute was founded by the Henry Lester Trust, and it gave technical advice to the hospital and conducted scientific research and experiments.[77] Until its own building was completed in 1932, the research institute was located within Renji Hospital.[78] Later it took over the hospital's laboratory and conducted research and examination on bacteriology, serology, clinical chemistry, tissue pathology, pharmacology, electric cardiology, clinical photography, and the like.[79] The adoption of new technologies and the development of bacteriology did not immediately improve clinical outcomes. As Charles

74. *Lester Annual Report* (1940).
75. *North China*, May 16, 1940 (filed in SMA U1-16-822).
76. *Report of Annual Meeting of Subscribers*.
77. Ruan Renze and Gao Zhennong, eds., *Shanghai zongjiaoshi*, 899.
78. Wong and Wu Lien-teh, *History of Chinese Medicine*, 584–85; *Lester Annual Report* (1933).
79. *North China*, May 30, 1940 (filed in SMA U1-16-822).

Rosenberg notes, "The alliance between science and clinical medicine remained shaky and ambiguous."[80] Still, the introduction of new technologies and laboratories transformed hospitals into a special places. Hospitals could provide special therapies and treatments that were not feasible or available at home or in shelters. Hospitals were now regarded as places where doctors could give proper diagnoses and carry out research based on "scientific" measures. In fact in 1933, Renji used radiation therapy to treat breast cancer patients.[81] It was the latest medical technique at that time.

If we understand Renji's partnership with the Lester Institute as indicative of the shift in the hospital's operation from evangelism and charity to science and research, similarly, Tongren's connection with St. John's University exemplifies its commitment to medical education and training. To secure the quality and quantity of medical staff at the hospital, Dr. Boone offered a training course at the hospital in 1880 to teach Chinese assistants necessary medical knowledge and skills. Believing they were responsible for disseminating Western medical knowledge among the Chinese, many medical missionaries in China began training Chinese assistants and opened schools related to hospitals.[82] Many of these missionary medical schools remained small, but the courses attached to Tongren expanded quickly. They eventually became part of the medical school at St. John's University, and Tongren became a teaching hospital associated with St. John's and provided a training ground for interns.[83]

St. John's was founded in 1879 by a bishop from the Episcopal Church in Shanghai. Spreading the word of God was at the heart of its mission, and most of its students at first were from poor Christian families. But St. John's quickly shifted its emphasis from evangelism to Western-style education, and English was adopted as the language of instruction. With these changes, it attracted students from affluent families who aimed at establishing successful careers in Shanghai. By the 1920s and 1930s, along

80. Rosenberg, *Care of Strangers*, 159.

81. *Shanghai Evening Post*, November 8, 1933 (filed in SMA U1-16-822).

82. Zhu Jianping, *Zhongguo yixueshi yanjiu*, 173–74.

83. Xu Yihua, ed., *Shanghai Sheng Yuehan daxue*, 47; Xiong Yuezhi and Zhou Wu, eds., *Sheng Yuehan daxueshi*, 11.

with its business and engineering schools, the medical training at St. John's had evolved into one of the best educational programs in China.[84]

Tongren was where St. John's medical students received on-site training. In their sixth year, in addition to taking regular classes, students were required to attend hospitals as externs to observe actual cases. It was mandatory for them to work as resident interns in their seventh year and to attend different departments in rotation.[85] In the course of their training, they met "farmers and others from the villages nearby" and "saw accident cases of many kinds, as well as other medical and surgical cases, for the hospital was in what soon became a very busy industrial section of the city where laborers and factory workers congregated."[86] Presumably patients in the third-class rooms were the ones most often observed and examined by student-interns. In the 1930s, internship was a standard feature of medical school curricula in China.[87]

The histories of Renji and Tongren illustrate the range of their functions; they provided free or inexpensive care to the city's poor for the purpose of evangelism, and their services attracted a considerable number of patients. Even with rising Chinese nationalism, neither Renji nor Tongren became an important target of antiforeign demonstrations.[88] Although bitter confrontations erupted between supporters of Chinese medicine and proponents of Western medicine, these confrontations did not directly affect the operation of the missionary hospitals in Shanghai. The

84. On St. John's University, see Yeh, *Alienated Academy*, chap. 2; Lamberton, *St. John's University*; Xiong Yuezhi and Zhou Wu, eds., *Sheng Yuehan daxueshi*; Xu Yihua, ed., *Shanghai Sheng Yuehan daxue*; Xu Yihua and Han Xinchang, *Haishang fanwangdu*; Kaiyi Chen, *Seeds from the West*; Yip, *Health and National Reconstruction*, 147–48.

85. Guo Dewen, "Mingyi de yaolan," 338. In the United States, there was a demand for clinical education and bedside teaching for medical students since the nineteenth century, and clinically oriented education and internship became standard by the 1920s. Rosenberg, *Care of Strangers*, 190–211.

86. Lamberton, *St. John's University*, 18–19.

87. On the curricula of medical schools in China, see Yip, *Health and National Reconstruction*, 132–61.

88. On Chinese reactions to Western medical missions, see Shang-jen Li, "Healing Body, Saving Soul."

general popularity of missionary hospitals is indicative of the flexible and practical attitudes toward Western medicine and Western hospitals held by Shanghai residents. Importantly, the missionary hospitals were not completely new institutions. Rather, they augmented the extensive social welfare network already in place in the city. Shanghai residents did not experience missionary hospitals as completely "foreign." This is evident in another *zhuzhici*, composed around 1906, that exemplifies the popular perception of hospitals as a whole. The author seems to be thankful for hospitals' medical services and their charitable nature. Here, again, she or he places Chinese and Western hospitals side by side and does not differentiate them from each other:

> Hospitals
> Chinese and Western hospitals are opened and run by big businesses.
> Numerous indigents are grateful for their beneficence and care.
> Hospitals can cure diseases and heal wounds,
> They help people and do not take their money.[89]

Over time these missionary hospitals diverged from their role as strictly charitable institutions and began to broaden their activities. By the 1930s, a hospital was no longer a modest station that accommodated the poor. A hospital was an institution with an imposing building in which patients received diagnosis and treatment by medical professionals; it was a residence where those who could afford to pay could find a comfortable environment in which to heal; it also continued to be an institution that provided medical and other services to those of more modest means. At the same time, a hospital was a classroom in which medical students observed patients and learned about advanced medical technologies. Saving human lives, Christian evangelism, charitable work, medical education, and scientific research were all part of the mix.

89. Gu Bingquan, ed., *Shanghai yangchang zhuzhici*, 106. This verse originally appeared in *Hujiang shangye shi jingci* (The Poetry of Scenes of Commerce and Market in Shanghai), which was compiled around 1906.

Seasonal Diseases and Elite Activism:
Summer-Disease Hospitals

Renji and Tongren owed much of their success to their abilities to adapt to Shanghai's society. Though they both had Western origins and were centers of Western medical practice, they were not radically different from preexisting Chinese charities. At the same time, Shanghai's traditional charity clinics also responded to the growing popularity of Western-style hospitals and Chinese interest in Western medicine. Seasonal disease hospitals (*shiyi yiyuan*), which opened only in the summer, best illustrate the fusion of traditional charities and Western medicine. Summertime in Shanghai was a dangerous time of year. The heat and humidity encouraged the propagation of germs that infected food and water; gastrointestinal diseases—including cholera, dysentery, and food poisoning—were common among Shanghai residents. Outbreaks of communicable disease often swept through the city. These summer diseases were collectively called *shiyi*. Literally translated as "seasonal diseases," the term often refers to summertime gastrointestinal disorders—particularly cholera. To help patients with such diseases, local elites in Shanghai regularly held short-term hospitals. Such venues dispensed free medical treatment and drugs for visitors and provided a place to stay for the seriously ill.[90] These hospitals usually opened in May or June, when the first summer-disease cases were identified, and closed in early fall once the outbreaks had subsided.

These summer hospitals, called *shiyi yiyuan,* were set up to provide temporary relief to a particular crisis. Based on the Confucian principle of benevolence and the associated sense of responsibility of elites, the operation of such hospitals was one of the routine services of the city's nongovernmental social welfare system. Many of them did not have stable endowments; they tended to be small and did not open every year. Some were run by persons who had very little knowledge of bacteriology or infection; as a result, they might not have offered appropriate treatment for infectious disease patients. Yet, such seasonal hospitals at least provided separate shelters for patients and helped prevent the spread of

90. Kohama, "Minkokuki Shanghai no toshi shakai to jizen jigyō," 73–77.

disease to an extent. The Settlement authorities commented that the Chinese were reluctant to avail themselves of the isolation hospital run by the Settlement, because Western institutions tended to enforce stricter quarantine regulations. They criticized Chinese summer-disease hospitals for impeding the normal development of municipal isolation facilities.[91] In spite of these criticisms, *shiyi* hospitals were well accepted by Chinese residents; moreover, in the twentieth century, these hospitals also followed the development of bacteriology. They employed Western-style doctors and provided treatment based on biomedicine. Some of them grew into general hospitals that remained open throughout the year.

Chinese Infectious Disease Hospital (CIDH) (Shanghai shiyi yiyuan) is a case in point.[92] Located on Tibet Road, CIDH was one of the major hospitals throughout the first half of the twentieth century. It was taken over by the Shanghai Branch Office of the Chinese Red Cross Society in 1953, and it is now part of Huangpu District Central Hospital (Huangpu Qu zhongxin yiyuan).[93] The history of CIDH illustrates the combination of elite activism, charitable sponsorship, and bacteriological knowledge.

CIDH was founded by a group of Shanghai's leading businessmen. Since 1908, Zhu Baosan (1848–1926), Shen Dunhe (1866–1920), and other Shanghai notables pooled their money and rented a Chinese property on Tianjin Road every summer. They used the premises as a seasonal hospital to treat summer-disease patients. This hospital was named Chinese Infectious Disease Hospital. Over the years, the building became run down, and the owner was no longer willing to rent it. Zhu and others were not able to find appropriate alternative premises for rent and decided instead to purchase a parcel of land on Tibet Road for the construction of a new hospital building. In 1929, they requested financial support from the SMC for this initiative. Health officers of the SMC gave positive recommendations in support of CIDH: it treated a large number of cholera patients using a saline transfusion method, and it was preferred

91. SMA U1-16-520, 377. Stevens, *In Sickness and in Wealth.*

92. Although the original Chinese name of this hospital literally means "Shanghai Seasonal Disease Hospital," English contemporary documents usually call this hospital "Chinese Infectious Disease Hospital."

93. SMA B241-1-502-30. For this hospital's official website, see http://yyk.39.net/sh/zonghe/4ef4c.html.

by Chinese patients over the isolation hospital run by the SMC. On the grounds that the hospital was serving the public, the SMC agreed to subsidize the construction of the new building.[94]

The hospital was first established as a summer hospital. However, as Shanghai developed, its population increased. In particular, a large number of working-class people (*pingmin laogong*) settled in the city. With its short-term arrangement as a summer hospital, it was not able to satisfy the medical demands of the commoners. Thus, when they constructed their own building, hospital managers decided to open it throughout the year.[95] From summer to early fall, the hospital functioned as a traditional seasonal hospital. It employed extra doctors and nurses and added more beds, and treated exclusively summer-disease cases—including cholera (*huoluan*), dysentery (*liji*), emesis (*tuxie*), and other acute diseases (*jisha*). When the epidemic season was over, CIDH downsized the staff and accepted non-summer-disease patients—including both surgical and medical cases.[96] In the spring, fall, and winter, it functioned more like a general hospital. Doctors, nurses, and clerks were on duty twenty-four hours a day and accepted patients throughout the day and night.[97] During the summer, all summer-disease patients received free treatment and accommodations, and in other seasons, non-summer-diseases patients were charged according to a class-ranking system. The hospital had first-, second-, and third-class rooms, and patients were asked to pay for drugs, injections, and accommodations.[98] According to the 1941 report, CIDH accepted 134,621 outpatients, out of which 40,949 (30 percent) were summer-disease patients, whereas 82,727 (61 percent) were general cases; others included non-specified acute cases and those who received vaccinations. In the same year, the total bed days for inpatients were divided into 14,809 days (42 percent)

94. For the correspondences between the CIDH and the SMC, see SMA U1-16-738; SMA Q6-9-190-12.
95. SMA Q113-4-1; Q6-9-190; Q6-9-190-12.
96. For example, in 1941, the hospital employed six regular doctors and twenty-one nurses in offseason, and in summer, their numbers increased to fourteen and thirty-six respectively. *Sanshi nian fen.*
97. *Shanghai shiyi yiyuan zhangcheng*
98. SMA Q113-4-1; Q6-9-190-13.

of summer-disease cases and 20,603 days (58 percent) of general cases.[99]

Because of its free treatment and convenient location, CIDH was popular, and it attracted a large number of patients in the summer. In the 1930s, it had 140–300 beds to accommodate summer-disease patients and treated 25,000 to 35,900 outpatients and 3,000 to 3,970 inpatients every summer.[100] It was listed on the "medical map" created in 1930 by the SMC as a "key" hospital of the city.[101] In 1934, it was also on Pang Jingzhou's list as a "public hospital."[102] In 1941, the hospital enlarged its building and added another floor to accommodate a larger number of patients.[103] The commissioner of public health of the Settlement commented that Chinese people generally preferred to go to this hospital during the epidemic season of 1942 and that this hospital was doing "valuable work in accommodating a large number of cholera patients and served as a great relief."[104]

Like missionary hospitals, CIDH was financed by three major sources: grants-in-aid from the SMC and the French Municipal Council (FMC), individual subscriptions, and fees paid by patients. Based on the financial statements of the hospital in the 1930s, subscriptions and grants-in-aid accounted for 36 to 57 percent of the entire annual income. In the 1940s, this support accounted for some 56 to 75 percent of its income. The SMC and the FMC provided the largest source of income. Other major contributors included the British-American Tobacco Company, the Jiujiang Match Company, and the Zhabei Water and Electric Company. Along with these firms, two gangsters-cum-businessmen, Du Yuesheng (1888–1951) and Huang Jinrong (1868–1953), were also named on the subscription lists. Finally, many obscure individuals gave small donations.[105]

---

99. *Sanshi nian fen.*

100. The numbers of patients vary depending on their source. For example, see Chinese Medical Association, ed., *Chinese Medical Directory* 1932, 60; 1934, 148; Pang, *Yiyao niaokan,* 25.

101. "Foreign Settlement of Shanghai, Census 1930."

102. Pang, *Yiyao niaokan,* 25.

103. *Sanshi nian fen.*

104. Minutes of Grand-in-Aid Committee meeting, June 10, 1943 (filed in SMA U1-4-213).

105. In the fiscal year of 1931, the CIDH received 2,000 taels and 500 taels from the SMC and the FMC, respectively. Zhabei Water and Electric Company and Neidi

The hospital invited amateur and professional actors and broadcast a radio program for fund-raising purposes.[106] The hospital also charged non-summer-disease patients fees for accommodation and treatment. Later on, the hospital also opened "special" rooms, above the first class, that garnered higher fees. These fees increased according to inflation, and their proportion to the entire hospital costs also increased. In 1940, the gross sum of patient fees (including outpatient fees, inpatient fees, drugs, and outcall fees) accounted for 25 percent of the entire hospital income.[107] It rose to 40 percent in 1940 and 37 percent in 1941. Still the needy were exempted from paying, and all summer outpatients and third-class inpatients were treated free.[108] Thus CIDH carried on its tradition as a seasonal hospital of charitable nature.

In the 1930s, as CIDH had become one of the major hospitals in the city, it set two goals: protecting human lives (*baowei shengming*) and curing gastrointestinal diseases (*jiuzhi yili*).[109] In pursuing these goals, CIDH identified itself as a modern hospital that practiced scientific medicine. It was staffed with properly trained doctors, nurses, pharmacists, and chemists. Though simple and lacking microscopes, it was equipped with a chemical laboratory and kept a supply of distilled water, glucose, and various types of saline solution to cure summer-disease patients. The primary treatment provided at the hospital was the injection of physiological saline to prevent dehydration. The hospital proudly remarked that since everything was well prepared there, once patients were admitted, they could receive intravenous and hypodermic injections promptly. All instruments as well as patients' bedding and tableware were completely disinfected, and patient discharges were properly disposed of. CIDH

Waterworks Company donated 100 yuan each. Huang Jinrong donated 100 yuan, and Du Yusheng donated 500 yuan. Many unnamed Shanghai residents donated one to six yuan each. Shanghai shiyi yiyuan, ed., *Shanghai shiyi yiyuan ershi nian baogao jian zhengxinlu* (CIDH Report 1932).

106.   SMA U1-4-220.

107.   "Statement of Receipts and Disbursement for the Year of 1940," "Statement of Receipts and Disbursement for the Year of 1941," and "Statement of Receipts and Disbursement for the Year of 1942."

108.   *Shanghai shiyi yiyuan zhangcheng*; Shanghai shiyi yiyuan, ed., *Shanghai shiyi yiyuan shiqi nian baogao jian zhengxinlu* (CIDH Report 1929); Letter from CIDH to the SMA, June 16, 1930 (filed in SMA U1-16-738).

109.   *Shanghai shiyi yiyuan zhangcheng.*

criticized massage, acupuncture, and phlebotomy as "wrong" treatments and drew a clear distinction between the treatment it offered and other "old" healing methods.[110] CIDH also equipped modern facilities to treat non-summer-disease cases. It opened an X-ray department, purchased an American X-ray instrument, and invited a radiologist. The hospital also purchased a state-of-the-art electric therapy machine made in Germany.[111] During non-epidemic seasons, the hospital performed surgeries.[112] CIDH proclaimed that it owned the newest medical facilities and employed scientific technologies to help the sick. In the early twentieth century, all Chinese intellectuals championed science, and those who sponsored CIDH were familiar with this intellectual discourse. They were convinced that scientific therapy was the best and only way to cure diseases.

Even after CIDH began accepting all cases, it still served as a traditional *shiyi* hospital that specialized in *liji*, gastrointestinal disorders in the summer. The hospital often featured treatment of acute gastrointestinal disorders, cholera in particular, as the main therapy it offered. According to CIDH reports, the hospital treated two-thirds of all the cholera patients in the city in 1931. It went on to treat 1,843 cholera patients in the summer of 1932. Yan Fuqing (1882–1970), then the hospital's director, asserted that the CIDH was the largest cholera-treatment center in Shanghai and that each year it treated nearly 50 percent of all cholera cases in the city. The hospital accepted summer-disease patients in the spring and fall as needed.[113] Settlement authorities endorsed Yan's remarks and usually gave favorable references in support of the hospital's request for grants-in-aid. They acknowledged that CIDH treated a large number of cholera patients with little means and thus significantly reduced the financial burden on the Settlement.[114]

110. Shanghai shiyi yiyuan, ed., CIDH Report 1929.

111. X-ray instruments were highly regarded as a tool of science. Sometime in the 1930s, the International Settlement created a list of institutions within the Settlement that owned X-ray and physical therapy equipment. This list contained only twenty-two institutions, including Renji, Tongren, and the Lester Institute. CIDH was not on the list. SMA U1-16-542.

112. *Sanshi nian fen;* Shanghai shiyi yiyuan, ed., CIDH Report 1929; *Shanghai shiyi yiyuan zhangcheng.*

113. SMA U1-16-737.

114. The correspondences between the International Settlement and CIDH and the hospital reports of CIDH are filed in SMA U1-16-737.

As a charitable organization run by Chinese, CIDH was open to all city residents regardless of their residency, age, or economic status, and it was committed to helping their lives in many ways. In 1932, the hospital took in the wounded after the Japanese attack with help from Red Cross Society staff.[115] CIDH also provided services other than medical treatment. According to its general regulations, if patients died in the hospital and were too poor to afford burial, CIDH purchased coffins and took care of the burial for them. If patients recovered and were willing to go home but did not have sufficient resources, CIDH also provided them with train or boat tickets.[116] Clearly, these services exceeded ordinary hospital work; they were reminiscent of the poverty relief provided by benevolent halls or native-place associations. Here "protecting life" did not mean simply providing medical care and giving saline injections to cholera patients. Lei Hsiang-lin (Sean Hsiang-lin Lei) argues that, in 1930s China, even those who were familiar with bacteriology still believed that life concerned more than the physiological body or physical health. "Life" included the body, mind, and emotion, and "life" should be based on China's sociocultural conditions and moral community.[117] His points are relevant here. CIDH helped its patients return to their native places; it also helped the deceased go through proper death rituals. In Chinese society, it was critical for sojourners to maintain and cultivate their physical and spiritual ties with their native place. It was also critical to perform prescribed death rituals for the needs of souls. Thus, the hospital helped the living and the dead conform to Chinese sociocultural norms and protected them from being deviant and deracinated. It protected not only corporeal but also the social and spiritual lives of patients; by extension, it protected Chinese culture itself.

The membership of the Board of the Trustees of CIDH reflected the new commercial and intellectual development of Shanghai. Board members in the 1930s included Liu Hongsheng (1888–1956), Shi Liangcai (1880–1934), and Yan Fuqing. Liu was nicknamed "the king of the match industry" and "the king of the concrete industry." He was one of the

115. SMA U1-16-737.
116. Shanghai shiyi yiyuan, ed., CIDH Report 1929; Shanghai shiyi yiyuan, ed., CIDH Report 1932.
117. Lei Hsiang-lin, "Weisheng weihe bu shi baowei shengming?"

leading entrepreneurs in the city. After quitting St. John's University, he first worked as a translator and legal assistant. Then he engaged in business as a comprador for a British company. In the 1920s and 1930s, he owned and managed several firms.[118] Shi Liangcai, a well-known liberal journalist, worked as editor-in-chief of *Shenbao*, a leading paper in the city. He was also a prominent member of the League for the Protection of Human Rights. Until he was allegedly assassinated by Chiang Kai-shek in 1934, he owned a couple of publishing houses and served on the municipal council of the Chinese city.[119] Yan Fuqing was a graduate of the medical school of St. John's and held a medical degree from Yale. He had also studied tropical medicine at Liverpool. After returning to China, he held several important posts, including director of the Chinese Medical Association and vice president of Peking Union Medical College. In Shanghai, he was president of the Medical School of Zhongshan University, and one of the founders of Zhongshan Hospital and the Shanghai Sanatorium.[120] The backgrounds of these people reflect the modern aspects of Shanghai society: connections with the West, entrepreneurship, liberal journalism, and higher education. These modern trustees who had received Western educations gave all-out support to Western medicine, but they ran CIDH in a manner similar to that of charitable clinics: saline injections and X-ray images were new, but elite-sponsored charitable organizations that admitted poor patients were not. In this hospital, these Chinese elites adopted Western medical concepts and technology to protect not only Chinese bodies but also Chinese cultural values and norms, and they did so without much intellectual effort or cultural anxiety.

The story of Chinese Infectious Disease Hospital presents another case of "hybridity." It was managed by Shanghai's elites, was financed by both private and public money, and responded to and fulfilled the medical and social needs of the general public. As such, it was neither strictly

118. On Liu Hongsheng and his business career, see for example, Zhang Qifu and Wei Heng, *Huochai dawang Liu Hongsheng*; He Kuang, *Huochai dawang Liu Hongsheng*; Cochran and Hsieh, *Lius of Shanghai*.

119. On the assassination of Shi Liangcai, see Wakeman, *Policing Shanghai*, 257–59.

120. On Yan Fuqing and his life, see, for example, *SWZ*, 647–48; Yan Zhiyuan, "Yixue jioyujia"; Keren, "Woguo gonggong weisheng."

"private" nor strictly "public." Likewise it was neither strictly "traditional" nor strictly "modern." The name of the hospital is particularly revealing. Although its English name identified it as a Chinese Infectious Hospital, its Chinese name identified it as a *shiyi yiyuan*, a hospital for seasonal diseases. The hospital trustees were knowledgeable of bacteriology and infection, but they chose to use the familiar term, *shiyi*, not *chuanranbing*, infectious disease, a new etiological category brought from Japan, to describe the hospital.[121]

Whereas the history of CIDH illustrates the fusion of elite activism, charity, and science, other summer-disease hospitals represented the combination of business and medicine. Shanghai Emergency Hospital (Shanghai jijiu shiyi yiyuan) (SEH) is a case in point. Originally, Huang Chujiu (1872–1931), a prominent businessman in Shanghai, opened this hospital on Tibet Road in 1926 to respond to the cholera outbreak of the year and to admit patients with little means.[122] Huang was a son of a Chinese-style doctor. When he was young, he made his living as a street vendor of Chinese drugs and herbs. He then engaged in various businesses and made a fortune. By the 1920s, Huang owned several drugstores and other enterprises, including the Great World Entertainment Hall.[123] Since he had little knowledge of Western medicine, he recruited Pang Jingzhou as director and Zang Boyong as chief doctor of SEH. Zang was Huang's son-in-law and had studied medicine in Japan.[124] The history of SEH in the 1930s is undocumented, but it had two hundred beds and was relocated in 1940 to the International Settlement in light of the increased population of the area. This time, SEH was supported jointly by the Shanghai Red Cross Society and the Shanghai Pharmaceutical Association (Zhiyaoye tongyehui).[125] SEH's board of the trustees consisted of prominent Shanghai businessmen, including Yu Qiaqing (1867–1945), Yuan Lüdeng (1879–1954), and Xu Xiaochu (1900–1998). Among them, Xu Xiaochu

121. On the concept of *chuanran*, see Sean Hsiang-lin Lei, *Neither Donkey nor Horse*, 21–44.

122. Yang Yun, "Huaxia xiyao zongshi."

123. On Huang Chujiu, see, for example, Cochran, "Marketing Medicine"; Cochran, *Chinese Medicine Men*, 38–60; Qin Lüzhi, *Haipai shangren*; Zeng Hongyan, *Shanghai jushang*; Yang Yun, "Huaxia xiyao zongshi."

124. Qin Lüzhi, *Haipai shangren*, 57–60; Yang Yun, "Huaxia xiyao zongshi," 232.

125. Letter from SEH to the SMA, July 16, 1940 (filed in SMA U1-4-259).

deserves special attention. He was another son-in-law of Huang Chujiu and inherited Huang's pharmaceutical business after Huang's death in 1931. At that time, he was also president of the Great Eastern Dispensary. The management of SEH, like that of CIDH and other summer hospitals, was similar to that of charitable clinics. It was open in the summer to admit summer-disease patients, and its primary goal was poverty relief: SEH charged some fees, but most patients were treated for free. SEH not only provided medical treatment but also arranged funerals for the dead. In 1940, the hospital treated more than sixty thousand patients from July to September. The directors proclaimed that the hospital was staffed by well-qualified doctors and nurses and that it was not like other ordinary charitable hospitals.[126]

However, SEH diverged from other summer hospitals in that Huang Chujiu and Xu Xiaochu were involved in its management. They represented not only Shanghai's business world but also its new medical industry. Neither of them had formally studied Western medicine, but through successful hospital management they had gained reputations as philanthropists and had created solid connections with medical professionals. Huang also expanded the market for his company's pharmaceutical product, Bailingji (Machine for Long Life). When patients recovered and left SEH, the hospital staff recommended that they take Bailingji as a nutritional supplement.[127] As Huang gained fame as a hospital manager, many doctors were willing to cooperate with him and voluntarily invested in his companies. They also offered their own prescriptions to Huang, hoping that he would manufacture and commercialize new drugs based on their formulas and that this would lead to profits.[128] SEH was a charitable institution open to the public mostly supported and financed by local elites. But it also conferred benefits on Huang and his company and helped doctors create commercial connections. The hospital promoted public welfare, scientific medicine, and private interest all at once.

In addition to CIDH and SHE, there were other small summer-disease hospitals. All were sponsored by local elites and businessmen,

---

126. On the management of SEH, see Jijiu shiyi yiyuan shiwuchu, ed., *Shanghai jijiu shiyi yiyuan gongzuo baogao fu zhengxinlu*; SMA U1-16-749.

127. Qin Lüzhi, *Haipai shangren*, 172.

128. Yang Yun, "Huaxia xiyao zongshi," 231–42.

and all provided medical as well as nonmedical services to their patients. Along with missionary hospitals, they were a part of the city's nongovernmental social welfare network. Although these institutions adopted the methods of Western medicine and some of them developed into general hospitals, they were still, on the whole, charitable organizations, and their primary target was the city's poor. In the 1920s and 1930s, when missionary hospitals constructed new wards and buildings, the Chinese-sponsored summer-disease hospitals remained relatively simple and modest. Missionary hospitals took Chinese names and followed the example of China's charitable institutions, while Shanghai's seasonal hospitals adopted Western medicine and used Western medical instruments. They both accommodated local social needs, influenced and inspired each other, and offered services to the general populace.

Chinese Medicine and Western System: Traditional Chinese Hospitals

Missionary hospitals and summer-disease hospitals both embraced Western biomedicine. However, even though Western-style doctors had gained state support and elite status, Chinese-style doctors were greater in number and remained popular among city residents. Since they received a proper Confucian education and were well versed in medical canons and classics and their commentaries, they were also called scholar-physicians.[129] They were further divided into different schools, specializations, and native-place origins. Shanghai and its suburbs produced several medical lineages, and each of them established their own school of medical theories. In addition to these local schools, since the mid-nineteenth century, a large number of scholar-physicians from the Jiangnan area migrated to Shanghai. Some of them were already well

129. In addition to these scholarly elites, various groups of nonliterate healers gave medical therapies, including shamans, exorcists, diviners, acupuncturists, and herbalists. In this book, I use the term "Chinese-style doctors" to mean primarily scholar-physicians. Although the majority of these practitioners were male, female healers who specialized in midwifery, gynecology, and pediatrics were also on practice. See Andrews, *Making of Modern Chinese Medicine*, 25–50.

established, while some were young and hoped to make their career in Shanghai.[130] Together these doctors strove to enhance the status of Chinese medicine, to attract patients, to counter challenges posed by Western medicine, and to create "a respectable, modernizing Chinese medicine."[131] As part of such efforts, scholar-physicians also opened hospitals. The emergence of hospitals run and supported by those who practiced Chinese medicine represented the combination of Chinese medicine and Western system.

In pre-1949 Shanghai, the majority of Chinese-style doctors practiced individually. Some well-off doctors owned or rented clinics with consultation rooms. Some saw outpatients at their own residences. They might also employ one or two assistants or apprentices and make house calls. Some did not have a place to practice and saw their patients at teahouses. Still other doctors worked in pharmacies. Patients consulted them there, and doctors gave out medical advice and prescriptions in storefronts. Besides practicing on their own, some of these Chinese-style practitioners participated in charitable clinics sponsored by the local elites.[132]

The concept of a general hospital—an institution complete with multiple departments and inpatient facilities that employed several doctors, nurses, and other staff—was new in itself to Chinese-style practitioners. However, as Western-style hospitals became increasingly popular, abundant, and too conspicuous to ignore, supporters and practitioners of Chinese medicine also undertook hospital management. Few Chinese-style practitioners had adequate connections and resources to construct a hospital, and so, compared with their Western counterparts, their hospitals were few in number and generally small in scale.[133] Still, the presence of Chinese-medicine hospitals is significant. Their presence sheds light on ways supporters of Chinese medicine appropriated the concept of a hospital for their own needs and purposes. Hospitals provided an arena for showcasing their skill and competence, projecting their concerns and values, and appealing to the desires and expectations of the general public. Some believed that Chinese medicine could readily

130. Scheid, *Currents of Tradition*, 175–88.
131. Andrews, *Making of Modern Chinese Medicine*, 46.
132. *SWZ*, 139; Scheid, *Currents of Tradition*, 182–83.
133. *SWZ*, 141.

coexist with Western medicine in the same institution. Although this intellectual eclecticism gradually lost popularity in the 1920s, some Chinese practitioners remained confident in the usefulness of hospitals for the practice of Chinese medicine and opened hospitals that adopted exclusively Chinese medicine.

The early history of Shanghai Public Hospital (Shanghai gongli yiyuan) (SPH) embodies the ideal of a hospital in which both Chinese and Western medicine are practiced. SPH started as Nanshi Shanghai Hospital (Nanshi Shanghai yiyuan) in 1909 and was located in the Chinese sector of the city. It was the first Chinese-sponsored general hospital in Shanghai. In 1916 the management of this hospital was placed under the jurisdiction of Shanghai *xian* (county), and it was renamed Shanghai Public Hospital. Unfortunately, because of a lack of sources, we do not know anything about this hospital's development during the 1920s. We only know that by 1933 it had several departments and some 145 beds; we also know that it was regarded as one of the most comprehensive hospitals in the Chinese sector of the city.[134] In 1934, the Chinese municipal government took over the management of this hospital. Today it is known as the Shanghai Municipal Number Two Hospital.[135]

The central figure in the founding of SPH was Li Pingshu (1854–1927). Li was one of the leading elites in Shanghai and was engaged in various businesses and civic activities in the Chinese sector of the city, including public health works.[136] He studied for the civil exam and was well versed in Chinese medical classics. In 1904, through introduction by a friend, Li became acquainted with Dr. Zhang Zhujun (1879–?), a female doctor who had studied Western medicine in Canton. After working at a couple of medical schools in Canton, she arrived in Shanghai and opened a school for women in the city. When Li learned that Zhang was having financial difficulty running the school, he immediately offered help and became a strong supporter of her school. To express her gratitude, Zhang performed a ritual to transform her into a fictitious daughter of Li and his wife. After getting to know Zhang Zhujin, Li became interested in combining Chinese and Western medicine. In 1905, Li and Zhang jointly opened the

134. Pang, *Yiyao niaokan*, 24.
135. Lu Ming, "Shanghai jindai xiyi yiyuan gaishu," 23.
136. On Li Pingshu's career, see Elvin, "Administration of Shanghai," 248.

Chinese-Western Medical School for Women (Nüzi zhongxi yixuetang), the first modern medical school open to females. Dr. Zhang taught Western medicine at the school; Li taught Chinese medicine, and he invited other teachers to lecture in the natural sciences (including chemistry and mathematics), English, and Chinese. Li and Zhang also opened a hospital specializing in obstetrics, Chinese-Western Hospital for Women (Nüzi zhongxi yiliaoyuan), which they attached to the school.[137]

This hospital was well accepted, but it was small and had only modest equipment. Thus Li entertained the idea of opening a larger hospital in Nanshi with better facilities that would adopt both Chinese and Western medicine. To collect necessary funds, he lobbied and met friends at a New Year's party in 1908, and brought up the plan for the hospital construction. According to Li, everyone there supported the idea and offered help. The same year, with financial help from local notables, Li opened Nanshi Shanghai Hospital and Zhang Zhujun became the president.[138] This hospital consisted of two buildings—a three-story structure in the front with a two-story structure in the rear. It also had inpatient facilities, operation rooms, and a kitchen. Li describes the hospital in his autobiography:

> While there are a quite a few hospitals in the foreign settlements, they are all founded by foreigners. When Chinese patients enter [one of these foreign-run] hospitals, the food, drink, and lifestyle there are unsuitable to Chinese [custom]. Most of all, foreign hospitals are not appropriate for [Chinese] women. In 1904, in consideration of the scarcity of women doctors in China, I opened the Chinese-Western Medical School for Women independently. I signed a six-year contract with Dr. Zhang Zhujun to train women doctors. Next to this school, we also opened a women's hospital. In these four or five years, some fifty women have entered this hospital and given birth to children. I am sorry that our ability is insufficient, and the hospital too small to admit [as] many women [as we would like]. I apologize for this. In light of this situation, we began a construction plan for a hospital in Nanshi in 1907. We organized raffles to raise money so we could cover expenses.[139]

137. Li Pingshu, *Qishi zixu*, 52; Shi Meijun, "Shanghai dianye juxing."
138. Li Pingshu, *Qishi zixu*, 54.
139. Ibid.

Nanshi Shanghai Hospital was another elite-initiated hospital, but it was unique in its eclecticism. Li studied and taught Chinese medicine. As a strong supporter of Chinese traditional medicine, he was engaged in the management of a company that sold traditional Chinese drugs; he also was affiliated with Southern Shanghai Chinese Hospital (Hunan Shenzhou yiyuan), which practiced Chinese medicine exclusively.[140] However, he never doubted the efficacy of Western medicine. In Li's understanding, Chinese medicine was based on the transformation of the vital energy (*qihua*) and Western medicine was based on the circulation of blood (*xuelun*). Those who studied Western medicine believed that, because *qihua* did not have a shape and was invisible, it was false. They did not understand that, even though *qihua* was shapeless, it was certainly reliable for diagnostic purposes. At the same time, he realized that those who spoke only about *qihua* were clinging to Five Phases theory, which was abstract and obscure.[141] He believed that those who practice medicine should study *qihua, xuelun*, and physiology (*tigong*) carefully, as well as *Neijing, Nanjing, Shanghanlun*, and other medical classics. By taking this all-embracing approach, they could make correct diagnoses and provide proper treatment to patients. He also believed that Chinese medicine and Western medicine could be "melted in the same pot." Zhang agreed with Li. Even though she studied Western medicine, she did not discredit nor reject Chinese medicine. Rather she believed that Chinese and Western medicine offered different insights about the human body and that they could complement each other. According to her, Chinese medicine hypothesized the function and disorder of the "inside" of the body through observations of the "outside." By contrast, Western medicine examined the body through anatomy and characteristic forms of organs (*zangqi de xing tezheng*). In sum, Chinese and Western medicine both investigated physiology and pathology but from two different perspectives. Knowing only one, the understanding of the body would be one-sided (*pianmianxing*).[142] Li wrote that Western hospitals were unsuitable for Chinese customs, but he never discredited them. The following

---

140.   Shi Meijun, "Shanghai dianye juxing," 465–67.

141.   On Chinese conceptions on *qi* transformation and blood, see Sean Hsiang-lin Lei, *Neither Donkey nor Horse*.

142.   Shi Meijun, "Shanghai dianye juxing," 454–56.

statement by Li exemplifies the syncretism in Chinese medical discourse of the late Qing and early Republican periods.

> Many of the hospitals in Shanghai were founded by Westerners. Thus, they generally use *xifa* (Western methods) to treat diseases. On the other hand, when benevolent halls treat patients, they only use Chinese medicine; they do not use Western medicine. Now that the whole world is opening up, we should not stick to old methods. Therefore in Shanghai Hospital, we use Western medicine and Chinese medicine together. In the morning, we use Chinese medicine . . . and in the afternoon, we use Western medicine . . . and prescribe Western drugs. For those who stay in the hospital, we cannot help but treat them exclusively with Western methods. Because [we require] various [medical] procedures, it would not be safe not to use Western medicine.[143]

Li's optimism about the possibility of the coexistence between Chinese and Western medicine in part reflects his background. Though he was born to a doctor's family, he was a businessman and activist. He had served as a director of the Shanghai General Affairs Office (Shanghai chengxiang neiwai zong-gongchengju) and Shanghai City Hall (Shanghai zizhi gongsuo); in addition he was involved in the city's public works and other affairs. He also participated in the Revolutionary Alliance (Tongmenghui). Since Li was not a medical professional and thus did not have to compete with Western-style doctors, he was able to maintain a flexible attitude toward Western medicine and Western-style hospitals.[144] Li left for Japan in 1912 after the failed second revolution, and soon after, Zhang Zhujun also left the hospital. The departure of Li and Zhang marked the end of this eclecticism. When Yu Yunxiu (1879–1954) took the position of chief medical director of the hospital in 1916, Shanghai Public Hospital dropped Chinese medicine and became a strictly Western-style hospital.

Other Chinese-style doctors opened hospitals to practice Chinese medicine exclusively as a strategy for survival and prosperity. It is estimated

143. Ibid.
144. On Chinese medical eclecticism, see Xiaoqun Xu, " 'National Essence' vs. 'Science,' " 849–50.

that some forty hospitals of Chinese medicine were in operation during the Republican period.[145] Although many of these hospitals in the city were small and obscure, some of them were organized by well-known doctors, supported by local elites, and gained excellent reputations. Volker Scheid reports that between 1917 and 1940, nine such hospitals were established in Shanghai by Chinese-style doctors and wealthy businessmen.[146] Of these, the two Guangyi (Broad Beneficence) Chinese Hospitals (Guangyi zhongyiyuan) were the best documented. These were Hubei (northern Shanghai) Guangyi Chinese Hospital and Hunan (southern Shanghai) Guangyi Chinese Hospital. Both of these hospitals survived the 1940s and were restructured under Communist rule. Hunan Hospital merged with Gongji Benevolent Hall (Gongji shantang) and three other halls in 1953 under the guidance of the Chinese People's Social Welfare Society (Zhongguo renmin jiuji fulihui). It became the Shanghai Social Welfare Society Number One Clinic for the Sick (Shanghai Shi jiuji fulijie di-yi bingmin zhensuo), and provided medical care to the old and the handicapped.[147] Hubei Hospital was smaller, and its building was an old Chinese bungalow.[148] The Communist Party decided to close this hospital in 1955, but this decision met strong opposition from local residents. Though the hospital was open only in the morning, it examined some 200 to 350 patients a day and offered inexpensive medical care. The hospital was not just self-reliant; it was actually turning a small profit. For these reasons, the Communists reversed the original decision. In 1956, the People's Committee took over the hospital and reorganized it into a clinic station (*zhenliaozhan*).[149]

Ding Ganren (1865–1926) led the group of Chinese-style doctors who set up the Guangyi hospitals. Ding hailed from Menghe in Jiangsu and

---

145. *SWZ*, 141.

146. Scheid, *Currents of Tradition*, 194–95.

147. SMA B242-1-476-1; SMA B242-1-476-3.

148. Settlement inspectors remarked that this hospital was "only a clinic" but "everything appeared satisfactory excepting the urinals and [water] closet" (August 8, 1934). But on November 5, 1941, the commissioner of public health commented that "it was a poor place run by unregistered practitioners," and rejected the hospital's request for rate remissions. SMA U1-16-549.

149. SMA B3-1-12-1; SMA B242-1-899.

was the founder of the Ding school of medical thought.[150] After practicing medicine in Wuxi, Suzhou, and other places, he settled in Shanghai in the late nineteenth century. Initially he was not financially prosperous, but he became closely acquainted with other sojourner doctors in Shanghai. Ding soon became famous for his successful treatment of fever and throat diseases. As his fame grew, he created social connections with Shanghai's elites and celebrities and accumulated wealth. While practicing on his own, he also became involved in some charitable clinics. As a leader of Chinese-style doctors in the city, he played a central role in organizing their professional and academic organizations.[151] In 1917, as a part of their efforts to enhance the status of Chinese medicine, Ding and other doctors, including Xia Yingtang (1871–1936) and Xie Guan (1880–1950), opened Shanghai Chinese Medical School (SCMS) (Shanghai zhongyi zhuanmen xuexiao).[152] Before the twentieth century, Chinese medicine was often a family business, transmitted from generation to generation. Sometimes doctors took apprentices and trained them. Some studied medical treatises as part of their classical studies.[153] Yet except for small private tutorials, few medical schools were open to the public. In light of this situation, the idea of opening a full-time school and recruiting students from the general public was itself relatively novel.

The original curriculum of SCMS consisted of a two-year preparatory course and a three-year regular course. Later the entire course was shortened to four years. In the preparatory course, students were required to study physiology, pathology, pharmacology, and diagnoses based on Chinese medical theory. In the regular course, students were required not only to take classes on specific subjects, including internal medicine, surgery, obstetrics, and pediatrics, but also to study the medical classics.

---

150. Today Menghe is a small town in Jiangsu. But it had been a significant medical site until the late nineteenth century and produced famous medical families and physicians. On a history of Menghe and Menghe doctors, see Scheid, *Currents of Tradition*, 17–172.

151. On Ding Ganren, see Scheid, *Currents of Tradition*, 223–48; He Shixi, *Jindai yilin yishi*, 1–17; He Shixi, "Menghe Dingshi," 1–4; Mingyi yaolan bianshen weiyuanhui, ed., *Mingyi yaolan*, 15–16.

152. In 1931, it was renamed "Shanghai zhongyi xueyuan."

153. Chao, *Medicine and Society*, 25–52.

Students were also required to take Chinese, ethics, and calisthenics.[154] In the 1930s, classes about Western medicine, public health, and party doctrine (*dangyi*) were also taught at the school.[155]

In addition to classes, practical training at the hospital was a significant part of the regular course curriculum. Thus, upon opening the school, Ding Ganren employed professors who could direct clinical practice. Ding and others also planned to build related hospitals so that students could gain practical training as interns. To cover the expenses of building and running the hospitals, Ding asked directors of Guangyi Benevolent Hall for financial help. Guangyi Benevolent Hall was founded in 1888 and was one of many social welfare organizations in the city. Its directors, including Zhu Baosan and Chen Gantang, agreed to fund the hospital construction, and two of the directors each donated a parcel of land for the sites—one in the north and the other in the south of the city. Ding and other directors of the hall opened Hunan Hospital in 1917 and Hubei Hospital in 1918.[156]

These hospitals were attached to the medical school and served as teaching hospitals for students and interns. Of the two, Hunan Hospital was the larger, and it was located on the same site as the school buildings and student dormitories.[157] Until Hualong Hospital was built in 1930 by Ding's grandson, Hunan Hospital served as the primary teaching hospital for SCMS. In clinical practice, students usually assembled in a consultation room of the hospital.[158] A teacher, one or more patients, and student-scribes worked on a platform placed at the center of the consultation room. Senior students usually worked as the scribes assisting the teacher. As the teacher examined the patient, he recited his diagnoses and prescriptions. All the students in the room watched the teacher work and took notes. Students were also required to fill out clinical records for each

154. Mingyi yaolan bianshen weiyuanhui, ed., *Mingyi yaolan*, 27–28, 128–30.
155. Ibid., 58–65.
156. Ibid., 28–29.
157. Ibid., 30–31.
158. Hualong Hospital was built in 1930 by Ding Jiman, a grandson of Ding Ganren. Like the two Guangyi Chinese Hospitals, Hualong Hospital was closely related to SCMS. Most of the staff of Hualong Hospital were graduates of SCMS, and the hospital served as a teaching hospital of SCMS. Ibid., 65–68.

patient and to review their notes and records.[159] The consultation room served as a classroom, and students received firsthand experience observing patients.

Though no match for missionary hospitals in size, the two Guangyi hospitals were the largest among Chinese medical institutions. Hunan Hospital was the main hospital of the two. Its administrative body was the board of directors (*dongshihui*), which consisted of Wang Yiting, Zhu Baosan, and other local notables, as well as those who made substantial donations. The board selected the president, chief medical officer (*yiwu zhuren*), and chief general officer (*zongwu zhuren*).[160] The hospital was open every day to provide medical care and drugs to outpatients. As of 1953, it consisted of three two-story buildings. The first floor of the first building had examination rooms, prescription rooms, and offices; the second floor had eight inpatient rooms with a total of sixty beds. In the second building were storage rooms, decoction rooms, and bathrooms on the first floor, and bedrooms for the staff on the second floor. The first floor of the third building had a kitchen, dining hall, and mortuary; additional inpatient rooms were on the second floor. The hospital operated a comprehensive range of departments, including pediatrics, gynecology, medicine, surgery, and acupuncture. Six doctors, five pharmacists, and three assistants worked there.[161] Hubei Hospital was small, but it still employed four doctors, two pharmacists, a clerk, and a custodian. It was open only in the morning and did not have inpatient facilities.[162]

Although these Guangyi hospitals were affiliated with a medical school and inaugurated as teaching hospitals, they had, according to their charters (*zhangcheng*), two primary missions: First, they were charitable institutions and committed to helping the needy. Second, they aimed at developing national medicine as an academic discipline and advocated for the efficacy of national drugs.[163] Similar to many other charitable clinics, the goal of the Guangyi hospitals was "broadening and promoting

159. Ibid., 82–88.
160. SMA Q6-9-192; SMA Q113-4-1.
161. SMA Q113-4-1; SMA B242-1-476-3.
162. SMA B242-1-899; SMA B242-1-899-1.
163. During their existence, the Guangyi Chinese Hospitals issued several versions of their charters, and each version contained slightly different contents. They are filed in SMA Q113-4-1. Also see SMA Q113-4-4.

public interest and helping the sick" (*tuiguang gongyi liji bingren*). The management of the hospitals was closely related to Guangyi Benevolent Hall: their financing depended primarily on donations from this civic group, while other subscriptions came from Chinese-style doctors across the city. The hospitals always emphasized their charitable nature, and in 1930, they registered with the Social Affairs Bureau of the city—not the Public Health Bureau.[164] Responding to a Communist inspection, Lu Jiesun, who was in charge of Hunan Hospital in 1953, said that originally the primary intent of the hospital was to provide outpatient care. Because it was inconvenient for the old and the handicapped to visit the hospital, and taxies were expensive, the hospital staff arranged for on-site rooms to provide lodging and food to accommodate the needs of such patients. Lu mentioned that though the hospital was staffed by medical personnel, it was more like a relief organization than a medical institution.[165] Although not completely consistent with the stated original goals, Lu's comments are indicative. The two Guangyi hospitals retained many features of traditional charity shelters. Initially the hospitals did not charge fees, but later on, Hunan Hospital opened first-, second-, and third-class inpatient rooms for fees to help cover its expenses.[166] Still, all outpatients were required to pay only a nominal fee and their medicine was provided for free. Moreover, the needy and those who were sent to the hospital by Guangyi Benevolent Hall could stay at no charge.[167] Most of the patients in these free rooms were the aged, the handicapped, or opium addicts with chronic diseases. Since these patients were not in critical condition, doctors usually treated them with "defensive" (*shou*) techniques rather than giving them specific medical therapies.[168] During the bitter winter, the hospitals dispensed cotton jackets to those who had no clothing. If patients died in the hospital and did not have a family in Shanghai, the hospital helped take care of their encoffinment.[169] Clearly, the sponsorship, management, and function of the hospitals were similar to those of

164. SMA Q113-4-1.
165. SMA B242-1-476-3.
166. SMA Q113-4-1.
167. Mingyi yaolan bianshen weiyuanhui, ed., *Mingyi yaolan*, 30; He Shixi, "Menghe Dingshi," 2; He Shixi, *Jindai yilin yishi*, 5.
168. He Shixi, "Menghe Dingshi" 6–7.
169. SMA Q113-4-1.

charitable shelters. In this regard, missionary hospitals, summer-disease hospitals, and the two Guangyi hospitals all shared the same goal: serve the public through medical care and other social services.

However, the Guangyi hospitals were established and operated by Chinese-style doctors. They practiced traditional Chinese medicine, and their pharmacies prescribed and decocted drugs based on traditional formulas. Through successful therapy and medication as well as competent hospital management, they sought to demonstrate the potency and authenticity of Chinese medicine. Though their hospitals emulated missionary hospitals in style and management, their accounts and records were full of Chinese medical terms. To judge patient conditions, doctors examined the tongue coating (*shetai*) and pulses (*maixiang*) of patients and kept clinical records based on their observation.[170] The hospitals always had multiple departments, and one version of the charters listed twelve departments: internal medicine (*nei*); surgery (*wai*); throat (*hou*); boil (*ding*); gynecology (*fu*); poison (*du*); pediatrics (*you*), including acute diseases (*sha*) and smallpox (*dou*); ophthalmology (*yan*); acupuncture (*zhen*); wound (*shang*); and wind (*feng*). Later, Hubei Hospital also opened a separate isolation ward that admitted seasonal-disease patients exclusively, called *shiyi bingfang*. Doctors and nursing staff on this ward were urged to leave the premises frequently so that they could exhale "polluted energy" (*huiqi*) and inhale "pure energy" (*qingqi*). They were also encouraged to eat well to fill up their stomach with vital energy before entering the ward. These accounts indicate that Guangyi's doctors conceptualized body, health, and disease in a traditional way. Instead of using X-ray technology, they examined tongues and checked the pulses of patients. Instead of adopting bacteriology, they understood the cause of seasonal diseases in terms of *qi*, or vital energy. In sum, Guangyi practiced what progressive intellectuals would call "old medicine." Yet they were not anti-Western. One of Guangyi charters mentions that "Western medicine was a study of surgery and was already well established."[171] Doctors at Guangyi recognized that Western medicine had its own strengths, and in caring for patients, they readily sought advice from Western-style doctors when needed and appropriate. It is also noteworthy that some of

170. See various versions of Guangyi charters filed in SMA Q113-4-1.
171. Ibid.

their sponsors, such as Wang Yiting and Zhu Baosan, also supported Western hospitals.

The opening of these hospitals that practiced Chinese medicine was in part a response to the introduction of Western medicine. Some intellectuals, including Li Pingshu, believed that Chinese medicine could easily coexist with Western medicine, but this optimism would gradually fade in the 1910s and 1920s. When the Republican state began to promote educational reforms, Western-educated elites and administrators sought to exclude Chinese medicine from the mainstream of the nation's educational curricula. The harshest attack on Chinese medicine came from May Fourth intellectuals. They viewed modernization as necessarily involving Westernization and regarded Chinese medicine as "backward" and "unscientific."[172] Practitioners of Chinese medicine began to organize and make political connections to counter these assaults. Using this logic to defend themselves, they would refer to Chinese medicine (zhongyi) as national medicine (guoyi), in an effort to appeal to nationalist feeling. The opening of the two Guangyi hospitals was another way to refute attacks. By constructing large hospital buildings, admitting inpatients, administrating separate specializations, and opening rooms for a variety of classes of people, Chinese-style doctors demonstrated their presence and ability to accommodate people from different classes; in these institutions they provided effective medical care and helped people. Along with professional organizations and medical schools, hospitals provided Chinese-style doctors with a means for gaining popular support and increasing their share in the "market for cure." Yet, these hospitals did not simply cling to "traditional ways." They aimed at "developing national medicine into an academic discipline and advocated for the efficacy of national drugs" (fayang guoyi xueshu tichang guoyao gongneng).[173] Doctors of the Guangyi hospitals were convinced that Chinese medicine was a legitimate area of scholarship, not an old, obscure craft. The two Guangyi hospitals provided

172. On the conflicts between Chinese and Western medicine, see, for example, Sean Hsiang-lin Lei, "When Chinese Medicine Encountered the State"; Sean Hsiang-lin Lei, Neither Donkey nor Horse; Xiaoqun Xu, " 'National Essence' vs. 'Science' "; Croizier, Traditional Medicine in Modern China.

173. "Gongyi cishan tuanti dengjibiao."

them a venue in which they could be engaged in serious research on Chinese medicine and enhance its value.

Conclusion

The stories of these hospitals present several interesting combinations of ideals, values, and social realities. Doctors and directors of the hospitals all shared the humanitarian ideals of helping the sick and needy and pursuing public welfare through medicine. Medical care was a significant form of social welfare, and the hospitals discussed in this chapter supplemented the work of the state or local authorities. However, the same institutions also served more specific interests of specific groups—the interest of Christian missionaries, medical researchers, local businessmen, pharmaceutical companies, and practitioners of traditional Chinese medicine. In running their hospitals, these groups strove to meet growing public demand for medical and nonmedical services; simultaneously, they pursued their own interests. Accordingly, the hospital had multiple functions and served social as well as economic purposes. It was a place in which Western missionaries spread Christianity and Chinese elites expressed their benevolence and fulfilled social responsibility. It served as a laboratory in which doctors used X-ray machines and microscopes to study pathology as well as a classroom in which students received training. It was also a site in which Chinese-style doctors organized themselves to strengthen their social status, and a market in which pharmaceutical companies promoted their products. Hospital management cannot be separated from its material basis, and all these hospitals made every effort to secure financial resources to support their activities. They appealed to foreign authorities and Chinese elites for subsidies and subscriptions, used radio programs to solicit public donations, and offered better treatments and accommodations so they could charge higher rates. In the end, they were all able to capitalize on the material wealth that Shanghai and the city's elites possessed.

Historians of modern China often find "syncretic intertwinings of social forms and values"[174] in the same institution, place, and space. They

174. Shue, "Quality of Mercy."

emphasize that "new" practices did not simply replace "old" ones: they intertwined with each other. In analyzing these intertwinings, instead of using conventional dichotomies of "China and West," "science and superstition," and "Confucian tradition and global modernity," historians pay close attention to the hybridity and fluidity of China's modernity and suggest synchronic coexistence of various values.[175] As this chapter has illustrated, a hospital could represent different meanings and values simultaneously. Some of the processes of changes that the hospitals discussed above went through—expanding and professionalizing, switching from free to fee-based consultation, adopting new technology, and commercializing—can be associated with "modernity"; importantly, such processes cannot be divorced from Shanghai's social contexts. The presence of wealthy elites who were willing to donate, a local tradition of charitable services, an increased number of clientele, growing interest in Western medicine, and a strong network of Chinese-style physicians all fashioned the way these hospitals developed. Hospitals were introduced to China by Westerners, but they quickly became part of the city's medical arsenal. Those who operated hospitals in Shanghai injected Western modes of healing and Western styles of management into already accepted institutions. There was no radical break from "traditional" or "old" social arrangements. These hospitals pursued public welfare and private interests as well as traditional benevolence and Western biomedicine simultaneously through medical care. Though they had different goals, these hospitals did not challenge or seek to overturn each other. None of them imposed uniform authority over notions of health, healing, and therapies. Rather, they coexisted in the city and collectively reflected, generated, and embodied medical culture, thus helping structure Chinese attitudes toward, desire for, and expectations of medical care, technology, and professions.

Moreover, Shanghai's general public did not seem to be particularly concerned about the incongruities and contradictions of various elements of these hospitals. By frequenting and staying in these hospitals, Shanghai people indirectly participated in their management and became a component of the medical culture. They learned what medicine was and experienced how it worked in the body while at hospitals. They were not aware of a need to make clear choices between "new" and "old," or

175.   Ibid.; Poon, *Negotiating Religion*; Nedostup, *Superstitious Regimes*.

"Chinese" and "Western" in seeking medical-care institutions. Their primary goal was protecting their corporeal, social, and even spiritual lives; what they were mostly interested in was the quality and cost of medical treatment and other social services that a hospital would offer—not the hospital's sponsorship or mission statement.

Although there existed a wide range of medical agencies in Shanghai open to the public, once the Nationalist government established its authority, personal health was directly connected with municipal administration. In the next chapter, our discussion shifts away from nongovernmental organizations to formal administrative systems and we consider the origins and mandates of the municipal Public Health Bureau of Shanghai.

CHAPTER 2

Protecting Life, Controlling the City

The Origins and Development of the Shanghai Municipal Public Health Bureau

On July 7, 1927, Chiang Kai-shek declared the opening of the Shanghai Municipal Government to control the Chinese sector of Shanghai. The next day, Chiang and other top Nationalist leaders held an inauguration ceremony at the former office of the Shanghai *daotai* (circuit intendant). At this ceremony, Chiang made a speech, declaring,

> We must establish in Shanghai a real municipal government, a municipal government which can compare favorably with, if not be better than, the foreign settlements, so that when the time arrives, we will be prepared to [*sic*] the Settlements back. Foreigners then cannot object to their return on the old ground that we are unprepared to administer affairs.[1]

Likewise, Huang Fu (1883–1936), who was sworn in as mayor of the city at this ceremony, proclaimed that "the whole body of Shanghai people should double their efforts and do their very best to help in the success of the municipal government so as to pave the way for the eventual restoration of the foreign settlements."[2]

As these remarks evinced, expelling foreign imperialists from China and restoring Chinese sovereignty were high on the Nationalist agenda, and China's top leaders were convinced that Shanghai should serve as a

1. *North China Herald*, July 9, 1927, 58.
2. Ibid., 59.

showcase and vanguard to demonstrate Chinese capability to create an effective and competent municipal administration. On the same day, Chiang and Huang attended the second ceremony held at the General Chamber of Commerce. At this ceremony, Huang identified public health, increasing production, and public order as "three movements" that would bring about civil order and modernization to Shanghai.[3] A messy and polluted city would justify the presence of imperialists in China; sanitation, cleanliness, and orderliness were prerequisite for a modern city and a key to successful recovery of foreign concessions.

With this background, the Nationalist regime opened the Shanghai Municipal Public Health Bureau (PHB) (Weishengju) in April 1927. This bureau was in charge of *weisheng* administration—various works and services related to public health and hygiene—in the Chinese sector of the city. In this chapter I trace the origins and evolution of this bureau and discuss what Shanghai's Chinese administrators did to improve the city's environment and to promote people's well-being. In their efforts to bring order to the city, they connected private bodies to public health and placed personal habits under public gaze and political control.

Shanghai's modern public health administration stemmed from the convergence of two sources: state imperatives and local initiatives. This convergence was further facilitated and complicated by the presence of Western powers. Commencing from the turn of the twentieth century, the Qing state, the Republican-warlord state, and the Nationalist state all tried to build a bureaucratic system that would improve the nation's health. Their efforts were not always effective or successful, and they were significantly assisted and supplemented by outside agencies, such as the League of Nations and the Rockefeller Foundation. In spite of various obstacles, however, the Nationalists "made the greatest, although still incomplete, progress towards their announced goals of state reintegration, institution building and national development"[4] during the Nanjing decade (1927–37), and conceived central and local administrative plans for a modern health system.[5] The Shanghai PHB was part of this nationwide

3. Wakeman, *Policing Shanghai*, 45–46.
4. Strauss, *Strong Institutions in Weak Polities*.
5. Yip, *Health and National Reconstruction*; Yip, "Health and National Reconstruction," 395.

scheme. Those who took charge of the Shanghai PHB and those in Nanjing shared the same goals: creating a sanitary city, establishing a strong
nation, and restoring Chinese sovereignty.[6] Chinese elites were well aware
that Western colonialists were aggressors and invaders that needed to be
expelled. Yet, they also acknowledged that Westerners provided a "catalyst"
and "conduit" for scientific knowledge of medicine and sanitation.[7] In creating Chinese public health, they were eager to learn from the West. They
also borrowed Japanese systems, styles, and terminology. In fact, *weisheng*, a term that originally appeared in the ancient text of Zhuangzi, was
reimported via the Japanese term *eisei* as a translation of the German term
Gesundheitspflege.

However, the Shanghai PHB was not a product of top-down directions from the state. Nor was it a simple imitation of Western or Japanese
models. It had local origins, evolved from a number of local institutions,
and developed in response to local affairs and problems. In carrying out
their duties, Shanghai's Chinese administrators designed their own public health measures and techniques based on socioeconomic conditions
particular to the city and in light of preexisting local organizations.
The bureau provided necessary services to clean the city and promote
health; it also issued and imposed laws and regulations. An examination
of the history of the PHB illuminates some important aspects of Chinese
society in the Republican era, including the relationship between the state
and society, the role of Western science in legitimizing coercive public
health measures, and the balance between colonial powers and Chinese
authorities. In this chapter, I first outline the rise of China's state medicine since the late Qing period, then closely look into specific features
associated with Shanghai.

The Japanese occupation contributed to changes and continuities in
Shanghai's public health administration during the Second Sino-Japanese
War. After the heavy fighting of 1937, the prewar PHB ceased its operation, and those who remained in Shanghai reopened the Chinese PHB to
resume their work with the backing of the Japanese military. The wartime
PHB carried out public health programs that were very similar to those
of the prewar period; it also adopted similar slogans on national strength

6.   Andrews, "In Republican China."
7.   Lewis and MacPherson, "Introduction."

and racial hygiene. The discussion of wartime public health that follows calls attention to the issue of collaboration. In wartime Shanghai, Chinese public health employees, doctors, and community leaders who worked with and received assistance from Japanese personnel were unintentionally helping the Japanese occupation. Yet, they probably did not perceive their activities as collaborating with Japan. Rather, they embraced medical science as a marker of universal modernity and transnational value. Identified with science, they worked together with the Japanese occupiers in an effort to address their greater concern for establishing a modern public health administration.

The Public Health Administration of the Nanjing Government

INTRODUCTION OF WESTERN MEDICINE
AND PUBLIC HEALTH SYSTEM

In the nineteenth century, medical missionaries and returned students who had studied medicine in Japan and the West brought a steady stream of information on Western medicine to China. However, the Qing state itself did not take much interest in Western biomedicine, nor was it actively involved in health-related work until the turn of the century. In 1905, as a consequence of internal and external pressure, the Qing launched the New Policy Reforms and opened a sanitary bureau (Weishengsi), which was placed under the jurisdiction of the police. This was the first official attempt by the Qing to create an administrative institution that would address public health at the national level. Unfortunately, the bureau did not have a well-trained medical staff, and its activities were far from adequate.

The 1910–11 outbreak of pneumonic plague in northeastern China that killed more than sixty thousand people marked a turning point in the Qing's medical policy.[8] The ferocity of the epidemic terrified the Chinese

8. On the Great Plague of 1911, see, for example, Carl Nathan, *Plague Prevention and Politic*; Liande Wu, *Plague Fighter*; Benedict, *Bubonic Plague*; Sean Hsiang-lin Lei, "Sovereignty and Microscope."

people as well as the Qing state. In addition to raising health concerns, the crisis gave Japan and Russia a pretext for military interference in the northeast. Responding to the disaster, the Qing asked Wu Lien-teh (Wu Liande) (1879–1960), a Cambridge-trained physician, to take charge and launch various antiplague measures.[9] The Qing government set up systematic cordons and quarantines to stop the further spread of the plague. Corpses of the dead were cremated in large quantities; state-authorized autopsies, which to date had been performed only infrequently, were also performed. The Qing also undertook coercive antiplague measures, including isolation and forced hospitalization of patients and prohibition of travel. Though there was resistance and opposition to these measures, overall the Qing was successful in containing the plague, and its effort denied Japan and Russia the opportunity to intervene in the northeast.[10]

As a result of the Great Plague, the Qing accepted germ theory and recognized that the state had a responsibility to become involved in disease-control activities. After the fall of the Qing, the new Republican government opened central administrative organizations to oversee nationwide health services. In 1912, the Sanitary Bureau in the Ministry of Internal Affairs (Neiwubu) was created. Lin Wenqing (1869–1957), a Singaporean Chinese who had received his medical degree in Great Britain, was appointed as its first chief.[11] The next year, the Sanitary Bureau was downgraded to the Division of Sanitation (Weishengke) of the Police and Security Bureau (Jingbaosi) under the Ministry of Internal Affairs. But the Sanitary Bureau was reinstated in 1916.[12] On paper, these organizations were charged with various kinds of public health work.[13] However, because of political disintegration exacerbated by a lack of proper personnel and inadequate funding, little was achieved to improve national health until 1928.

9. Later, Wu held a series of positions in the national government; he went on to become one of the most prominent public health administrators in Republican China. For Wu's career, see Liande Wu, *Plague Fighter*.

10. *Report of the International Plague Control*, 4.

11. Zhang Zhikang, "Gonggong weisheng," 198.

12. Chen Haifeng, ed., *Zhongguo weisheng baojianshi*, 17.

13. Ibid.

In contrast to the slow moves of the central government, the Rockefeller Foundation and Peking Union Medical College made significant contributions to the development of China's medical world. In 1914, John D. Rockefeller Jr. invited a number of educators and intellectuals to a meeting to discuss the foundation's involvement in China. This meeting resulted in the formation of the China Medical Commission. The members of the commission, including American medical professionals and the former consul general in Hankou, stayed in China in the summer of 1914 to study local medical conditions. In November of the same year, they established the China Medical Board (CMB) to implement a modern medical program. The first imperative of the CMB was the training of elite medical professionals to lead the nation. To this end, the CMB decided to open a completely Western-style medical school of outstanding quality. The CMB purchased the property of Union Medical College from the London Missionary Society, reorganizing it into Peking Union Medical College (PUMC), which was formally dedicated in 1921. Using an American model, the CMB upgraded the curriculum of PUMC to meet international standards of medical science. Many PUMC faculty members were Americans, and instruction at PUMC was conducted completely in English. Admitting only a small number of highly select students, PUMC was considered the best medical school in China in the late 1920s. Although the PUMC was often criticized as "too comfortable" and "separated from ordinary life," it produced many leading figures of Chinese medical science, including several world-class researchers. PUMC graduates came to occupy the best positions in the health administration of the Nanjing government.[14]

The overall emphasis of PUMC education was on training researchers and teachers of the best quality, but it also introduced the concept of preventive medicine and promulgated the idea of community-based health care. This was largely thanks to the efforts of John Grant (1890–1962), one of the best-known figures involved in public health activities at PUMC. Grant created the school's Public Health and Preventive Medicine Department. Born in China as a son of a Canadian missionary, he had firsthand knowledge of Chinese customs, lifestyles, and sanitary

14. Bowers, "American Private Aid," 86–96; Yip, "Health and Society in China," 1200–1201.

conditions. He was interested in preventive medicine and used his depth of understanding to adapt Western medicine to China. In the interest of providing local residents with health-related services and education and providing students with a venue for training in the department, Grant opened a health station (*weisheng shiwusuo*) in Beijing in 1925. Under the supervision of the Beijing police, the station took charge of the public health work and collected vital statistics of the Second Inner Left District of Beijing. This was the first public health center in China to serve a specifically designated community. When other municipalities and rural areas began opening their own health service centers, they adopted the model established by the health station in Beijing.[15]

Grant's idea to build community-based public health services was shared with his colleagues and students at PUMC. The Public Health and Preventive Medicine Department produced several well-known public figures, including Chen Zhiqian (C. C. Chen) (1903–2000) and Yang Chongrui (Marion Yang) (1891–1983)—two of the famed rural reformers of Dingxian.[16] More relevant to the case of Shanghai, Hu Hongji (Hou-ki Hu) (1894–1932) and Li Ting'an (Ting-an Li) (1898–1948), two commissioners of public health in prewar Shanghai, both acquired their training at PUMC. Hu Hongji worked as the chief of the Division of Vital Statistics in Beijing's health station until 1926. Li Ting'an, a PUMC graduate who specialized in public health under John Grant, also worked as a student at the station in the late 1920s.[17]

CREATING THE CENTRAL AND LOCAL PUBLIC
HEALTH ADMINISTRATION

In 1928, after negotiating with the left-wing Nationalists and with Zhang Xueliang, a northeastern warlord, Chiang Kai-shek formally announced the opening of his government in Nanjing. Embracing Sun Yat-sen's Three

15.   Bullock, *American Transplant*, 144–51; Bu, "Beijing First Health Station."
16.   Dingxian is a name of the county in North China. From the late 1920s through the 1930s, Yan Yangchu (James Yen), an American-educated reformer, carried out rural reconstruction programs, including education and public health. Concerning James Yen and Dingxian, see, for example, Hayford, *To the People.*
17.   Bullock, *American Transplant*, 134–89.

Principles of the People, the Nanjing government launched a comprehensive program of national reconstruction.

The newly created Nanjing government faced an enormous task as it set out to improve the sanitation of the nation and the health of its people. The physical state of the Chinese people in the pre-1949 period was generally poor. The crude death rate was estimated to be twenty-five to thirty per thousand; that of infants was higher than two hundred per thousand. The average life expectancy was around thirty-five years. Plague, cholera, smallpox, tuberculosis, malaria, and various parasitic diseases were prevalent among the population. In some areas where minorities lived, the infant death rate was as high as 78 percent. Even in large cities, health conditions were not much better. For example, in 1934–35, Nanjing's crude death rate was eighteen per thousand and that of infants was 123 per thousand. As of 1935, male life expectancy in Nanjing was 39.8 years, and that of females was 38.22 years.[18]

In April of 1928, against this bleak background, the Nanjing government opened the Department of Public Health (Weishengsi) under the Ministry of Internal Affairs (Neizhengbu). Chen Fangzhi (1884–1969), who had a medical degree from Tokyo Imperial University and hailed from the same province as Chiang Kai-shek, assumed the directorship.[19] After seven months, the department was upgraded to Ministry of Public Health (Weishengbu) and Xue Dubi (1892–1973) took the position of minister of health. This new ministry was created in part to give Xue Dubi the status of a minister. Xue was the mayor of Beijing when PUMC's health station was created; he was on good terms with several prominent medical leaders at PUMC, including John Grant.[20] He appointed Liu Ruiheng (J. Heng Liu) (1890–1961) as a technical vice minister. Liu had a medical degree from Harvard and was the president of PUMC at the time of his appointment. Moreover, as a classmate of Song Ziwen (T. V. Soong) (1894–1971) at Harvard, Liu had a strong political connection with Song and Kong Xiangxi (H. H. Kung) (1881–1967), who were related by marriage to Chiang Kai-shek. Liu Ruiheng became the de facto

18.   Chen Haifeng, ed., *Zhongguo weisheng baojianshi*, 15–16; Yip, *Health and National Reconstruction*, 9–10; Watt, *Saving Lives in Wartime China*, 17–34.

19.   Fu Hui and Deng Zongyu, "Yixuejie de yingmeipai yu deripai zhi zheng," 66.

20.   Yip, *Health and National Reconstruction*, 47.

leader of the new Ministry of Public Health. Under Liu's leadership, most of the ministry's positions were filled by men associated with PUMC.[21] Liu stayed at the top of the Chinese public health administration until 1939 and continued to play a significant role in the national health program.[22]

At the outset, the Ministry of Public Health had two advisory boards, and five administrative departments: the Department of General Affairs (Zongwusi), the Department of Medical Administration (Yizhengsi), the Department of Health and Sanitation (Baojiansi), the Department of Epidemic Prevention (Fangyisi), and the Department of Vital Statistics (Tongjisi). In addition, the Central Hygiene Laboratory (Zhongyang weisheng shiyansuo) and the Central Epidemic Prevention Bureau (Zhongyang fangyichu) were placed under the purview of the ministry. These two institutes conducted chemical and bacteriological research and experiments.[23]

However, the independent Ministry of Public Health did not survive very long. The Nanjing government streamlined its entire administration in 1930, and, as a result, the ministry was downgraded to the National Health Administration (NHA) (Weishengshu) in 1931. It was placed under the Ministry of Internal Affairs. When the ministry was downgraded to the NHA, its original five departments were reduced to three (the Departments of General Affairs; Health and Sanitation; and Epidemic Prevention). In 1932, with help from the League of Nations, the Nanjing government opened the Central Field Health Station. The NHA functioned mostly as an administrative and supervisory organization, while the Central Field Health Station was assigned to take up technical matters and scientific work.[24] From 1932 until the outbreak of the war, the National Health Administration and the Central Field Health Station were the two key organizations in charge of national health.

21. Ibid; Fu Hui and Deng Zongyu, "Yixuejie de yingmeipai yu deripai zhi zheng," 66–67.

22. For Liu's career, see Irene Ssu-chin Liu Hou, *Dr. J. Heng Liu.*

23. This organizational structure is prescribed in *Fagui* (1929). Also see Yip, *Health and National Reconstruction*, 47; Zhang Zhikang. "Gonggong weisheng," 198–219; J. Heng Liu, "Ministry of Health," 289–90.

24. J. Heng Liu, "Chinese Medical Association," 304

With this administrative framework in place, the Nationalist state assumed responsibility for nationwide public health activities. According to the First Sanitary Code, issued in December 1928, these activities included collecting statistics; inspecting food and water; and providing school, maternal, and industrial health care.[25] To implement these projects at the local level, the Nanjing government promulgated the "General Outline of the Public Health Administration System" (Weisheng xingzheng xitong dagang).[26] The "Outline" stated that each province should have a public health division (*weishengchu*), each municipality should have a public health bureau (*weishengju*), and each *xian* (county) should also have a public health division under its Department of Public Security.[27] According to this "Outline," the public health division of each province (*sheng weishenchu*) and the public health bureaus of each special municipality (*tebieshi weishengju*)—including Shanghai—were under the direct jurisdiction of the Ministry of Public Health. In practice, however, the Nanjing government controlled only the eastern part of the country. Even in provinces dominated by the Nationalists and their allies, the influence of the ministry was slight, and the actual implementation of health-related projects was left to local agencies. It was the responsibility of each local agency to secure necessary funds and personnel for its operation.[28]

These accounts point to the emergence of a state-sponsored public health administration during the Republican period. Nationalist leaders and Chinese elites increasingly saw medicine and sanitation as among the most basic functions of a modernizing government, and concern for national strength was a powerful impetus for shaping state public health policies. However, although Shanghai's PHB was within the purview of the Nationalist government, the bureau emerged from the city's local traditions; it developed within and adapted to its specific environment. The goal of making a healthy city and defending city people from disease

25. Lucas, *Chinese Medical Modernization*, 63.
26. *Fagui* (1929). Also see Zhang Zhikang, "Gonggong weisheng," 199–203.
27. J. Heng Liu, "Ministry of Health," 292–93.
28. Yip, *Health and National Reconstruction*, 49.

brought administrators, local elites, and police forces together and put them into a network of collaboration.

Public Health Administration in Prewar Shanghai

THE INTERNATIONAL SETTLEMENT AND
THE CHINESE "DEFICIENCY"

Although the Qing did not open a sanitary bureau until 1905, Shanghai's public health administration already existed in the nineteenth century in the International Settlement. British settlers created the administration in response to the city's "dirty" environment and "unsanitary natives." Shanghai's earliest public health administration began as nuisance-removal work in the Settlement. In 1861, the Shanghai Municipal Council (SMC) appointed a health inspector (*weisheng jichayuan*) to oversee the general sanitation within the Settlement. The following year, the SMC employed one more inspector and created a *fenhuigu*—literally "division of human waste and dirt"—to supervise waste removal and street cleaning. In 1863, this division was upgraded to the Office of Hygiene (Qingjiebu) to deal with other health-related activities in the Settlement. In 1898, Arthur Stanley became the first full-time medical officer of the Settlement. At that time, the Office of Hygiene was reorganized into the Public Health Department (PHD) (Weishengchu).[29] In the early years, the work of the PHD focused mostly on cleaning the environment, educating the Chinese, and issuing and enforcing regulations.[30] This department gradually expanded. By the 1920s it had become a comprehensive public health administration that covered not only street cleaning but also other medical and technical matters.[31] Until the Japanese took over the Settlement in 1941, all the commissioners of public health were British; the PHD

29. *SWZ*, 534; Jordan, "Shanghai Municipal Council," 93; Xinzhong Yu, "Treatment of Night Soil," 58–64.

30. *Shanghai Municipal Council Public Health Department Annual Reports* (*Shanghai Municipal Council*), 1898 and 1900. For a chronological development of the PHD, see Peng Shanmin, *Gonggong weisheng*, 38–54.

31. Peng Shanmin, *Gonggong weisheng*, 55–82.

was staffed by inspectors who had come directly from England and had received special training there.

The formation of this department in the Settlement reflected the concept of "state medicine," which originated in England in the late nineteenth century.[32] As summarized by Carol Benedict, the central tenets of this concept are "that the state had primary responsibility for protecting the public's health and that it therefore had the right, even the duty, to impose hygiene and sanitation regulations on private citizens for the public good."[33] In doing so, the British were not so much concerned about improving Chinese health as protecting themselves from an unclean environment, unhealthy food, and "an immense alien population whose ways are obfuscated with prejudice."[34]

Chinese elites were well aware that the goal of the public health department in the Settlement was to serve the foreign population—not the Chinese.[35] Yet the British were successful in improving the city's appearance. From the 1860s through the twentieth century, Chinese, Western, and Japanese observers unanimously praised the cleanliness and orderliness of the Settlement. In contrast, the Chinese sector was unclean and odoriferous.[36] For Chinese elites, the lack of modern urban hygiene was a clear marker of Chinese backwardness and weakness. After the loss of the First Sino-Japanese War, the realization that urban sanitation involved something more than a simple matter of aesthetics and appearance became evident; the Chinese saw a close connection between public health and national strength.[37] Public health, or *gonggong weisheng*, was a comprehensive system charged with carrying out policies and projects to improve the city's sanitation and people's health.

The contrast between the Settlement and the Chinese sector reminds us of what Ruth Rogaski has called the discourse of "Chinese deficiency."

32. Lucas, *Chinese Medical Modernization*, 49–50.

33. Benedict, *Bubonic Plague*, 138.

34. For British remarks on Shanghai's sanitary conditions, see various issues of *Shanghai Municipal Council*.

35. Chen Fangzhi, "Shanghai Shi de gonggong weisheng wenti," 106–24.

36. Peng Shanmin, *Gonggong weisheng*, 38–41; Mine Kiyoshi, "Shin koku Shanghai kenbun roku," 27–28. Also see MacPherson, *Wilderness of Marshes*.

37. Xingzhong Yu, "Treatment of Nightsoil," 58–64; Peng Shanmin, *Gonggong weisheng*, 38–41.

Many Chinese reformers in the early twentieth century embraced the notion that China was not as modern or civilized as the West, and regarded the poor health and hygiene of the Chinese as directly related to that deficiency. Even though Chinese elites were aware of the imperial nature of the public health in the Settlement, they were also convinced that they needed to institute a similar system to overcome Chinese deficiencies in cleanliness, order, and medical knowledge, and by extension, modern civilization. Shanghai's elites, inspired by the British model, embarked on public health measures.[38] In doing so, they also employed disciplinary methods to educate and regulate the urban masses, who lacked proper understanding of hygiene.

THE ORIGINS OF THE SHANGHAI MUNICIPAL PUBLIC HEALTH BUREAU

In spite of intellectual concerns, the development of the public health administration in the Chinese sector was slow and only sporadic. In the first two decades of the twentieth century, the Chinese city itself consisted of a number of different entities.[39] Each entity created its own administrative organizations in charge of sanitation.[40] These organizations were small and, in practice, simply supervised street cleaning.

Finally Sun Chuanfang (1887–1936) consolidated his rule over Zhejiang, Jiangsu, Anhui, and Jiangxi. He also unified several local districts of Chinese Shanghai in 1925. In the following year, he invited Ding Wenjiang (1887–1936), a May Fourth intellectual who had studied geology at Glasgow University, to serve as the director general of the city.[41] Like many intellectuals of this time, Ding hoped that Sun's military power and authority would offer stable local rule and that successful administration could lead to the recovery of Chinese sovereignty. During his tenure as the director general, from April to December 1926, he strove to

---

38. On Chinese deficiency, see Rogaski, *Hygienic Modernity*, 4–9, 165–92.

39. Henriot, *Shanghai, 1927–1937*, 7–18.

40. For a chronology of early public health administration in the Chinese sector, see Peng Shanmin, *Gonggong weisheng*, 89–90.

41. On Ding Wenjiang, see Furth, *Ting Wen-chiang*; Lei Qili, ed., *Ding Wenjiang yinxiang*; Song Guangbo, *Ding Wenjiang tuzhuan*.

build a modern administration.[42] He also unified three existing organizations associated with sanitation: the sanitary division of the Songhu Police Hall (Songhu jingchating), located in Wusong, northeast of the city; the patrol section of the Hubei Bureau of Industry, Patrol and Taxation (Hubei gongxunjuanju), located in Zhabei, north of the city; and the health office of the Shanghai City Council (Shanghai Shi gongsuo), located in Nanshi, south of the city.[43] The result of this amalgamation was the Public Health Bureau of the Wusong-Shanghai Commercial Port (Songhu shangbu weishengju). This office was renamed the Wusong-Shanghai Public Health Bureau (Songhu weishengju) (Songhu PHB) in 1927.[44] This was the first unified public health administration in the Chinese sector. Ding invited Hu Hongji, a medical doctor who had studied in the United States, to be the deputy director of this bureau.

The Songhu PHB presented an interesting mixture of various elements. As Hu Hongji has described it, this bureau was created "due to Dr. Ting's [Ding Wenjiang] effort together with the enthusiasm of Messrs. T. Y. Yen [Yan Chunyang], the former commissioner of police, and Li Pin Sze [Li Pingshu], a prominent local gentleman . . . to consolidate the [sic] existing nominal health departments of both the police and civil authorities under the Directorate General Sun Chuanfang, and with the cooperation of the former police."[45] In keeping with this tradition, Yan Chunyang, the commissioner of police for the Port of Shanghai and Wusong district was concurrently appointed commissioner of health, and a number of local businessmen, including Li Pingshu and Lu Bohong (1875–1937), joined the bureau's advisory committee.[46] In addition, distinguished medical doctors, such as Niu Huilin (1889–1937), Yu Fengbin (1884–1930), and Wang Qizhang (1885–1955), were also members of the advisory committee.[47] Although Ding Wenjiang and Hu Hongji were both Western-trained scientists brought in from elsewhere, they were supported by these local

---

42. Zhu Peilian, "Ding Wenjiang, Huang Fu."
43. *SWZ*, 540. Also see Elvin, "Gentry Democracy."
44. Zhang Zhikang, "Gonggong weisheng," 199.
45. Hou-ki Hu, "New Department of Health," 429.
46. Ibid., 432–38.
47. Ibid., 429, 434–35; Peng Shanmin, *Gonggong weisheng*, 90. Although no Chinese-style doctors were listed as board members, Li Pingshu was a supporter of Chinese medicine. See chapter 1.

personnel in organizing the bureau. Also, because of their academic backgrounds, Ding and Hu were favorably accepted by the British in the city. The former British consul general, the former commissioner general of the SMC, and John Grant introduced Ding and Hu to officials at the Public Health Department of the Settlement and helped them acquire documents and reports on regulations, license conditions, notices, and other materials relevant to their work.[48] Ding and Hu used these British materials as templates to create their own. Other cities, too, separated public health services from police duties and created an independent administration to oversee health-related matters in the 1920s. Many of these administrative bodies were soon transferred back to the jurisdiction of the police because of a lack of proper funding and unskilled management.[49] By contrast, the Songhu PHB survived and maintained its independent status. According to "Regulations of the Wusong-Shanghai Public Health Bureau," as of 1927, the bureau had three divisions (the Division of Sanitation and Street Cleaning; the Division of Vital Statistics, Regulation of Medical Practices, and Meat Inspection; and the Division of Communicable Disease Control) and a laboratory.[50] Even after the Nationalists arrived in the city and took over the bureau, the organization did not expand significantly. The three divisions of the earlier Songhu PHB remained in 1928, and the municipal PHB retained them until 1934.[51]

During the two years of its existence, the Songhu PHB achieved some success in improving the physical appearance of the city. Over 65 percent of the PHB budget was spent on street sweeping and night-soil removal. The PHB employed 430 full-time garbage collectors, and divided the city into several sections to promote efficiency in the cleaning work. Hu Hongji wrote that "the conditions of the streets are greatly improved" and that the removal of feces "may be considered satisfactory from a hygienic view in respect to the present living standard of the Chinese." The Songhu PHB also opened eleven clinics and gave free vaccinations against smallpox to city residents.[52]

48.   "Relationships between the Municipal Public Health Department."
49.   Wong and Wu Lien-teh, *History of Chinese Medicine,* 740.
50.   Hou-ki Hu, "New Department of Health," 433–34.
51.   Kim, "Brief Survey," 175–76.
52.   Hou-ki Hu, "New Department of Health," 431–32.

Western observers gave mixed evaluations to the Songhu PHB. According to an article in the *China Weekly Review*, "Dr. Hou-ki Hu, an American returned student, who in the brief space of a few months and in the face of complications produced by the disturbed political situation, was however, able to get his department going in pretty good order. Health stations and dispensaries were established and considerable progress was made in the dissemination of health propaganda, particularly from the standpoint of vaccination against smallpox."[53] Yet, between 1926 and 1928, British inspectors from the Settlement were still making strongly negative remarks about the sanitation of the Chinese sector. The water supply was inadequate and sometimes contaminated. Food factories used improper production methods and did not come close to meeting present-day public health requirements. The conditions of dairies were poor, and slaughterhouses were the "most disgusting." Innumerable ordure pits and accumulations of refuse were left around in the city—both bred flies. Ponds and creeks bred mosquitoes. There was no system of vital statistics to measure progress. Chinese districts did have refuse removal and ordure collecting systems, but these were not supervised by the health department. No system of notification of infectious disease was in place. Stray dogs wandered the streets and rabies was prevalent. In all, the British inspectors concluded that the Chinese sector did not have a public health organization equal to what had been established in the Settlement.[54]

Hu Hongji admitted that the work of his bureau was still very limited and many of the new plans were still in rudimentary stages as of 1926. The PHB did not have trained personnel who could collect accurate vital statistics in a systematic manner; since there was no isolation hospital, it was not feasible to cordon off communicable disease patients.[55] In spite of many deficiencies, however, the Songhu PHB's presence meant that the Nationalist government did not have to create a public health administration from scratch. It simply took up where the Songhu PHB had left off.

53.   *China Weekly Review*, April 16, 1927, 178.

54.   Letters and reports of British inspectors regarding the public health conditions in neighboring Chinese districts are filed in SMA U1-16-319.

55.   Hou-ki Hu, "New Department of Health," 432.

FROM THE SONGHU PHB TO THE MUNICIPAL PHB

Although 1928 marked the beginning of the Nanjing government, the municipal government of Chinese Shanghai under the Nationalists was inaugurated in 1927. In March of 1927, the General Labor Union in Shanghai organized a general strike and armed insurrection in support of the Northern Expedition led by Chiang Kai-shek. When the National Revolutionary Army entered the city, union members welcomed them, but this "Shanghai Spring" did not last long. On April 12, Chiang launched a coup against the union members who led the strike. He ordered Green Gang members to attack, kill, and arrest them; unions and strikes became illegal; and "leftist" elements were completely driven from the city. On April 18, 1927, six days after the coup, Chiang Kai-shek formed his own regime in Nanjing opposed to the powers in Wuhan. On July 7, Chiang's regime established the Special Municipality of Shanghai. This new government unified various political powers and organizations in the Chinese-administered sector of the city. In doing so, the municipal government rearranged several preexisting organizations that had been created by local notables. Consequently, the municipal Secretariat (Mishuchu) and nine bureaus (*ju*) were newly opened and placed under its jurisdiction. The Songhu PHB was transformed into the Shanghai Public Health Bureau.[56]

In June 1927, under Huang Fu's direction, after a three-month interval, Hu Hongji reassumed the position of the commissioner of the PHB.[57] After Hu's death in 1932 in a traffic accident, Li Ting'an, who was teaching at PUMC at that time, succeeded to the position based on the recommendation of Liu Ruiheng, Yan Fuqing, and others. Li retained this position until 1937. Hu Hongji and Li Ting'an shared similar backgrounds. Hu received his medical degree in 1916 from the National Medical College in Beijing. After serving in France with the British Expeditionary Force during World War I and working as a physician several years in China, he received a fellowship from the Rockefeller Foundation to study in the United States. He earned a doctoral degree in public health from

56.   Tang, Shen, and Qiao, *Shanghaishi*, 651; Xiong Yuezhi, ed., *Shanghai tongshi*, vol. 7, *Minguo zhengzhi*, 237–238; *Shanghai shizheng gaiyao* (*SSGY*), chap. 1, 11.

57.   When the municipal government first opened, Liu Xuzi took the position for three months. Hu resumed his position in July 1927. See *SWZ*, 540; Henriot, *Shanghai, 1927–1937*, 245; "Shanghai Health Department," 469–70.

Johns Hopkins University and studied locally based public health work in the United States for several months. After returning to China in 1924, he worked at the health station in Beijing with John Grant in 1925 and 1926 as a chief of the Division of Vital Statistics.[58] Li was a graduate of Peking Union Medical College and held a doctoral degree in public health from Harvard. He had once worked at the Gaoqiao Health Station, located in the northeastern suburb of Shanghai.[59] Like Liu Ruiheng and several other public health officials of the central government, Hu and Li had received American educations and had empirical knowledge of American public health. They were both products and champions of Western medical science.

Similar to many Republican elites, both Hu and Li were devoted nationalists and believed that healthy individuals were the foundation of national strength. In his *Introduction to Public Health* (*Gonggong weisheng gailun*), Hu wrote that public health was the key to the rise and fall of a state and, ultimately, to national survival.[60] Likewise, Li wrote that public health was not a simple matter of putting lids on night-soil carts or cleaning streets; public health included the strength and weakness of the state (*guojia qiangruo*) and the happiness of individuals (*geren xingfu*). Li also discussed connections among public health, mortality rates, socioeconomic loss, and national power.[61] At the same time, Hu and Li were also well aware that intellectual discourse on individual bodies and national health should be translated into the social reality and local setting of Shanghai.

Even though Republican Shanghai was the center of Chinese commerce and industry, the wealthiest part of the city was under foreign control. The Chinese sector always suffered from a lack of financial resources, and the public health bureau had only limited funds at its disposal.[62] As of 1934, whereas the annual public health facility budget

58. Hu Hongji, *Gonggong weisheng gailun*.
59. "Health Commissioner in Shanghai," 1220.
60. Hu Hongji, *Gonggong weisheng gailun*.
61. Li Ting'an, "Shenme shi 'gonggong weisheng?'"; Li Ting'an, "Guomin huiyi yinggai zhuyi weisheng shiye," 43–44.
62. Li Ting'an, "Shanghai Shi weishengju gongzuo zhi gaikuang"; Li Ting'an, "Shenme shi 'gonggong weisheng?'"; Li Ting'an, "Shanghai Shi zhi gonggong weisheng xingzheng."

(*weisheng shebeifei*) per person was 2.24 yuan in the International Settlement, it was only 0.19 yuan in the Chinese sector. This amount was even smaller than that of several other Chinese cities, such as Guangzhou (1.09 yuan), Shantou (0.55 yuan), and Nanjing (0.54 yuan). Li Ting'an commented that at least 1.5 yuan per person should be allocated for public health; he also noted that the current amount was way below what it should be.[63]

Shanghai also experienced health and sanitation problems that were unique to large cities. Though hard statistics are not available, the crude death rate in Shanghai was estimated at around twenty-five per thousand—not much better than the national average.[64] As the city attracted increasing numbers of immigrants, it became overcrowded. The urban infrastructure—including the maintenance of a clean water supply, sewage systems, and public latrines—could not keep up with the rapid population growth. Even in peaceful times, many people died and were abandoned on the street and in vacant areas.[65] In addition to the hazards posed by abandoned corpses, people often retained the bodies of deceased relatives in coffins for extended periods between death and burial.[66] These practices contributed to the pollution in the city and were believed to cause serious health problems. Shanghai, moreover, had a large slum population. It is estimated that around two hundred thousand households and close to a million residents lived in shantytowns in pre-1949 Shanghai.[67] These shantytowns were regarded as (or imagined to be) hotbeds of communicable diseases, and such diseases frequently hit the city. Confronting these problems with limited resources, and motivated by the desire for the recovery of national sovereignty, the new PHB was pressed forward to implement reforms and carry out health-related works. In doing so, the bureau was supported and supplemented by the police force. Early on, the police were responsible for supervising

63. Li Ting'an, "Woguo zhongyao dushi weisheng xingzheng jingfei zhi xiankuang."
64. Hu Hung-chi, "Plans and Ideas," 4.
65. Hauser, *Shanghai: City for Sale*, 36; Henriot, "'Invisible Deaths, Silent Deaths.'"
66. Ting-an Li, "Report on the Bureau of Public Health"; Xiong Yuezhi, ed., *Shanghai tongshi*, vol. 9, *Minguo shehui*, 37.
67. Shanghai shehui kexueyuan jingji yanjiusuo chengshi jingjizu, ed., *Shanghai penghuqu de bianqian*, 7, 32. Also see Hanchao Lu, "Creating Urban Outcasts"; Lamson, "The Problem of Housing," 147–48.

environmental sanitation. Even after the public health bureau became independent from the police, the duties of police and public health officers were often related and overlapped. Physically and metaphorically, officers from both departments aimed at "sanitizing" the city and defending it from pollution. To carry this out, they exerted their control over the bodies and behavior of residents.[68] In doing so, the public health bureau also took full advantage of other preexisting institutions and facilities; it also negotiated and addressed issues with Westerners in the city. Three areas of public health illustrate these points: taking care of the sick and dead; regulating water and food; and controlling epidemic diseases.

TREATING THE SICK AND DISPOSING
OF THE DEAD

One of the significant tasks of the public health administration was taking care of the sick and dead. To this end, the Shanghai Public Health Bureau relied significantly on the city's preexisting private institutes.

With its establishment, the bureau declared that it would provide medical care to all residents in the city regardless of their economic status.[69] Accordingly, Hu Hongji published a grand plan to build a general hospital with 1,500 beds, a few branch hospitals, and district clinics, in the city.[70] This ambitious plan was never realized because of lack of funding. Although the city had purchased private hospitals and turned them into municipal institutions, it was not able to build a large general hospital until 1937.[71] Throughout the first half of the twentieth century, Shanghai people sought medical help mostly from nongovernmental institutions and individuals, and the municipal government was largely content to leave curative medicine in the hands of private institutions. However, instead of building full-scale hospitals, the PHB opened health

68. Wakeman, *Policing Shanghai*, 84–85.
69. *SSGY*, chap. 7, 7; Hu Hung-chi, "Plans and Ideas," 13; Hu Hongji, "Shanghai Shi wunianlai zhi weisheng xingzheng huigu," 12; Ting-an Li, "Report on the Bureau of Public Health," 15.
70. Hu Hung-chi, "Plans and Ideas," 13; Hu Hongji, "Shanghai Shi wunianlai zhi weisheng xingzheng huigu," 5.
71. Henriot, *Shanghai, 1927–1937*, 209.

stations (*weisheng shiwusuo*) that were in charge of local public health matters.[72]

Health stations were designed to be the core unit of health care for designated districts. The PHB planned to set up one station in each of the seventeen districts in the city, but only four stations, in Hunan, Jiangwan, Gaoqiao, and Wusong, were actually built during the Nanjing decade.[73] These stations were in close communication with local residents and in charge of various tasks related to public health, such as collecting vital statistics; supervising environmental sanitation (street cleaning, inspecting the quality of food and water, eliminating mosquitoes and flies, removing garbage and feces, etc.); administering anti-epidemic vaccinations; isolating and treating communicable disease patients; taking care of maternity and school health; and providing popular health education.[74] In addition, these stations offered free or inexpensive medical treatment to residents at their attached clinics.[75] Reflecting their experience and expertise, Hu and Li applied a community-based public health system to Shanghai. According to the statistics of 1935, each health station had the following total number of clinic visits: 112,139 (Hunan), 29,041 (Jiangwan), 27,298 (Wusong), and 24,127 (Gaoqiao). Compared with the number of patients that major hospitals in the city treated per year, these numbers are modest, and these four stations played only a limited role in providing medical care to Shanghai people.

However, health stations served as the center of community health and promoted sanitary services. It is particularly noteworthy that two out of four stations were built not in the city proper but in the suburban rural areas of Gaoqiao and Wusong. These two stations were more or less independent, and practically took charge of all health-related matters for each district. Moreover, the medical schools of Central University and Tongji University sent their professors and students to these rural stations

72. Li Ting'an, "Shanghai Shi zhi gonggong weisheng xingzheng," 24.

73. Ibid; Hu Hongji, "Shanghai Shi wunianlai zhi weisheng xingzheng huigu," 12; Li Ting'an, "Weishengju ji ge qu weisheng shiwusuo zhi zuzhi ji gongzuo," 460.

74. Li Ting'an, "Weishengju ji ge qu weisheng shiwusuo zhi zuzhi ji gongzuo," 460–61.

75. Li Ting'an, "Shanghai Shi zhi gonggong weisheng xinzheng," 23; Ting-an Li, "Report on the Bureau of Public Health," 14; *SSGY*, chap. 6, 7.

for practical, hands-on training in public health.[76] The stations of Gaoq-iao and Wusong exploited the human and financial resources of the two medical schools. Additionally, the Gaoqiao Health Station employed fifteen Chinese-style doctors as its staff.[77] It is unclear what duties these Chinese-style doctors actually performed at the station, but the fact that they were included in the municipal health program is noteworthy. Presumably the presence of Chinese-style doctors improved the popularity and approachability of the station. In light of the insufficient numbers of medical facilities in the suburbs, residents in Wusong and Gaoqiao areas benefited the most from the services provided by the health stations.[78]

In addition to these stations, the PHB also organized "mobile teams" and "traveling clinics." Mobile teams were dispatched to schools in remote areas;[79] "traveling clinics" were most useful in crisis situations. When Japan attacked Shanghai in 1932, the northeastern part of the city suffered considerable damage. Since neither the Jiangwan nor the Wusong Health Station was in operation in the wake of the battle, the PHB organized three "traveling clinic" vehicles. These vehicles traveled across the war-afflicted zones to provide medical relief to residents. From June 1932 to June 1933, these three traveling clinics saw a total of 78,641 patients.[80]

Health stations, traveling clinics, and mobile teams were all beneficial for Shanghai people and promoted Shanghai's welfare; they were particularly useful for rural health and emergency care. They did not replace or displace the preexisting institutions, however, and mostly responded to crises and disasters and provided auxiliary support to private services.

Another area of public health in which private organizations took a leading role was the disposal of corpses. Abandoned bodies and coffins raised serious health problems and damaged the city's appearance. In keeping with long-standing Chinese customs, coffins were often placed in a field or a temporary shelter pending burial, and a considerable number

76. Hu Hongji, "Shanghai Shi wunianlai zhi weisheng xingzheng huigu," 7–8; *SSGY*, chap. 7, 4; Shimose, "Shanghai no igaku oyobi byōin sankanki," 27.

77. Yip, *Health and National Reconstruction*, 76.

78. On Gaoqiao Health Station, see Shanghai Shi weishengju Gaoqiao weisheng shiwusuo, ed., *Shanghai Shi weishengju Gaoqiao weisheng shiwusuo*.

79. *SWZ*, 100.

80. *SSGY*, chap. 7, 7–8.

of coffin shelters existed in the city. According to Li Ting'an, as of 1934 and 1935, over one hundred thousand coffins had been deposited around Shanghai.[81] Often, coffined corpses were left unburied because of an insufficient number of grave sites; many simply abandoned their dead. Wu Lien-teh commented that "within one mile of the Bund, one may notice hundreds of ugly, foul-smelling, corpses in all stages of decomposition. Some coffins were actually empty, the contents having been removed by dogs or the ravages of time."[82] A high percentage of the abandoned bodies were those of infants and young children. Still others fell dead in the street with no one to look after them. To improve the situation, the PHB prohibited retaining corpses without burial. The PHB also opened two new municipal cemeteries in 1934 and 1935 so that corpses could be promptly disposed.[83]

The PHB was not the only or the primary agency that took care of abandoned corpses. Before the opening of the bureau, the police were in charge of street cleaning; throughout the 1930s, they were still assigned to pick up abandoned bodies from streets and alleys. Collected bodies were sent to a benevolent hall (*shantang*). As discussed in chapter 1, since the Ming period, local elites had voluntarily established numerous benevolent halls and performed charity work. Along with medical care, disposal of the dead was a significant part of such work.[84] Among these charitable organizations, Mountain Villa of the Universal Philanthropy (Pushan shanzhuang), which was opened in 1914, was the largest institution that provided free or inexpensive coffins and disposed of the dead. Mountain Villa owned sixty burial grounds and employed forty workers to bury abandoned bodies. This charitable organization not only collected corpses from the street, but also accepted unclaimed bodies from other institutions and hospitals. In 1930 Mountain Villa performed simple burial ceremonies for more than thirty-five thousand unidentified

81.   Ting-an Li, "Report on the Bureau of Public Health," 13; Ting-an Li, "Activities of the Bureau of Public Health," 991.

82.   "Shanghai Crematory," 995.

83.   *SSGY*, chap. 7, 5; Li Ting'an, "Weishengju ji ge qu weisheng shiwusuo zhi zuzhi ji gongzuo," 460; Shanghai Shi weishengju, *Brief Survey*, 13.

84.   Kohama, "Minkokuki Shanghai no toshi shakai to jizen jigyō"; Kohama, "Minkokuki Shanghai no minkan jizen jigyō to kokka kenryoku"; Kohama, *Kindai Shanghai no kōkyōsei to kokka*, 76–83.

bodies.[85] The primary goal of Mountain Villa and other similar institutions was to protect the community from the untended dead.[86] Yet, by taking care of corpses, these organizations also helped clean up the city and eliminate pathogens.

Hospitals and charitable halls were not completely autonomous; they had to register with municipal bureaus. However, the degree of governmental control was slight, and these civic organizations remained vital and useful actors in Shanghai society. The municipal government recognized and relied on them as semipublic organizations to perform necessary services related to the sick and dead. The municipal PHB did not take over tasks already carried out by preexisting local organizations. Rather, the municipal administration and charitable institutions supplemented each other.

WATER, FOOD, AND NATIONAL SOVEREIGNTY

Having a healthy life is impossible without potable water and safe food. Gastrointestinal disease was prevalent in the city, and Shanghai's administrators were concerned about the quality of water and food. Westerners often made negative remarks about the sanitation of food and drink in the Chinese sector, and they expressed anxiety about the safety of the food that entered the Settlement from surrounding Chinese areas.[87] For Chinese administrators, securing safe food and drink was not only a way to protect Chinese lives from sicknesses but also a way to restore Chinese pride and sovereignty.

In pre-1949 Shanghai, each sector of the city had its own waterworks companies; altogether five companies operated in the city. Early on, troubled by the quality of the water in the city, foreigners undertook the construction of waterworks. In the International Settlement, Shanghai Waterworks Company (Shanghai WC), run by the British, began operation in 1883.[88] Tasked mainly with supplying tap water to the foreign

85. Kohama. "Minkokuki Shanghai no toshi shakai to jizen jigyō," 72–73.

86. Henriot, "'Invisible Deaths, Silent Deaths,'" 420.

87. A letter from the commissioner of public health, dated July 25, 1927 (filed in SMA U1-16-319).

88. On the opening of the Shanghai WC, see MacPherson, *Wilderness of Marshes*, 81–122.

concessions, Shanghai WC was the largest waterworks company in pre-war Shanghai; in 1931 it provided more than two hundred thousand cubic meters of water per day. To provide local tap water, the French Municipal Council also started a company in its concession in 1897. This company was taken over by Compagnie Française de Tramways et d'Éclairage Électrique in 1909.[89]

These developments in the foreign sectors triggered Chinese interest in water service business, and local elites called for construction of a Chinese waterworks system. An early challenge was convincing the Chinese that paying for simple water was worthwhile. Some of them were concerned about the quality of water that came from underground pipes. Finally, in 1902, a group of Cantonese merchants was preparing for the launch of Shanghai Neidi Waterworks Company. Unfortunately, a lack of funds prevented them from proceeding. Just as they were about to sell the company to a French business, Li Pingshu and other notables stepped in and officially took over the management of the company. In 1909, Neidi Waterworks Company (Neidi WC) was formally opened in Nanshi and began providing tap water to the southern part of the city. The construction of its entire plant was completed in 1929.[90] Zhabei Water and Electric Company (Zhabei WEC), the second water supplier in the Chinese sector, completed its plant and began to supply tap water to residents of the northern part of the city in 1911. Although Li Pingshu initiated the formation of this company, Zhabei WEC was financed not only by private capital but also by a subsidy from Jiangsu provincial funds.[91] The company was completely privatized in 1924.[92] Finally, in 1937, the Public Utilities Bureau (PUB) (Gongyongju) and a private company jointly opened a water plant in Pudong, providing pure water for the residents of Pudong.[93]

89. Xiong Yuezhi, ed., *Shanghai tongshi*, vol. 8, *Minguo jingji*, 211–13; Xiong Yuezhi, ed., *Shanghai tongshi*, vol. 9, *Minguo shehui*, 2–4; Ma Changlin, *Shanghai de zujie*, 124–29.

90. Shi Meijun, "Shanghai dianye juxing," 386–87.

91. Li Pingshu, *Qishi zixu*, 62.

92. On this transition, see Wang Shu-hwai, "Dispute over the Ownership," 205; Shi Meijun, "Shanghai dianye juxing," 390–91.

93. Zhao Zengjue, *Shanghai zhi gonggong shiye*, 54; Xiong Yuezhi, ed., *Shanghai tongshi*, vol. 9, *Minguo shehui*, 2–4.

Compared with the foreign companies, these Chinese enterprises were inaugurated with much less capital: whereas Shanghai WC and Compagnie Française began their businesses with a base of 22,217,000 yuan and 12,000,000 yuan, respectively, Zhabei WEC raised 8,641,000 yuan and Neidi WC raised only 2,500,000 yuan.[94] The volume of their water supply was also smaller: as of 1948, the average amount of daily water supply for each company was (in ten thousand cubic meters) Shanghai WC, 31.5; Compagnie Française, 10.0; Neidi, 9.3; Zhabei, 6.4; and Pudong, 0.4.[95] Moreover, until the opening of the municipal government, there was no supervising organization for tap water in the Chinese sector. In the 1920s, Westerners made unfavorable comments on the quality of Chinese water.[96] In particular, Zhabei WEC left poor records. In 1920, the company's six filtration pools were all old and of inferior quality. As the population grew and factories increased in size and number, Zhabei WEC was unable to keep up with demand. The shortage of the company's water supply caused serious challenges not only for private households, but also for street-cleaning operations, factories, and firefighting.[97] Moreover, in 1926, the company's water was contaminated and caused the spread of cholera in Zhabei.[98]

These problems raised concerns among Chinese elites. With the establishment of the municipal government, laissez-faire businesses gave way to governmental control and regulation. The PUB was first assigned to supervise the Chinese waterworks companies, and it urged these companies to evenly distribute water and to unify water pricing across the Chinese sector of the city. The PUB also inspected water plant installations and their operation to assure that the companies produced an adequate quantity of water. To improve the quality of water, Zhabei WEC, following instructions from the PUB, built a new water treatment plant in 1928. Likewise Neidi WC constructed new filtration basins, precipitation

94. Daitōashō, "Kōso, Sekkō, Anki sanshō no suidō jigyō narabini denki jigyō," 136–37.

95. Shanghai gongyong shiye guanliju, ed., *Shanghai gongyong shiye*, 165. Cited in Peng Shanmin, *Gonggong weisheng*, 237.

96. SMA U1-16-319.

97. Wang Shu-hwai, "Dispute over the Ownership," 171–72.

98. A letter from chief health inspector, dated July 13, 1927 (filed in SMA U1-16-319).

tanks, and pipes in 1930.[99] Consequently, the water supply in the Chinese sector increased considerably during the Nanjing decade. In 1937, Zhabei WEC and Neidi WC together produced some 165,000 cubic meters of water each day for the Chinese sector.[100]

The PUB was mostly concerned with the management of the water-works companies and the quantity of the water supply; the Public Health Bureau (PHB) oversaw the quality of the tap water. In September 1927, the PHB consulted the PUB, and the two bureaus jointly drew up the inspection standards for tap water. The PHB notified the waterworks companies of these standards and instructed them to set up laboratories. The companies were required to inspect the quality of water every day and report the inspection results to the PHB and the PUB. Moreover, the PHB took water samples from each company every week and carried out chemical and bacteriological examinations at the Municipal Laboratory. As a result, the overall quality of tap water in Shanghai during the Republican period proved to be suitable for drinking.[101]

It is difficult to estimate the diffusion rate of tap water in the city. The authors of *General History of Shanghai* (*Shanghai tongshi*) note that some 4,160,000 to 4,400,000 residents were using tap water at the end of the 1940s;[102] in contrast, a sociologist estimated that, as of 1936, only 15 percent of households within the business districts of the waterworks companies used tap water.[103] In his 1934 report, Li Ting'an also remarked that "a fairly large percentage of the population" still depended on wells and ponds for drinking water.[104] On the whole, in spite of the increased water supply, it is possible to conclude that many people still had no access

99.   Hu Hongji, "Shanghai Shi wunianlai zhi weisheng xingzheng huigu," 5; Henriot, *Shanghai, 1927–1937*, 73–74; *SSGY*, chap. 9, 5.

100.   Xiong Yuezhi, ed., *Shanghai tongshi*, vol. 8, *Minguo jingji*, 212; Xiong Yuezhi, ed., *Shanghai tongshi*, vol. 9, *Minguo shehui*, 3.

101.   Hu Hongji, "Shanghai Shi wunianlai zhi weisheng xingzheng huigu," 5–6; Li Ting'an, "Shanghai Shi zhi gonggong weisheng xingzheng," 22; Ting-an Li, "Activities of the Bureau of Public Health," 991; *SSGY*, chap. 6, 1; *SSGY*, chap. 7, 5; Ting-an Li, "Report on the Bureau of Public Health," 11.

102.   Xiong Yuezhi, ed., *Shanghai tongshi*, vol. 8, *Minguo jingji*, 213; Xiong Yuezhi, ed., *Shanghai tongshi*, vol. 9, *Minguo shehui*, 4.

103.   P. Y. Jen, "Survey of the Water Supply Companies," 284.

104.   Ting-an Li, "Report on the Bureau of Public Health," 13; Ting-an Li, "Activities of the Bureau of Public Health," 991.

to tap water. Sometimes people dug artesian wells for drinking water. To secure the safety of well water, the PHB and the PUB revised the inspection standards for tap water and drew up new regulations outlining the hygienic standards for drinking water, which would apply not only to the tap water but also to well water.[105] When a new well was drilled, the well's owner was required to submit a sample of the water to the PHB.[106]

Other residents—notably shantytown dwellers—were not able to afford tap water. To provide safe water to the city's poor, the PHB urged waterworks companies to open fire hydrants so that the poor would have access to cheap or even free water. Li Ting'an reported, in 1934, that "nine water stations from which people can get any amount of city water free of charge have been recently installed in the slum districts,"[107] and by 1935, "fifteen free water supply stations have been built . . . in different parts of the city."[108] The PHB also periodically disinfected wells, ponds, and rivers with chemicals. According to Li, 22,000 pounds of disinfectant powder were used for this purpose in 1934, and in 1935, 150,000 pounds were used.[109]

The PHB also supervised the food supply; the inspection of meat was a particular concern. According to Hu Hongji, foreign veterinarians conducted only nominal meat inspection before 1927. When the municipal PHB was opened, the meat trade and livestock inspection in the Chinese sector were completely under Chinese control. In 1927, the PHB inaugurated pre- and post-slaughter inspection of hogs; in 1929, it extended this to include cattle and sheep. The PHB also conducted the pre-slaughter inspection of cattle whose meat would be sold in the foreign concessions. As of 1934, the bureau hired twenty-one veterinarians. When sick animals were discovered, they were not permitted to be sold as food. Instead, they were sent to oil factories to be rendered for industrial use. Anyone who sold meat of inferior quality was penalized. According to Hu and Li,

105. Hu Hongji, "Shanghai Shi wunianlai zhi weisheng xingzheng huigu," 6.
106. "Public Health Laboratory," 865.
107. Ting-an Li, "Report on the Bureau of Public Health," 13.
108. Ting-an Li, "Activities of the Bureau of Public Health," 991.
109. Ting-an Li, "Report on the Bureau of Public Health," 13; Ting-an Li, "Activities of the Bureau of Public Health," 991; *SSGY,* chap. 6, 1; Li Ting'an, "Shanghai Shi zhi gonggong weisheng xingzheng," 22.

some cattle traders at first complained of these arrangements, but their complaints gradually subsided. From the first inspection to 1932, the PHB examined altogether 3,819,898 hogs, 258,204 sheep, and 304,249 cattle. Of these, the PHB identified 21,054 hogs, 364 cattle, and 208 sheep as sick and unsuitable for human consumption.[110]

In addition to supervising abattoirs and meat sales, the PHB set up a registration system to monitor food-related businesses including restaurants, food shops, meat shops, and milk bars. All were required to register with the PHB, and the PHB often sent inspectors to examine the sanitary condition of the shops. When staff was inadequate, the PHB relied on the police to inspect the shops. If certain kinds of food were suspected of being unsanitary, their samples were immediately sent to the Municipal Laboratory for testing. The number of registered shops increased each year. Only 1,200 food shops were registered in 1927, but the number grew to 4,079 in 1928, 8,387 in 1930, and 10,010 in 1932. Likewise, 355 meat shops were registered in 1929, and 831 in 1932.[111]

Setting up regulations and testing the quality of water and meat certainly benefited many Shanghai residents, and supervising food-related businesses helped improve the general sanitation quality of the food sold in the city. By controlling the water and food supply, the Shanghai PHB reduced the likelihood of gastrointestinal disorders among the population. The PHB also monitored and inspected various local businesses, ranging from waterworks companies to the livestock trade and petty food shops. The bureau set hygienic standards, based on modern chemistry and bacteriology, that these businesses were required to follow. It also imposed penalties on those who violated regulations. Having a checklist for water quality, sprinkling chemical disinfectant on rivers, requiring food shops to register, and certifying inspected meat with official stamps were all markers and vehicles of hygienic modernity. The PHB served as a provider of necessary services while also functioning as a supervisor.

110. Hu Hongji, "Shanghai Shi wunianlai zhi weisheng xingzheng huigu," 6–7; Ting-an Li, "Report on the Bureau of Public Health," 13; Li Ting'an, "Shanghai Shi zhi gonggong weisheng xingzheng," 23; Ting-an Li, "Activities of the Bureau of Public Health," 991; *SSGY,* chap. 7, 12–13; Shanghai Shi weishengju, *Brief Survey,* 48.

111. *SSGY,* chap. 7, 10-11; Li Ting'an, "Shanghai shi zhi gonggong weisheng xingzheng," 22; Ting-an Li, "Report on the Bureau of Public Health," 13; Ting-an Li, "Activities of the Bureau of Public Health," 991.

Importantly, PHB-certified "safe food" was also a manifestation of Chinese competence and a source of national pride. Several disputes over food sales that took place between the Chinese PHB and the health authorities in the International Settlement illustrate this point. In the winter of 1927, Hu Hongji raised the issue of reciprocal licensing of bakeries and confectioneries in the Settlement and the Chinese sector. After visiting licensed bakeries in the Chinese sector, however, Settlement inspectors determined that the sanitation of the Chinese premises did not meet their standards, and they postponed the reciprocal licensing. The Chinese registered a complaint, and negotiations were stalemated. Meanwhile, problems cropped up regarding pork sales. In 1928, the SMC started a new pork inspection system. According to the SMC, health authorities in the Settlement had provided the Chinese PHB with required information about inspection measures, and Hu Hongji also had agreed that the pork from the Settlement could be sold in the Chinese sector. However, when traders in the Settlement were about to transport their meat, all pork stamped by the Settlement was prohibited from entering the Chinese sector. Health authorities in the Settlement regarded this action as retaliation for the postponement of the reciprocal licensing. In 1929, another conflict broke out between Chinese and British authorities. The SMC and the Chinese Public Works Bureau (Gongwuju) agreed that the SMC could use a site on the Huangpu River for the disposal of residential waste from the Settlement. Hu Hongji opposed this project from a sanitation point of view. The SMC regarded Hu as "rude," "deceptive," and "hostile," and claimed that he and the Chinese PHB had sacrificed "the public health and welfare to the attainment of political ends."[112] On the other hand, Hu Hongji believed that "'sanitation' and 'safeguarding Public Health' constitute[d] an important excuse on the part of Imperialistic nations for encroachment on China."[113] From his perspective, when the SMC blocked the licensing of Chinese bakeries, it was a violation of Chinese jurisdiction. As a representative of the Chinese state, the highest public health officer of Chinese Shanghai, and champion of modern science, Hu Hongji believed that he was entitled to protest sales of pork that had not passed pre-slaughter inspection; he also

112. SMA U1-16-289, 37.
113. SMA U1-16-292, 4.

asserted that improper and unsanitary disposition of refuse violated Chinese health and welfare and, by extension, Chinese sovereignty.[114]

These stories about water and food also point to the complex relations between the Chinese and Settlement authorities and illuminate local experiences of semi-colonialism. Chinese elites were deeply sensitive to the colonial nature of the British public health. The British promoted public health programs in the Settlement not for the good of the Chinese, but for the benefit of themselves and their economic viability: to experience hygiene was to experience colonialism and racism. However, because the majority of the residents in the Settlement were Chinese, it was impractical and impossible to strictly segregate colonialists from local Chinese. Moreover, British colonialists did not monopolize the command of biomedical knowledge and practices. Such knowledge exerted influence on Chinese elites, and they knew that public health could serve as grounds for criticism and resistance to the British presence in the city. Protecting Chinese lives, inspecting bakeries and meat, and claiming Chinese sovereignty were all closely related.

PREVENTING COMMUNICABLE DISEASES

Although the overall standard of living and sanitary conditions in Shanghai were better than those of the countryside, several serious communicable diseases—including cholera, smallpox, typhoid, diphtheria, and meningitis—were still common in Shanghai. Communicable diseases in Shanghai generated fear and anxiety among medical workers and public health administrators for several reasons. Shanghai had evolved into a commercial and industrial center—an outbreak of a disease there could easily and quickly be transmitted to other domestic and international locations. Shanghai could, in effect, become a distribution center for the disease. Shanghai was also an international port with two foreign concessions; prevalence of an epidemic in the city easily attracted the attention of foreigners and thus could damage China's international reputation. Of various communicable diseases, cholera and smallpox were the two most significant targets of the public health administration. Hu Hongji noted

114. On the conflicts between the Chinese PHB and the Public Health Department of the Settlement, see SMA U1-16-290; SMA U1-16-318; SMA U1-16-319.

that cholera and smallpox had caused the greatest harm to Shanghai residents, and that bringing these two diseases under control was a top priority of the municipal government.[115] Cholera and smallpox in Shanghai were also a concern of the central government. The Ministry of Public Health identified them as major epidemics in Shanghai.[116]

To prevent the outbreak and spread of these two diseases, the PHB implemented citywide free vaccination programs. The bureau designated May through September as the cholera prevention period; during these months, the bureau conducted educational programs to teach residents about the benefits of vaccination and offered general information about the prevention and treatment of cholera. Similarly, the PHB designated October through April as the smallpox prevention period; during these months, the PHB provided free vaccinations against smallpox.[117]

These two vaccination programs had different medical outcomes. It was widely recognized by the early twentieth century that vaccination was effective in preventing smallpox, and there was little opposition to smallpox vaccination among Shanghai residents. The number of vaccinations that the PHB gave increased each year: from 67,131 in 1927–28 to 246,013 in 1933–34. By contrast, the clinical efficacy of the cholera vaccination was unproved. Hu Hongji himself admitted that the cholera vaccination could only strengthen people's resistance to the disease—it did not prevent cholera outright. Since cholera was a waterborne disease, controlling the quality of drinking water and food was more efficacious than vaccination.[118] In spite of its uncertain efficacy, cholera vaccination was the only medical strategy taken to prevent cholera outbreaks, and the PHB organized extensive injection drives on various occasions. In the spring and summer, the PHB set up simple injection booths on the street, and staff called out to passers-by imploring them to get a vaccination. Street injections became a common feature of Shanghai life. They were thoroughly carried out during citywide hygiene campaigns. The bureau also sent injection teams (*zhushedui*) to schools, factories, and prisons, so that a

115. Hu Hongji, "Shanghai Shi wunianlai zhi weisheng xingzheng huigu," 10.
116. *Fagui* (1930).
117. *SSGY,* chap. 7, 4–5; Ting-an Li, "Activities of the Bureau of Public Health," 992; Hu Hongji, "Shanghai Shi wunianlai zhi weisheng xingzheng huigu," 10–11; Li Ting'an, "Shanghai Shi zhi gonggong weisheng xingzheng," 22–23.
118. Hu Hongji, "Shanghai Shi wunianlai zhi weisheng xingzheng huigu," 10.

sizable number of people could be vaccinated at once. The PHB even mobilized the police force to ensure that shantytown residents received vaccinations.[119] Whereas only 48,906 cholera vaccinations were administered in 1927–28, the number increased to 280,941 in 1929–30; 562,479 in 1931–32; and 710,692 in 1932–33.[120]

The PHB carried out citywide cholera vaccination drives not only for medical purposes but also to prove the strength and effectiveness of its public service. These drives provided an opportunity for Chinese administrators to demonstrate their administrative capability to foreigners. Injection booths, with their syringes, cotton balls, vaccines, and doctors and nurses in white coats embodied modern biomedicine and administrative authority. These were the tangible means by which the Republican municipal government protected its citizens and the city from the devastation of disease. After 1937, the anti-cholera injection drive was taken over by the wartime public health administration.

THE CHOLERA OUTBREAK OF 1932

In spite of these measures, periodic outbreaks of cholera continued from the 1920s through the 1940s. The prevalence of outbreaks of cholera is confirmed by several sources. The *China Weekly Review* and *Chinese Medical Journal* (*CMJ*) frequently carried articles and reports on cholera cases in Shanghai; Wu Lien-teh provides a chronological record of cholera outbreaks in the city in the 1920s to the 1930s to substantiate his claim that "Shanghai occupies a predominant position in cholera history."[121] The Ministry of Public Health pointed out that in 1930, fifteen cholera outbreaks had taken place in the city over the last twenty-five years.[122] The cyclical appearance of cholera in Shanghai generated much concern among medical workers.

In particular, in the summer of 1932, a severe and extensive cholera outbreak—the worst in the prewar period—swept China. The cholera outbreak of this year hit at least 21 provinces and 303 large cities, including

119.   Henriot, *Shanghai, 1927–1937*, 206.
120.   Shanghai Shi weishengju, *Brief Survey*, 50; *SSGY*, chap. 7, 5.
121.   Wu Lien-teh et al., *Cholera*, 33–34.
122.   *Fagui* (1930).

Shanghai. Some one hundred thousand people became sick, and nearly thirty-four thousand died. In Shanghai, the first case was confirmed on April 26. Thereafter, the number of daily cases steadily increased until August 21, when the maximum of sixty cases was recorded. As the weather became cooler, the epidemic declined and eventually disappeared altogether on October 22.[123]

Unfortunately for Shanghai, the city suffered from two other disasters in 1931–32: a great flood and the attack of the Japanese. The flooding of the Yangzi River in 1931 was one of the most severe in modern times. It struck Hunan, Hubei, Anhui, and parts of Jiangsu. Ping-ti Ho estimates that more than twelve million people were affected.[124] Though an accurate figure is unavailable, the flood brought a large refugee population to Shanghai. The Japanese attack on Shanghai in January 1932 destroyed part of the city. The war dragged on until March, and the Japanese army did not withdraw until May. The city administration fell into disorder, and the financial situation of the municipal government became desperate. Japanese bombing had destroyed many of the city's medical facilities and institutions.[125]

In spite of these unfavorable conditions, records show that, compared with other cities, Shanghai weathered the cholera epidemic of 1932 well, with a relatively low mortality rate. Even though the number of patients was large, the number of cholera deaths was small and symptoms were mild. Table 2.1 shows figures from *The China Yearbook* of 1933.

An article written in 1932 in *CMJ* also commented that "the unusually low death rate of [sic] Shanghai even among an enormous poor population is in striking contrast with that in other cities."[126] Another article from *CMJ* also noted that the overall death rate among Chinese in Shanghai was even lower than that among the Westerners. Generally, this low mortality rate was attributed to the vaccination of city residents and the early hospitalization of patients.[127]

In spite of the social and political chaos, and its limited budget for public health services, Shanghai succeeded in minimizing the damage

123. *China Year Book* 1933, 173; "Cholera in 1932," 1207.
124. Ping-ti Ho, *Studies on the Population of China*, 233–34.
125. "Medical Aftermath."
126. "Cholera in 1932," 1208.
127. "Hygiene and Public Health," 932.

Table 2.1
The Cholera Outbreak of 1932

Locality	Estimated Population	Total Cases	Total Deaths	Mortality Percentage
Shanghai	3,124,212	4,291	318	7.4
Nanjing	619,745	1,555	388	24.82
Hangzhou	529,862	551	56	10.16
Xiamen	164,087	1,614	746	46.22
Guangzhou	812,241	1,093	386	35.31
Shantou	161,087	541	80	14.78
Hankou	777,993	777	125	16.09
Qingdao	367,410	165	30	18.19
Qifu	130,575	503	216	42.94
Tianjin	1,388,747	100	16	16.00

Source: China Year Book 1933, 173

caused by cholera in 1932. The city went on to celebrate a "cholera-free year" in 1933. Whereas other gastrointestinal diseases—typhoid and dysentery in particular—were still common in the city, few cases of cholera occurred in the city from 1934 to 1936.

Although imperfect, Shanghai's municipal PHB made notable progress with respect to urban sanitation. This was not generally the case in other Chinese municipalities. Students of Peking Union Medical College conducted nationwide surveys of the urban public health conditions between 1924 and 1931 for nineteen cities with over one hundred thousand residents. For reasons unknown, Shanghai was not included in this survey. After reviewing the results of the surveys, John Grant and T. M. P'eng of PUMC concluded that the public health administration in urban areas in China was still very rudimentary. Above all, they emphasized the serious lack of medical experts. In fifteen out of the nineteen cities surveyed, the public health administration was run by the police, and most of their workers were garbage collectors and police inspectors. Instead of providing appropriate medical services based on science, street cleaning was still the main business of most public health administrations. None of the cities surveyed performed bacteriological inspections of water and food; education of the general populace about health and sanitation was minimal at best. None of the municipalities had set up specific regulations for notification and isolation of communicable disease patients. Only four cities—Shaoxing, Nanjing, Suzhou, and Changzhou—distributed free vaccination for both cholera and smallpox. Grant and P'eng concluded that "the problem of public health in China is more a question of competent personnel than of finance."[128]

The history of the Shanghai Public Health Bureau (PHB) reflects the complex and synergic relations between the state and society as well as between medicine and power. On the one hand, local elites and private institutions were actively involved in health-related works through medical and social services. The PHB approved of these nongovernmental initiatives, and saw them as a major force for taking care of the sick and dead. On the other hand, the PHB was a state organization, and administrators endeavored to manage and monitor personal sanitation and private businesses on a constant basis. They were well aware that public health was a vehicle for the expression of power. Chinese elites and administrators were advocates and champions of Chinese sovereignty and assumed the responsibility for protecting Chinese people. To achieve their goals, they supervised and controlled people's lives. The level of such intervention and regulation significantly intensified under the Japanese occupation.

Shanghai Public Health Bureau during the War

The breakout of the war in 1937 brought the development of the PHB to a halt. The Marco Polo Bridge Incident on July 7, 1937, led to an all-out war against Japan; from 1937 to 1945, Shanghai was under Japanese military occupation. Wartime memories of the people are full of hardship, misery, suffering, and terror. The battle of 1937 destroyed the city and devastated the populace. Human and economic losses were enormous. In occupied Shanghai, terrorist attacks and political corruption were

128.   Grant and P'eng, "Survey of Urban Public Health," 1079.

rampant; soaring commodity prices created further challenges.[129] Sanitation in the city deteriorated considerably during the war years, resulting in several cholera outbreaks. However, to protect the city and its residents from the threat of cholera, Chinese public health administrators and the Japanese occupation forces worked together and took various measures to control the cholera epidemic.

THE REOPENING OF THE CHINESE
PUBLIC HEALTH BUREAU

The prewar municipal PHB ceased functioning in November 1937. The public health department of the two foreign concessions continued to operate until 1941, but the Chinese sector did not have a unified public health administration for forty months. During this interregnum, the police and the Great Way (dadao) Government, one of the early puppet governments of the city, each created public health sections (*weishengke*), but the removal of debris, refuse, and corpses was their main focus.[130] Epidemic prevention was a serious concern among the occupation forces, but they were simply too busy looking for appropriate personnel to organize a strong puppet government. Finally, in February of 1941, Chen Gongbo (1892–1946) stepped in as mayor; Chen launched a reorganization of the city government and ordered Yuan Jufan to open a preparation office (*choubeiju*) for a public health bureau. After two months of preparation, Yuan reopened a municipal PHB on March 26, 1941, and assumed the position of acting commissioner.[131] Yuan, a native of Anhui and hitherto an obscure man, had graduated from the Nanyang Medical School and Forensic Medicine Institute. Prior to this appointment, he held positions in several medical schools and hospitals, including a midwifery school.[132]

Under Yuan's commissionership, the PHB took on the necessary personnel to resume its business. The staff of the temporary health sections

129.   Wakeman, *Shanghai Badlands;* Poshek Fu, *Passivity, Resistance, and Collaboration*, 120–29.

130.   SMA R1-12-15; Shanghai tebieshi weishengju, *Yewu baogao*, 1, 16.

131.   Xiong Yuezhi, ed., *Shanghai tongshi*, vol. 7, *Minguo zhengzhi*, 370; *SWZ* 35; Shanghai tebieshi weishengju, *Yewu baogao*, 1.

132.   Yuan Jufan's resume is listed on SMA R50-1151, 8.

who were still in the city were transferred to the wartime PHB and reappointed.[133] In addition, the wartime PHB also recruited youths, ages eighteen to twenty-five, with a minimum of a junior high school education, to be its lower-level staff. These youths were first enrolled in free training courses; after two months of general public health administration training and the successful completion of exams, they went to work for the PHB and associated institutes.[134] Finally, an officer of the Special Agency Organization (Tokumu kikan) of the Japanese military was appointed as a liaison to the PHB.[135]

At least nominally, the wartime PHB was designed to comprehensively cover various public health activities across the city. As of 1942, it consisted of four sections (*ke*) with thirteen divisions. The PHB also had four administrative offices (*shi*): the Secretarial Office (Mishushi), the Technical Staff Office (Jizhengshi), the Clerical Staff Office (Zhuanyuanshi), and the Accounting Office (Kuaijishi). In the same year, the PHB had altogether 105 staff members—a figure similar to that of 1931–32 (107). In addition, the Nanshi Health Station (Nanshi weisheng shiwusuo), the Huxi Public Health Office (Huxi weisheng banshichu), and municipal hospitals and clinics all fell under the PHB's jurisdiction.[136] At least on paper, the wartime PHB had an organizational structure similar to that of the prewar PHB.[137]

Although the wartime PHB was able to expand its jurisdiction to the suburbs, in fact it commanded fewer resources. Some of the key facilities had been destroyed in the fighting or converted for the use of the Japanese military. Most importantly, both the prewar Municipal Laboratory and the Municipal Communicable Disease Hospital were turned into Japanese military hospitals. Because the Municipal Laboratory never reopened during the war, the wartime PHB was forced to depend on laboratories in the International Settlement and on the Dōjinkai, a Japanese medical organization, to carry out necessary chemical and bacteriological

133. SMA R1-12-15, R1-12-105, R50-1151, R50-1142, and R50-1254 all provide information on the transferred personnel, documents, and office fixtures.

134. On the selection of the youths and these training courses, see SMA R50-872 and SMA R50-1183.

135. *SWZ*, 545.

136. Shanghai tebieshi weishengju, *Yewu baogao*, 1–4; SMA R1-12-11.

137. *SWZ*, 545.

tests and manufacturing. With limited resources and finances, the wartime PHB focused on cholera-control work and citywide hygiene campaigns.

CHOLERA PREVALENCE IN SHANGHAI

The Japanese occupation forces and the wartime PHB could not afford to spend either time or resources on reconstructing the city's infrastructure, but they gave considerable attention to *fangyi* or *bōeki*—the control of communicable diseases—and cholera continued to be one of the main targets. The PHB archives created during the Japanese occupation period are full of records and documents associated with their cholera-control work. Similar to prewar administrators, wartime PHB and the Japanese occupation forces invested time and effort into vaccination programs in the city, and they left very detailed reports on the implementation of the vaccination drives. In carrying out mass vaccinations and other cholera-control work, Chinese administrators often took advantage of the Japanese presence. By using Japanese materials and relying on the assistance of the Japanese military, physical coercion brought to bear by the occupation forces was channeled into protecting the health of residents and saving the city from the disease.[138]

In the 1920s, cholera had been a great concern and outbreaks occurred frequently; by the early 1930s, morbidity and mortality rates from cholera in Shanghai were on the wane. After the cholera year of 1932, Shanghai had been spared from serious cholera attacks, but during the war, cholera returned to the city. Cholera outbreaks, to a greater or lesser degree, took place every year between 1937 and 1942. Available sources give the following accounts: In 1937, cholera broke out in Nanshi and the French Concession in August, and then spread to the International Settlement. Some 2,500 true cholera cases and some 2,000 suspected cases had been

138.　Reliance on mass vaccination was not unique to Republican Shanghai. Ruth Rogaski has noted the importance of epidemic control and injections in Japanese public health policies in Manchuria. Citing Iijima Wataru's study, she writes that "vaccination was the primary manifestation of *eisei* activity. The hypodermic needle was the medium that represented *eisei* in the common experience of Chinese in Manchuria." See Rogaski, "Vampires in Plagueland," 148–49.

identified across the city by the end of September.[139] With the influx of refugees, 1938 had the highest number of cholera patients during the war. The earliest patient was identified on May 20, and the disease soon raged throughout the city.[140] During the summer, 11,365 cholera cases occurred, and 2,246 individuals died.[141] In 1939, the first case appeared on June 7, and although the mortality rate was low, 455 cholera cases had been identified by the end of the season.[142] In 1940, the earliest cholera patients were identified in May among immigrants from Shaoxing; altogether there were 573 patients and 99 died.[143] In 1941, the total number of patients reached 834 by November, and 115 individuals died.[144] In 1942, the earliest cholera patients were found in July in Nanshi; by the end of October, the total number of cases had reached 2,986 with 560 fatalities.[145] Considering that not all cases were reported, the actual number of patients in these years was likely much higher. To fight cholera outbreaks, the Chinese and Japanese worked closely together.

DEVELOPMENT OF THE EPIDEMIC PREVENTION
COMMITTEE: COLLABORATION IN
CHOLERA-CONTROL WORK

During the war, the Epidemic Prevention Committee (Chinese, Fangyi weiyuanhui, Japanese, Bōeki iinkai) (EPC) took a leading role in anti-cholera work in Shanghai. At first, the EPC was a provisional organization created by and for the Japanese in 1938, and was engaged in mass injections and inspection and disinfection of food shops in the Japanese residential area. But this committee developed into a permanent organization that involved both Chinese and Japanese personnel after 1941. Eventually the Chinese Public Health Bureau and the EPC teamed up, shared

139. Dispatch from the Shanghai Consulate General to the Ministry of Foreign Affairs (DSCG), no. 2361 (November 28, 1937). This document is filed in *Gaimushō kiroku* (GK) H-4-1-0-18.
140. *Shūhō* 26, 27, 29, 31 (1938).
141. *SWZ*, 34.
142. "Kimitsu 1109"; *Shūhō* 41 (1939).
143. "Shōwa jūgo nendo Shanghai ni okeru korera ryūkō ni tuite."
144. "Chūshi ni okeru korera ryūko jyōkyō ni kansuru ken."
145. Shanghai tebieshi weishengju, *Yewu baogao*, 9–10.

information and resources, and jointly conducted cholera-control works. The history of this committee highlights a case of wartime collaboration between the Chinese and Japanese.[146]

On March 31, 1941, only four days after the inauguration of the wartime PHB, the EPC called for a meeting at the Cultural Bureau of the Asia Development Board (Kōain bunkakyoku) and summoned Yuan Jufan, the commissioner of public health, and Wu Yaodong, a PHB officer, to discuss cholera-control programs with Japanese.[147] At this meeting, the EPC set out a plan for cholera vaccination drives and divided up the tasks between Chinese and Japanese. According to the meeting resolution, the vaccination drives would be carried out from April 7 to 27; the Japanese would be in charge of Hongkou (the Japanese residential area); the navy, the Dōjinkai, and the Chinese PHB would jointly take charge of Nanshi; and the Chinese PHB would be in charge of all other occupied areas in the city.[148]

On April 5, the PHB convened a meeting, inviting delegates from municipal hospitals and clinics. Yuan and Wu delivered EPC directions to participants regarding how to organize the scheduled vaccination drives. It was decided at the meeting that staff from the municipal hospitals and clinics would organize injection teams and also that these teams would be stationed at traffic points throughout the city. The president of each hospital was assigned to secure an adequate number of injection certificates (*zhushe zhengshu*). If someone counterfeited certificates or issued one to someone who had not been vaccinated, both parties would be punished in accordance with Japanese military law. Technical matters, such as the amount of vaccine, alcohol, and cotton to be used and the proper part of the arm to be injected, as well as the proper way to sterilize uten-

146. On the EPC in Shanghai, see Fukushi, "Nicchu sensōki Shanghai ni okeru kōshū eisei to shakai kanri." Also see *Shūhō* 23.

147. The Asia Development Board was established in 1938 to manage and coordinate Japanese activities in occupied China except for diplomatic affairs. It was placed under the Cabinet and had three bureaus: Political Affairs, Culture, and Economy. It was abolished in 1942 when the Japanese government created the Greater East Asia Ministry. See Kubo, "Kōa-in."

148. SMA R1-12-343.

sils, were also discussed at the meeting.[149] Yuan Jufan attended the next EPC meeting in May. At this meeting, after making a report on the injection drive in April, he stated that the municipal PHB did not have enough financial and human resources to carry out future cholera-control work and requested subsequent assistance from the Japanese military.[150]

In administering injections, Chinese public health workers relied on the Japanese for necessary materials. Since the PHB did not have a facility for manufacturing vaccines, the Dōjinkai supplied the necessary doses.[151] The PHB also used injection certificates printed by the EPC. These were stamped with the seals of the PHB and of the doctor who gave the vaccinations. The EPC already had a large stock of certificates, which allowed the PHB to save on printing costs. By sharing the same form, the EPC and the PHB also avoided confusion and forgery. Moreover, these certificates were written partly in Japanese, making it convenient for the Japanese military personnel who inspected them. Chinese public health officers received three hundred thousand doses of vaccine and three hundred thousand certificates through the Asia Development Board and distributed them to medical institutes around the city.[152]

The EPC not only directed vaccination drives but also oversaw the citywide physical examination and inspection of injection certificates. According to an EPC directive, medical personnel from the municipal government and the Japanese Residents Association were assigned to pay home visits in the occupied area to conduct physical examinations. Contingents of the Japanese navy and the garrison headquarters, stationed at important traffic spots, stopped passers-by at random to verify that they had valid certificates. The Chinese PHB, the navy, the army, the West Shanghai Area Special Police Force, and the garrison headquarters of the military police were all mobilized to check the physical conditions of refugees.[153] As a result of these measures, from April through October 1941,

149. These meeting minutes are filed in SMA R1-12-133.
150. The minutes of the EPC meeting on May 20, 1941 (filed in SMA R50-299); "Shanghai tebieshi weishengju gaikuang."
151. Shanghai tebieshi weishengju, *Yewu baogao*, 9.
152. "Minguo sanshi niandu liuyuefen gongzuo baogao"; *Shūhō* 13 (1941).
153. The minutes of the EPC meeting on July 21, 1941, and the minutes of the EPC cadre meeting on July 25, 1941 (filed in SMA R1-12-133 and R50-299).

the PHB administered 1,284,309 vaccinations. Including the number of the vaccinations administered by the navy, the army, and the authorities of the two foreign concessions, the PHB estimated that 4,300,000 vaccinations were given overall.[154] Although these vaccinations included booster shots, clearly a considerable portion of the population in the city received vaccinations in 1941.

By 1942, the EPC had developed into an umbrella organization that supervised virtually all aspects of cholera-control work in Shanghai. According to "Shanghai EPC Regulations" (Shanghai fangyi weiyuanhui guicheng), drafted in August 1942, the EPC was composed of delegates from the army, the navy, the Asia Development Board Central China Liaison Office (Kōain kachū renrakubu), the Japanese Consulate General, the Dōjinkai, the Japanese Residents Association, the Shanghai municipal government, the SMC, the FMC, Customs, the Japanese Doctors Association, and the Central China Railway Company. The same "Regulations" stipulate that the head office of the EPC should be located at the Cultural Bureau of the Asia Development Board Central China Liaison Office.[155] The EPC was a Japanese-sponsored civic organization, but it came to involve military and medical personnel as well as other civilians, which included not only Japanese and Chinese but also delegates from the foreign concessions.

"The Regulations on the Enforcement of Cholera Prevention" (Huoluan fangyi shishi guicheng), drawn up in July of 1942, describe the EPC's work. The tasks assigned to the EPC can be summarized in three points: First, the EPC was a liaison center, responsible for data collection and public relations. It organized the anti-cholera education programs directed at the general populace. It also gathered disease statistics and made official announcements of the numbers of patients through newspapers and radio broadcasting. It circulated information among medical practitioners and public health administrators inside and outside Shanghai. Second, the EPC was in charge of performing cholera vaccination drives and issuing certificates. Some of the drives targeted passers-by in general, and some targeted specific groups of people, including those who

---

154.   Shanghai tebieshi weishengju, *Yewu baogao*, 12; the minutes of the EPC meeting on August 12, 1941 (filed in SMA R1-12-133).

155.   "Shanghai bōeki iinkai kitei."

lived on boats and in "cholera problem areas." When actually giving vaccinations, the EPC could be assisted by the Chinese and Japanese police forces. The EPC was also charged with the inspection of certificates. All Shanghai people were subject to random inspection; anyone could be stopped on the street, and those found to lack the proper certificate might be prohibited from purchasing a train ticket or receiving rice coupons. Third, when cholera patients were discovered, the EPC supervised their medical treatment and the sterilization of their neighborhoods. Cholera patients were sent to a designated isolation hospital in the city. Depending where patients were found, staff from the Japanese Residents Association, the SMC, the FMC, or the Chinese municipal government were responsible for drawing a sanitary cordon around the area and taking any necessary medical measures. In cases of death, each of these organizations monitored the disposal of corpses. Since the wartime PHB did not have a laboratory, the Dōjinkai, the SMC, and the FMC were responsible for bacteriological tests, and the navy and army also lent support.[156]

According to these accounts and EPC meeting minutes, the EPC functioned as if it were a governmental organization. In 1943, on the grounds that the Chinese Public Health Bureau had now obtained adequate personnel and resources, the PHB took over the EPC. As the Shanghai mayor and the commissioner of public health were appointed to be the chief committee member (*zhuren weiyuan*) and the vice-chief committee member (*fu-zhuren weiyuan*), the EPC became a Chinese organization. The EPC continued its routine work until 1945.

THE CHOLERA-CONTROL PROGRAM AND
THE NANSHI NEIGHBORHOOD

The cholera-control programs during the war were not drastically different from those of the prewar period. However, Chinese health workers and the occupiers commanded better enforcement capabilities in wartime. In carrying out epidemic control programs, they could penetrate into neighborhoods and intrude on the daily lives of residents. The cholera outbreak in 1942 in Nanshi was a case in point.

156. "Korera bōeki jisshi kitei."

In spite of the city's extensive vaccination drives, a cholera outbreak did take place in 1942, which turned out to be one of the severe "cholera years" during the war. On July 1, eight residents in Nanshi became ill and were admitted to a neighborhood hospital. On July 6, cholera bacilli were detected in these patients.[157] On July 7, the Nanshi Health Station received a report from the hospital and determined that these patients were all native residents of Huininglu and Jiandaoqiao Streets in Nanshi. The station notified the municipal PHB and asked for medical and clerical staff and necessary drugs and instruments for sterilization. The station also notified local police offices and the heads of the *baojia* mutual responsibility system in Nanshi about the cholera outbreak and instructed them to inform the station immediately of any cholera patients in their jurisdictions. Within a few days, policemen from local posts, military police from the Japanese Military Police Corp, and staff from the Epidemic Prevention Section of the Nobori Detachment of the Japanese army had collected stool samples from the local residents of the Huininglu and Jiandaoqiao area. Several cholera cases and carriers were identified, and they were sent to a hospital for isolation and treatment. Medical staff from the PHB examined the injection certificates of the local residents and gave vaccinations to those who did not have a certificate. Meanwhile a sterilization team disinfected residences in the neighborhood, and policemen drew a sanitary cordon around the area.[158] The cordon was not lifted until August 1942.[159]

In spite of all these measures, the disease spread beyond Nanshi. Cholera cases were also identified in Huxi and Wusong in July.[160] Through the summer and fall, cholera cases occurred throughout Shanghai. By the end of October, the total number of the patients reached 2,986.[161] Responding to the rampant cholera epidemic, the PHB designated several hospitals as isolation hospitals, to admit cholera patients only.[162] As some

157.   *Bōeki hō* 30; DSCG, no. 2061 (August 18, 1942). This document is filed in GK I-3-2-0-13, vol. 8.

158.   SMA R50-304; Shanghai tebieshi weishengju, *Yewu baogao*, 8–9.

159.   The minutes of the Nanshi Provisional Epidemic Prevention Committee Meeting on August 8, 1942 (filed in SMA R50-1203).

160.   SMA R50-305.

161.   Shanghai tebieshi weishengju, *Yewu baogao*, 9.

162.   Ibid., 4–8.

of the patients died, the PHB gave detailed instructions to caretakers and funeral homes in the city concerning the proper disposal of infected bodies.[163]

The cholera outbreak of 1942 originated in Nanshi, and 35 percent of all Shanghai cases occurred in that part of the city. Thus Nanshi became the target for control work. Since Nanshi was completely under the control of the Chinese government and occupation forces, the Japanese military readily participated in the work. On July 31, the Nanshi branch of the Japanese Military Police Corps issued an order to organize the Nanshi Provisional Epidemic Prevention Committee (PEPC) (*linshi fangyi weiyuanhui*). Following this order, the Nanshi PEPC was formally inaugurated on August 1.[164] This temporary organization carried out all cholera-control programs in Nanshi through the end of October.

The Nanshi PEPC embodied a combination of public health administrators, medical workers, policemen, and other local personnel in Nanshi, and it was backed by the Japanese military. Liu Zhenya, chief of the Nanshi Health Station, chaired the Nanshi PEPC, which consisted of three groups: the advisory board, the standing committee (*changwu weiyuan*), and general members (*weiyuan*). Of the seven board members, with the exception of one delegate from the Chinese police, all belonged to the Japanese military or police.[165] The standing committee consisted of six members. Of these six, two were presidents of local hospitals, three were chiefs of police stations in Nanshi, and the last was the chief of the Nanshi branch office of the Social Affairs Bureau. The standing committee was required to meet every week to make plans for all anti-cholera activities and to give instructions to general members. General members included chiefs of the Nanshi branch offices of municipal bureaus,

163. As a rule, cremation was preferred. When cremation was not feasible, the corpses could be buried. In these cases, strict rules applied. The interment location must not be close to any water source, the graves should be at least seven *chi* deep, and the inside and outside of the coffins should be filled with lime. SMA R50-1183.

164. The minutes of the Nanshi PEPC meeting on August 1, 1942 (filed in SMA R50-1203).

165. They were delegates from the Shanghai Fuji Detachment, the Nanshi branch office of the Shanghai Special Agency, the Nanshi branch of the Japanese Military Police, the Nanshi branch of the Consulate Police, the Nanshi Navy Garrison, the Nanshi Army Garrison, and a liaison officer from the Nanshi branch of the Chinese police.

presidents of local hospitals, district heads (*fangzhang*) of Nanshi, two delegates from the Central China Water and Electricity Company (CCWEC) (Huazhong shuidian gongsi), and a delegate from the Nanshi Health Station.[166] These general members and staff of the Nanshi Health Station were responsible for handling everyday duties, with the assistance of Japanese organizations and the Nanshi police.[167]

The Nanshi PEPC provides another example of wartime collaboration. Although local Chinese members were in charge of the actual work of the Nanshi PEPC, Japanese presence supported the management of this committee to a considerable degree. The municipal PHB was supposed to be responsible for administrative expenses, but the Japan Club actually paid these.[168] And, as mentioned above, with the Municipal Laboratory destroyed, the Dōjinkai stepped in to perform necessary bacteriological and chemical tests.[169]

The Nanshi PEPC set up and ran cholera-control programs, including administering vaccination drives, inspecting certificates, sterilizing public spaces, and gathering disease statistics in the Nanshi area. To carry these out, the Nanshi PEPC called on various nonmedical personnel, including not only the police and military forces but also local Nanshi leaders. In particular, the Nanshi PEPC incorporated neighborhood networks into its program by using the *baojia* system. The basic unit of this system was a household; ten households composed a *bao*, and ten *bao* composed a *jia*. The original purpose of this system was to register households and carry out mutual surveillance within the neighborhood. It had a long history, going back to ancient times, and even though it was not always effective, the *baojia* system survived until the 1940s and played an important role in cholera-control work in Nanshi. Working

166. When the Japanese military occupied Central China, the Japanese government and private investors jointly established Central China Development Company (Naka Shina shinkō gaisha) in 1938. CCWEC was a subsidiary of this company. It seized Chinese waterworks companies and took charge of water and electricity supply in Central China.

167. The minutes of the Nanshi PEPC meeting on August 1, 1942 (filed in SMA R50-1203).

168. The minutes of the Nanshi PEPC meeting on October 17, 1942 (filed SMA R50-1203).

169. SMA R50-1183.

from *baojia* units, health administrators divided the Nanshi area into five districts (*fang*), and each district had its own head (*fangzhang*). *Baojia* heads and district heads were assigned various tasks to help monitor and supervise local residents.

These nonmedical personnel assisted in the implementation of Nanshi's cholera-control work. When the Nanshi PEPC organized vaccination drives, injection teams were stationed in each of the five districts. Each district head was responsible for the smooth delivery of vaccinations in his district. When residents found a corpse in the street, they were instructed to contact the police through their *baojia* leader and to notify a local doctor. The police and staff of the health station inspected sales of fruits and vegetables and prohibited the dumping of trash and feces in the street. When a person who had died of cholera was to be interred, a district head followed PHB directives to determine how the interment was performed.[170] When there was a suspicious case of cholera in a district, local heads called the police and the Japanese military force. The police formed a security cordon; then, under military surveillance, medical personnel disinfected the neighborhood, gave injections to residents, and inspected their stool. That local residents experienced these measures as intrusive and troublesome would be unsurprising; tight cordons might have caused inconvenience, and disinfection may well have damaged personal property and belongings. The presence of the police and military could have been intimidating. Yet coercion and threats from the police and occupation forces as well as neighborhood networks facilitated the effective implementation of modern medical measures. All the measures taken were based on modern epidemiological knowledge and, in all likelihood, prevented the spread of the disease.

In addition to these tasks, the Nanshi PEPC was in charge of providing a safe water supply, and *baojia* heads were assigned to manage public water taps. Many Nanshi residents depended on a well or a river for their drinking water.[171] Yet the quality of the well or river water was questionable; after the outbreak of cholera, local wells that were suspect were closed. To provide safe drinking water to Nanshi residents, the

170. The minutes of the Nanshi PEPC meeting on August 8, 1942 (filed in SMA R50-1203).
171. Shanghai tebieshi weishengju, *Yewu baogao*, 28.

Nanshi Health Station and the Central China Water and Electric Company (CCWEC) agreed to open twenty-five water taps in Nanshi from August to October. The CCWEC was responsible for construction and repair of the water supply facilities, while the Nanshi Health Station was responsible for management of the facilities and meters. In light of the emergency, the CCWEC agreed to offer the water at a deep discount.[172]

Detailed rules were drawn up concerning the use of tap water. The company opened twenty-five taps throughout the five districts of Nanshi, from 8:00 a.m. to noon, and from 2:00 to 6:00 p.m. Only those who did not have a tap-water facility at home were eligible to purchase the cheap water. To purchase water, individuals had to present their household registration to the health station to be verified for the necessary amount of water. After these procedures, the health station issued a "water receipt certificate" (*lingshuizheng*). Individuals then brought their certificates to the designated tap to purchase and receive water in an orderly manner. The water was to be used only for drinking, and anyone who broke the rules was penalized. Local *baojia* heads were responsible for keeping the keys to the taps and for opening and closing them. They were also in charge of maintaining order around the taps and collecting payment. If local heads were found to be using the water for personal profit, they were penalized.[173]

Such detailed arrangements regarding the water supply reveal the connection between cholera-control work, everyday life, and the Nanshi local community. Safe drinking water is indispensable to human life, and access to tap water was a matter of life and death for Nanshi residents. By managing the drinking water supply, health administrators not only provided a necessary service for Nanshi residents but also controlled a crucial basic necessity. Protecting health, providing services, and controlling daily life were interrelated. Moreover, as agents of the Nanshi health administration, *baojia* heads and district heads linked the local community to the cholera-control programs. Throughout Chinese history, various

---

172.   SMA R1-12-341, 5–8. After 1942, the PHB negotiated with the CCWEC to offer the same kind of service. See *Gongzuo baogao* July 1944.

173.   Shanghai tebieshi weishengju, *Yewu baogao*, 28–29; SMA R1-12-341.

regimes found it difficult to control common people at the grassroots level. Mandatory house-to-house inspection and supervision of the drinking water supply in Nanshi in 1942 were among the few occasions when Shanghai residents directly felt the presence of the government in their local communities.[174]

Conclusion

Shanghai's administrators believed that having a sanitary environment and healthy people was a marker of civic order; acting on this understanding, they opened a public health bureau. In carrying out its tasks, the bureau was significantly assisted by local personnel and local institutions. At the same time, Chinese elites were always conscious of the foreign presence in the city. Shanghai's public health bureau emulated a British model, used British materials, and employed Western science and biomedicine as a basis to supervise and monitor urban life.

The connection of the Shanghai PHB to the British links this story to issues of colonialism. The corporeal nature of colonialism and the colonial nature of Western medicine are familiar themes in the history of medicine and disease in non-Western societies.[175] Shanghai's Chinese elites were well aware of the colonial nature of public health implementation and racial prejudice in the Settlement. At the same time, they believed in the benefits of Western medicine and hygiene and did not hesitate to request technical advice from experts in the Settlement. Even though the British opened the port of Shanghai with violence, the British had only limited capacity to transform the city and to scrutinize Chinese bodies. It was Chinese administrators—not British—who strove to enforce discipline and regulations to improve Chinese hygiene.

During the Japanese occupation, the coercive and disciplinary aspects of public health came to the fore. The Japanese occupation forces

174. Zhang Jishun, "Kindai ni ishoku sareta dentō."
175. Arnold, *Colonizing the Body*, 4. Also see, for example, Arnold, ed., *Imperial Medicine and Indigenous Societies*; MacLeod and Lewis, eds., *Disease, Medicine, and Empire*; Mark Harrison, *Public Health and Preventive Medicine*.

possessed bacteriological knowledge, financial resources, and the policing capacity necessary to implement various public health policies; they were actively involved in the city's cholera-control program and adopted the police-directed model of public health. In carrying out their work, Chinese public health workers and local leaders received technical and material support from the Japanese and complied with directions and instructions issued by Japanese authorities to effectively enforce coercive methods.

An examination of public health work during the war illuminates the ambiguity of wartime collaboration. It also raises the question of ethical responsibility among medical workers and administrators during the war. These individuals collaborated with the Japanese, followed Japanese directions, and took advantage of the presence of the Japanese military. Some of them enjoyed higher social status and more prestigious positions under the occupation. In fact, the two commissioners of public health in Shanghai during the war were accused of collaboration and treason. Each was sentenced to five years of prison.[176]

To lump all medical workers together as "traitors" and "collaborators" is problematic and too simplistic. In discussing the various motivations of those who worked with the Japanese during the war, scholars such as Keith Schoppa, Poshek Fu, Charles Musgrove, and Timothy Brook all present a more complicated picture. They suggest that the ultimate goal of many Chinese was survival—they did not particularly identify themselves with the Chinese state. Rather, they viewed themselves as members of a family, a local community, or a business. Some of them established their identity as bearers of an East Asian tradition that China and Japan shared.[177] It was inevitable, and sometimes even preferable, for them to work with occupiers in order to protect the interests of their communities and families. In considering the case of public health workers, no clear difference distinguishes the prewar cholera-control program from what was carried out during wartime. Cholera control was a trans-war

176. *SWZ*, 39. What happened to other health administrators during the war is unknown.

177. Schoppa, "Patterns and Dynamics"; Poshek Fu, *Passivity, Resistance, and Collaboration*; Brook, *Collaboration*; Musgrove, "Cheering the Traitor."

endeavor. Before and during the war, those who were engaged in anti-cholera programs administered injections and forced isolation based on modern biomedicine.[178] They believed that protecting their community and neighborhood was the key issue. They embraced the universal value of bacteriology, and their mission was teaching and offering the benefits and efficacy of modern medical science to the city's general populace. Their direct enemy was the cholera bacillus—not Japanese occupiers. Faith in biomedicine and the threat of an epidemic united the Chinese and Japanese. It also brought the people of Shanghai under governmental control in an unprecedented way.

The discussions in this chapter offer insights into issues around the operation of power. As Michel Foucault has discussed in various contexts, power can take different forms and act differently according to different means.[179] In creating and running Shanghai's public health administration, multiple agents wielded power and invented new technologies and rationalities by applying scientific methods to manage, monitor, and regulate urban residents and their bodies. Powerholders often resorted to surveillance and force. They imposed fees, rules, and penalties, watched and examined people's behavior, and mobilized the police and military forces, justifying such use of power on the grounds that it was their mission to civilize and lead the masses. At the same time, these powerholders, including medical elites, administrators, and even Japanese occupiers and their collaborators, also exercised their power to make individuals healthy and productive members of the society and to optimize and maximize their capabilities to contribute to the nation. The development of the public health bureau was situated at the juncture of these different modes of power operation. Shanghai's administrators deployed the knowledge of chemistry, biology, and other sciences to build health stations, collect vital statistics, inspect the quality of water and foodstuff, and conduct mass vaccinations. Through all these measures, they regulated and fostered the corporeal health of the Shanghai people.

178. On the cultural meanings of syringes, see Dikötter, "Cultural History of the Syringe."

179. For Foucault's conceptions of power, see, for example, Foucault, *Power*.

Power operates not only between administrators and citizens. Power is ubiquitous, and it can diffuse and circulate among population. Shanghai's hygiene campaign, the focus of the next chapter, provided an occasion in which the city's elites strategically utilized a diverse array of symbolic and cultural resources in the city to spread the knowledge on health and hygiene and mobilize the masses.

CHAPTER 3

Teaching about Health,
Mobilizing the Masses

Hygiene Campaigns in Shanghai

In April of 1928 the public health bureau (PHB) of the Shanghai municipal government organized its first hygiene campaign (*weisheng yundong*). The PHB held an opening ceremony at the public recreation grounds on April 28 to kick off the two-day program. Close to ten thousand people attended the ceremony. The mayor, commissioner of public health, and other notables all gave speeches; after the ceremony, attendees marched in a procession through the city. Some marchers carried banners and posters bearing slogans: "practice good hygiene" and "health saves the nation." Over the course of the campaign period, famous medical doctors delivered public lectures on summer diseases, local entertainers gave performances introducing hygiene practices, and students handed out handbills to passers-by. In keeping with the spirit of the celebration, Shanghai residents swept city streets, scrubbed the floors of their work places, and cleaned their residences.[1] In this chapter I explore this and other hygiene campaigns held in Chinese Shanghai in the early twentieth century. Hygiene campaigns were educational programs designed to teach the general populace proper knowledge of health and hygiene. They were also part of a mass movement organized by medical elites to involve the city's entire population. In designing and carrying out these campaigns, organizers exploited a wide assembly of cultural resources available in the city and borrowed styles and formats from other

---

1. *Shenbao*, April 28, 1928, 13; April 29, 1928, 13; April 30, 1928, 13.

social and political events to communicate with and mobilize Shanghai residents.

In their effort to build a modern nation-state, Republican-period Chinese reformers and administrators paid special attention to cities and strove to "remake" them. If the Republican period was "the starting point of the forceful modernization drive,"[2] cities were the engine of that drive and urban reform was "a fundamental part of the modernization agenda."[3] As we saw in chapter 2, Shanghai's Chinese elites came to see health and sanitation as a primary responsibility and basic function of the municipality, and they strove to provide potable water and safe food and to regulate markets and burial grounds. Yet, city administrators and reformers lacked the substantial financial resources necessary to build a new infrastructure to ameliorate workplace and living conditions in the city. As an alternative, Chinese elites allocated part of the responsibility for creating a sanitary city onto individual residents and initiated hygiene campaigns for educational purpose. Instead of "remaking the city," they targeted ordinary people and sought to remake their bodies, mentalities, and attitudes. They did this by giving them proper information on disease prevention and raising their consciousness about personal hygiene and environmental sanitation. In sum, through hygiene campaigns, they strove to transform the Shanghai populace into informed citizens who would be a cornerstone of a modern city and a strong nation.

The primary goal of hygiene campaigns was always providing information and guidance to laypeople, and the continuity and durability of Shanghai's hygiene campaigns was one of their most striking features. From the late Qing period to the twenty-first century, various organizers under several different regimes have administered such campaigns. In fact, one of the major themes of Confucianism is the perfectibility and educability of humans. Since ancient time, Chinese literati have believed that proper education and emulation could make people perfect. They also believed that literati should serve as teachers and role models for the masses. Late Qing reformers applied such understanding to the field of public health, and they put it into practice when they held a small-

2. Bergère, "Civil Society and Urban Change," 55.
3. Esherick, "Modernity and Nation," 5.

scale campaign as early as 1904.[4] As a greater number of Chinese learned Western medicine, and as the Nationalist Party became actively involved in the campaigns, this program significantly expanded and took a new form in the Republican period. In the mid-1910s, members of the YMCA and Chinese medical elites carried out larger hygiene campaigns.[5] When the Nationalists arrived in the city and opened the Shanghai Municipal Public Health Bureau (PHB), new administrators continued established hygiene campaigns. They elaborated on them, making them official events held twice a year. Even during the Second Sino-Japanese War, the wartime PHB continued their promotion, and the Communist government resumed citywide patriotic hygiene campaigns after 1949.

Regardless of organizers, hygiene campaigns consisted of similar events and activities. However, from the 1910s to the 1920s and through the 1930s, the campaigns underwent significant shifts in their emphasis and ideology. Early YMCA campaigns were voluntary educational movements, but after the Nationalist takeover of the city, hygiene campaigns became increasingly standardized and formulaic. They gradually developed into political events that connected the physical health of individuals and their mundane practices to larger social and national issues. Campaign organizers not only gave city residents knowledge and information but also taught them that it was their duty to practice good hygiene and clean their environment, and that their efforts would contribute to the building of a strong nation.

To effectively communicate with the city's populace and disseminate information and instruction among them, campaign organizers employed a wide range of methods and tactics. While intellectuals and YMCA reformers introduced educational programs from the West to China, the Nationalists further fleshed them out to mobilize the masses; in actuality, many campaign programs and strategies were variations, modifications, and refinements of other events and activities that were already in place in the city. Campaign administrators quickly assimilated their agenda into the city's dynamic medical and political culture. In doing so, they deftly utilized a diverse array of the city's symbolic and cultural

4. *SWZ*, 214.
5. Bu, "Public Health and Modernisation," 305–19.

capital for the purposes of education, inspiration, and mobilization. I argue that hygiene campaigns owed their durability and longevity to their capacity to adopt and incorporate the city's available cultural resources and assets into their programs. Hygiene campaigns were not created in a vacuum; they evolved from and adapted to Shanghai's cultural settings. In this chapter I analyze five major campaign programs: exhibitions and performances, texts and cartoons, lectures and talks, opening ceremonies and street sweeping, and monitoring and policing. Through an in-depth analysis of these campaign programs, I highlight some of the dominant themes and enduring motifs and examine how personal bodies, social etiquette, and state hegemony were all intertwined in hygiene campaigns.

An examination of hygiene-campaign programs calls attention to what Jeffrey Wasserstrom has called "collective action scripts." In his study of student movements, he compares student protests with other political and nonpolitical events, and finds close similarities among them. Using a theatrical metaphor, Wasserstrom argues that student protesters followed a set of "collective action scripts" abundant in the city.[6] Hygiene-campaign organizers were also attuned to these "scripts," which were designed to mobilize and draw the attention of the people. Accordingly, organizers used them completely to their advantage. Such scripts had various origins: some came directly from the past, some were used by religious workers and Confucian teachers, and some drew from antigovernment activities. Various organizers of hygiene campaigns refined preexisting scripts and devised their own strategies to move and unite the masses. In this way, Shanghai's hygiene campaigns augmented and enriched the repertoire of the city's collective action scripts.

After the rise to power of the Nationalist Party, hygiene campaigns offered a venue in which the Nationalist state interacted with and interfered in the everyday lives of Shanghai's populace. During the campaign, the state urged or even forced people to conform to good hygiene. The state also organized ceremonies in a respectful and disciplined manner by deploying national symbols and infusing state ideology into personal demeanor. In the end, Western ideas of health and medicine were annexed to state power, authority, and prestige. At the same time, however, not

6. Wasserstrom, *Student Protests*. Also see Esherick and Wasserstrom, "Acting Out Democracy."

only the state but also Shanghai citizens of various socioeconomic backgrounds looked at Western medical science and global public health to provide answers to Chinese problems. By the 1930s, hygiene practices had become an important element of indigenous conventions. Good hygiene was a reflection and indication of modernity and civility, and Shanghai people were eager to identify themselves and their nation with these values. Many Shanghai people participated in campaign programs of their own accord and took part in ceremonies and marches to make a public representation of modern citizenship.

From Community Service to State-Sponsored Event

THE EARLY CAMPAIGNS

Even before the inauguration of the Shanghai PHB, some nongovernmental institutions had organized educational activities to teach the city's general populace basic knowledge of medicine and hygiene and to improve urban sanitation. Late Qing reformers and educators, the Public Health Department of the International Settlement, and religious and social welfare organizations all organized such programs, calling them *weisheng yundong*, "hygiene campaigns."[7]

Of all pre-1928 hygiene campaigns, those organized by the YMCA were the most influential and best documented. Since YMCA campaigns served as a model for later campaigns and the YMCA provided educational materials on public health for other institutions, YMCA hygiene campaigns deserve special attention here.[8] The Chinese YMCA was established in Tianjin in 1895. Despite the political chaos of the 1910s, the

---

7. For a chronological list of these early hygiene campaigns, see *SWZ*, 216–17. On early campaigns in the International Settlement, see Gamewell, *Gateway to China*, 35–41.

8. The Public Health Department of Shanghai's International Settlement also used YMCA materials and sponsored a health exhibition at the YMCA building. China Contribution Committee, *Christian Occupation of China*, 434; Gamewell, *Gateway to China*, 41.

YMCA achieved considerable success in soliciting support from Chinese elites and recruiting urban youth. Although the original goal of YMCA programs was to provide information on modern Western life to the Chinese urban middle class and train them to be community leaders, public health soon became a key component of the YMCA's social reform programs.[9] In 1913, the YMCA established its health department and carried out a small-scale hygiene campaign in Hangzhou. The YMCA also organized lectures and exhibits on public health in other cities. By the mid-1910s, these experimental events had developed into hygiene campaigns that involved "all-day exhibits, meetings, lectures, and slide demonstrations,"[10] held in China's major cities. To disseminate basic knowledge on health and hygiene, YMCA leaders sought out effective methods to appeal to Chinese tastes and interests in their campaigns. To this end, the YMCA Lecture Department produced information materials on public health and Western medical science, including booklets on tuberculosis, health calendars, cartoons, films, and slides to be used in campaigns.[11]

The YMCA was also successful in coordinating with other Christian groups and medical organizations. In 1916, the YMCA, the China Medical Missionary Association (Zhonghua yixue chuanjiaohui), and the National Medical Association (Zhonghua boyihui)[12] founded the Council on Health Education (Weisheng jiaoyuhui) to promote health education in China.[13] (The YWCA and the Chinese Christian Educational Association also joined the Council in 1920.) The council produced various educational materials, which were distributed among missionaries and schools; in addition to these materials, it published a guideline for hygiene campaigns.[14] In promoting health education, the council worked

9.   Garrett, *Social Reformers*; Garrett, "Chamber of Commerce."

10. Garrett, *Social Reformers*, 145.

11. Ibid., 144–48; Peter, "Popular Health Education."

12. The China Medical Missionary Association was founded in 1886 by medical missionaries. The National Medical Association was founded in 1915 by Chinese doctors who trained in Western medicine to promote Western medicine in China.

13. Yip, *Health and National Reconstruction*, 21.

14. The Council on Health Education, "Gongzhong weisheng yundong chengxu," quoted in Lou, *Weisheng yundong*, 55–72.

with local organizations to carry out citywide hygiene campaigns in several Chinese municipalities. Thus, by 1920 the YMCA had already generated a considerable amount of educational material and had gained experience with campaign techniques. The council was suspended in 1929 because of financial difficulties, but many former council members received official appointments from public health departments of central and provincial governments under the Nationalists.[15] The YMCA continued publishing guidebooks and sourcebooks for campaigns until the 1930s.[16]

In Shanghai, the YMCA and the China Medical Missionary Association held a small health exhibition in 1915, and the YMCA organized its first hygiene campaign and staged a lantern parade in June 1920.[17] Between then and 1928, the YMCA carried out several hygiene campaigns on its own in the city.[18] Among these campaigns, the best-documented is the overall plan for the 1925 summer campaign.[19] A committee of four people led the campaign, recruiting and training thirty-six volunteers, who took charge of the actual work. According to this plan, the YMCA's hygiene campaigns had three goals: (1) improving the public health conditions of the society (*shehui weisheng zhuangtai*); (2) calling people's attention to information on hygiene; and (3) uniting YMCA members through carrying out their social missions. The main venue of the campaign was the YMCA building on Sichuan Road. During the campaign period, YMCA members displayed models, pictures, and books on hygiene and diseases. They also sold personal hygiene items, invited speakers to give lectures, and administered vaccinations at this venue.[20]

To mobilize people, the YMCA looked for cooperation from other social and public groups in the city, including the YWCA, the Boy Scouts,

15. Xu Yi, "Zuijin de jiaohui weisheng shiye," 156.

16. The March 1936 issue of *Qingnian jinbu*, a journal published by the Shanghai YMCA, carries a full-page advertisement for YMCA publications, including campaign guidebooks, collections of slogans, resources for performances, and other materials.

17. Garrett, *Social Reformers*, 145; *Shenbao*, June 19, 1920, 11; June 25, 1920, 11.

18. *SWZ*, 214.

19. For 1925 hygiene campaign programs, see *Shenbao zengkan*, May 21, 1; May 22, 1; May 23, 1.

20. Lou, *Weisheng yundong*, 14.

churches, and, most importantly, schools. Under the assumption that it would be easier and more effective to teach young people new information and knowledge, students played an important role in the YMCA plan, and schools were targeted as primary sites for health-related educational programs. The YMCA planned to involve school administrations in organizing "school hygiene campaigns" to fully mobilize students. Students were expected to participate in various school activities, such as cleaning school buildings, participating in fly-catching competitions, and writing compositions on the harm caused by flies, mosquitoes, and rats. Moreover, the YMCA deployed students as agents of the campaign and dispatched them to the neighborhoods to give lectures on the harmfulness of flies and mosquitoes, and to distribute handbills.[21]

In planning these campaigns for the YMCA, Christian reformers and Western-style doctors drew on their familiarity with public health movements in the West and invited Western advisers. As a result, YMCA campaigns in Shanghai shared many features of early twentieth-century American public health campaigns. Like their American counterparts, supporters of the Chinese hygiene campaigns embraced the idea that "the fight [against diseases] must be won, not by construction of public works, but by the conduct of individual life."[22] YMCA leaders purchased educational materials from the United States and produced similar items. Emulating American methods, they widely used mass media, such as movies and radio broadcasting, to circulate their ideas.[23]

Hygiene campaigns were a global phenomenon, and American models provided Chinese reformers with a touchstone. However, it is misleading to assume that the YMCA health campaign organizers simply imported and copied American methods. Strategies and techniques of health education flowed from the West to Chinese Shanghai not in a directly prescribed or imposed manner; rather, they were locally adapted and adjusted. YMCA leaders championed Western medical knowledge, but they were also sensitive to Chinese folk customs and tried to integrate

21.   Ibid., 16–17.

22.   Winslow, *Evolution and Significance*, 55.

23.   Bu, "Public Health and Modernisation," 308–9; Pernick, "Thomas Edison's Tuberculosis Films," 24.

indigenous traditions into their campaigns to facilitate acceptance by the Chinese. An example of this sensibility is reflected in the timing of the campaigns. According to the YMCA plan, one summer campaign and one winter campaign would be held in a year. The summer campaign would follow the Chinese folk customs of Duanwujie (Dragon Boat Festival), and the winter campaign would follow the Chinese New Year. On Duanwujie, people conducted family rituals to protect themselves from the communicable diseases of summer. A picture of Zhong Kui, a popular deity, was posted as a charm at the entrance of one's house, and *Calamus* (*changpu*) leaves were hung inside the house. Both Zhong Kui and *Calamus* leaves were believed to ward off harmful air and summer diseases. People drank a special kind of wine that was believed to drive out worms and detoxify poisons in one's body.[24] People also dusted their rooms and cleaned their residences on New Year's Eve. Although Chinese medical elites often criticized old Chinese customs, such as geomancy, fortune-telling, and prayer, as superstitious, and excluded traditional Chinese physicians from campaigns, they took advantage of certain popular customs to promote their programs.[25] Both the Nationalist government and the puppet governments during the war adopted these festivals for their hygiene campaigns as well. Moreover, as discussed below, campaign programs owed much in terms of styles, methods, and tactics to other events that were not directly related to health or medicine.

The YMCA paved the way and provided a "template" for later campaigns. When the Nationalists arrived in the city and the municipal government took over the sponsorship of the campaigns, the new organizers carried on and modified YMCA tactics that had been in place since the 1910s.

24. Hui Xicheng and Shi Zi, *Zhongguo minsu daguan*, 89–93. Xue Li, *Zhonghua minsu yuanliu*, 311–13.

25. Liqi Guangzuo, "Gonggong weisheng: shenme jiaozuo weisheng yundong," 12–13; You Qihua, "Shenme jiaozuo weisheng yundong," 110–11; Ye Juquan, "Weisheng yundong yu jiufengsu," 28–29.

THE MUNICIPAL HYGIENE CAMPAIGNS, 1928–1937

In 1928, the central government in Nanjing issued an "Outline for Implementing Summer Hygiene Campaign Meetings" (*xiaji weisheng yundong dahui shishi dagang*). According to this "Outline," every year, the capital city as well as all provinces, cities, and counties should simultaneously hold a summer hygiene campaign. The public health administration in each locality should invite other organizations and schools to create a preparation team (*choubeihui*) (PT) and the PT should lead the campaign.[26] In 1929, the central government issued another notice that one summer and one winter hygiene campaign would take place every year nationally.[27] Thus hygiene campaigns became official events.

Shanghai followed the directives from Nanjing. From 1928 through 1937 the municipal government sponsored a total of thirteen hygiene campaigns. Each time, the secretariat of the municipal government created a preparation team. The composition of the team differed from year to year, but delegates from the secretariat, municipal bureaus, and the Nationalist Party were always the core of the team. In addition to these delegates, preparation teams usually included members of Western-style medical professional groups, such as the China Medical Society, the Chinese Anti-Tuberculosis Association, the Shanghai Medical Practitioners Association, the Shanghai Dentist Association, the New Pharmacist Association, and the public health department of the Shanghai Railroad Administration.[28] Representatives of nonmedical public organizations came from the Chamber of Commerce, the labor union, the YMCA, and the YWCA. The public health departments of the two foreign concessions also participated.[29] As the task force for municipal hygiene campaigns, the PT was responsible for drawing up the overall budget and program. Usually under the chairmanship of the commissioner of public health, the PT was divided into several sections (*zu*). These sections were in charge of specific assignments, such as general affairs, book-

26.   Guomin zhengfu, "Xiaji weisheng yundong dahui shishi dagang."

27.   Yip, *Health and National Reconstruction*, 129–30.

28.   Traditional Chinese physicians were not invited. For a complaint from a Chinese-style doctor, see Yang Zhiyi, "Chi baoban weisheng yundong zhe."

29.   For an example of the organization of a campaign, see Changwu weiyuanhui, "Shanghai Shi di-shisan jie weisheng yundong baogaoshu," 405–14.

keeping, publicity, lectures, site arrangement, epidemic prevention, and monitoring.

Shanghai's administrators and medical elites were convinced that they had the privilege of teaching the masses proper knowledge and the responsibility for helping and guiding them, and they often underscored the significance of education. In his *Plans and Ideas for the Health of Greater Shanghai*, written in 1928, Hu Hongji, the first commissioner of public health, ranked "wide promulgation of health and hygiene education" as one of the urgent goals to be achieved by the PHB in its first two years. To carry out health administration properly, quickly, and economically, Hu argued, it was necessary "to inculcate personal hygiene and health habits, and tell of the methods of guarding against infection, and make known the principles of public health, to cause all the people of the city to take notice, and strengthen their faith and resolution in taking precautionary measures at once."[30] As for the methods of education, he listed "literature, of both literary and colloquial styles, slogans, large posters, cinematograph [*sic*], lectures, etc."[31] Likewise, Li Ting'an, Hu's successor, counted publicity as one of the top-priority jobs of the PHB.[32] Li also wrote that publicity should be "carried out in form of public lectures, radio broadcasting, motion pictures, home visiting by public health nurses, health posters, health monthly, and health exhibits."[33] Others concurred with them. Zhang Bingrui (1906–81), a supporter of Western medicine, commented, "If one wants the general populace to understand disease prevention, to cultivate hygienic habits, and to promote physical health, then one needs to pay attention to the implementation of health education. This is the responsibility of those of us who are in charge of public health. Every country in Europe and America is trying hard to carry out health education. In this way, they can save costs, and can gain great effects."[34] Believing that they were the designers and authors of hygienic modernity and the masses should be placed under their tutelage, Chinese elites promoted popular education through mass media.

30. SMA U1-16-293, 17.
31. Ibid.
32. Li Ting'an, "Shanghai Shi zhi gonggong weisheng xingzheng."
33. Ting-an Li, "Activities of the Bureau of Public Health," 991.
34. Zhang Bingrui, "Chengshi weisheng jiaoyu," 105.

Chinese public health administrators and YMCA leaders shared similar backgrounds and agreed on the necessity of public health education and usefulness of visual media, but not everyone was enthusiastic about the implementation of mass campaigns. Zhang cautioned in the same article that hygiene campaigns would only stir up temporary excitement and morale and that their lasting effects were questionable.[35] Likewise a *Shenbao* author pointed out that the urban poor struggled to make both ends meet, and they simply could not afford to keep their residential areas clean or practice good hygiene. He implied that campaigns were not an answer to the problem of poverty.[36] Another author wrote that fly-catching contests and cleaning efforts by schoolchildren were ineffective, if not harmful.[37] Yet, these voices were in the minority, and hygiene campaigns became part of the official business of the municipal public health bureau.

Some hygiene campaigns lasted only a single day, while some lasted for as long as ten days.[38] Two hygiene campaigns were planned each year, but, in practice, they were sometimes cancelled because of financial difficulties or the lack of adequate preparation. The Japanese attack of 1932, in particular, brought the sequence of hygiene campaigns to a halt. The northeastern parts of the city, including Zhabei, Wusong, and Jiangwan, were devastated by bombing, and important medical facilities and schools suffered severe damage.[39] In the summer of 1932, the city was able to administer a campaign to disinfect the areas destroyed by the battle; it would be the last to be held in the city for eighteen months. However, Shanghai quickly recovered from this setback. From 1934 to 1937, a summer hygiene campaign was held each year, though no winter campaign occurred during this period. Finally on July 6, 1937, a final prewar hygiene campaign was administered as a part of the tenth anniversary of the inauguration of the city government.[40] Ironically, on July 7, the very day of the anniversary, a clash between Japanese and

35. Ibid., 109.
36. Shouzi, "Wei benshi weisheng yundong yiyan," 1.
37. Chen Hanzhang, "Xianzai Zhongguo xuexiaozhong weishengshang liang da wumiu."
38. *SWZ*, 216.
39. "Damages to Medical Institutes in Shanghai," 332–33.
40. *Shenbao*, July 6, 1937, 11.

Chinese troops near the Marco Polo Bridge broke out that initiated the Second Sino-Japanese War. With the outbreak of war, the Shanghai municipal PHB was temporarily disbanded, and municipal health campaigns were brought to a halt.

NATIONAL SALVATION, GERM THEORY, AND PERSONAL HYGIENE

Chinese elites of every stripe in the Republican era, including YMCA leaders, medical doctors, social reformers, journalists, and educators, all participated in the discourse on racial health that presented individuals as components of the "race," and associated the rise and decline of a nation with the strength of its race. This link between the individual bodies, race, and nation was not new or distinctive of the Republican period. With the introduction of Social Darwinism, prominent reformers of the late Qing period, including Yan Fu and Kang Youwei, proclaimed the close connections between the wealth and power of the nation and the physical strength of the population.[41] However, it was during the Republican period that biomedicine and statistics increasingly replaced Confucian virtues in defining the "strength" of a body or a nation, and the creation of a healthy population became a target of state intervention and a focal point of public control.[42]

Hygiene campaigns reflected this intellectual discourse. Campaign organizers used morbidity and mortality as indicators of national strength and appealed to Chinese patriotism. Early on, YMCA leaders were also aware of the rise of Chinese nationalism, and they often emphasized the connection between national health, strength, and economy. For example, W. W. Peter of the YMCA delivered a lecture called "The Relation between National Health and National Strength," which used YMCA data to compare China's death rates with those of Western countries.[43] As hygiene campaigns became official events and Chinese elites reiterated and elaborated these points, national strength—rather than individual

41. Dikötter, *Sex, Culture, and Modernity,* 107.
42. Ibid.
43. Bu, "Public Health and Modernisation," 311; Peter, "Popular Health Education," 745.

health—became the goal of the campaigns. A Nationalist guidebook on hygiene campaigns warns readers that China is called "the sick man of East Asia," and that the Chinese are looked down on by foreigners. Because China is weak, imperialists encroach on China's sovereignty. The guidebook presents creating a healthy population as a basic step toward national salvation—a healthy, robust population will increase economic productivity and create the wealth of the nation. The consequences of a weak population are correspondingly dire: sick and frail people will not work productively or efficiently. Sickness will cause mental damage to the race, economic loss, and national poverty.[44] Some writers identified the short life expectancy of the Chinese as the root cause of economic loss. According to these authors, Chinese life expectancy at birth is about thirty years. Since it takes around fifteen years for a person to become self-supporting, a Chinese person can serve the nation for only fifteen years on average. They asserted that, if a person dies before the age of fifteen, all that he or she has consumed is completely wasted.[45] National salvation and economic prosperity were the two major goals that a healthy people could achieve. These arguments and figures were popular among Chinese elites, and reiterating them was a regular feature of hygiene-campaign literature.

Authors of campaign materials often identified germs and infectious diseases as the primary culprits causing most of these "unnecessary deaths." They also argued that individuals could prevent the spread of disease by eliminating and avoiding germs. In sum, they embraced what Nancy Tomes has called "the gospel of germs," which is "the belief that microbes cause diseases and can be avoided by certain protective behaviors."[46] Since the late nineteenth century, bacteriology had made remarkable progress in Western Europe, and scientists had learned how to isolate, track down, and even photograph various microbes. China's medical elites also became familiar with germ theory, and they transferred the theory from laboratories and classrooms to streets, homes, and shops.

44. These points were often made by public health administrators and the party politicians. See Zhongguo Guomindang zhongyang zhixing weiyuanhui, ed., *Weisheng yundong xuanchuan gangyao*; Hu Hongji, *Gonggong weisheng gailun*.

45. Jin Baoshan, "Weisheng yu jiuguo," 2–3. Also, Liu Ruiheng, *Xinshenghuo yu jiankang*.

46. Tomes, *Gospel of Germs*, 3.

How to locate, eliminate, and avoid germs in daily life became significant themes of hygiene campaigns.

Since germ theory was still relatively new in China in the 1920s, campaign literature often addressed the presence of germs, explicitly or implicitly, in a rudimentary manner for lay readers with little education in science. Germs are small and invisible to the naked eye, but they are discovered through a microscope. They are ubiquitous in the air, and water and foodstuff could be a source of germ-borne diseases. They spread through various venues and could cause serious harm to human bodies. Flies, mosquitoes, fleas, and other pests can be carriers of germs and infect people. Ideas and images about germs and infection were abundant in campaign materials. Aiming at popularizing germ theory among a wider audience, authors of campaign materials used simple language and vivid descriptions rather than providing comprehensive knowledge of bacteriology. In doing so, they often equated germ with dirt, filth, and bodily discharges and combined germ theory with everyday practices. By the 1930s, the focus of the campaigns gradually shifted from medical knowledge to personal conduct. Each individual should practice good hygiene and behave politely to avoid germs. Simple household chores, such as dusting, sweeping, and washing, were also significant means to prevent diseases. In sum, private bodies and homes became crucial sites to fight against germs and germ-carrying vectors. Poor hygiene would damage not only individuals but also the entire society, and it was uncivilized and ethically wrong. The pursuit of civility and decorum, betterment of domestic spaces, and fear of infectious diseases were combined in hygiene campaigns, and germ theory became a vehicle for moral lessons and social order.

The Nationalists further reinforced the connections between bacteriology, personal hygiene, and modern civilization and incorporated physical fitness into their state building program in the 1930s. Personal health evolved from something that indicated national strength into a symbol of state power and a feature of political slogans. This politicization of personal health and hygiene culminated in the New Life Movement. After several military campaigns against Communists, Chiang Kai-shek and his advisers were convinced that the Nationalist regime needed a new ideology to create a loyal and militant population and to rejuvenate the nation. Based on this belief, they developed the New Life ideology, a set

of doctrines that combined Confucian ethics, Sun Yat-sen's Three Principles of the People, and Christian reformist ideas. The New Life Movement
was launched in Nanchang (the capital of Jiangxi Province) in 1934 and
soon spread to other cities and provinces. From 1934, hygiene campaigns
were strongly influenced by the ideology of New Life, and in 1936, Shanghai's hygiene campaigns were subsumed under the New Life Movement.[47]
The Shanghai New Life Movement Promotion Association (Shanghai
xinshenghuo yundong cujinhui) was made up of members of the Blue Shirts
Society, a group of cadets devoted to Chiang Kai-shek.[48] This group took
the position of general secretariat of the campaign preparation team.
Under the influence of the Blue Shirts, the 1936 campaign was carried
out "in compliance with the spirit of New Life Movement to protect the
health of citizens and reduce their sickness."[49]

At first glance, the biomedicine and bacteriology embraced by progressive elites were at odds with the Confucian teachings and militarism
of the New Life Movement. Looking closer, however, it is evident that
many of the tenets of the New Life Movement were consistent with those
of hygiene campaigns. New Life was a complex movement that had various aspects, but it strongly advocated public health and looked for cleanliness and orderliness. New Life applied these values across the spectrum
of Chinese society, and concern for public health was linked to the improvement of individual practices and morality.[50] Many New Life instructions concerned trivial personal habits, such as to eat and drink
noiselessly, to cover one's mouth when coughing, to tie one's shoelaces
tightly, and to not laugh at funerals. Likewise, the hygiene campaigns
prescribed individual propriety as a requisite condition for a healthy population. New Life and hygiene campaigns both transformed private hygiene habits into public matters, and by doing so, raised the individual
consciousness of the "public," the community, and the state.[51] As the

47.   SMA U1-16-291.

48.   Eastman, "Fascism in Kuomintang China," 21.

49.   SMA U1-16-300, 11. On the influence of the New Life on hygiene campaigns in
different places, see various articles in *Xinyun yuekan* 34 (1936).

50.   Ferlanti, "New Life Movement"; Yip, *Health and National Reconstruction*,
36–37.

51.   Sean Hsiang-lin Lei, "Habituating the Four Virtues"; Hsiang-lin Lei, "Habituating Individuality." Also see Lei Hsiang-lin, "Weisheng weihe bu shi baowei shengming?"

hygiene campaigns became integrated into the New Life Movement, their focus further shifted from the promulgation of medical knowledge to instruction on maintaining a correct personal mentality and spirit. Moreover, campaigns were conducted in an increasingly ceremonial and formulaic manner and brought together personal habits and loyalty to the Nationalist Party.

HYGIENE CAMPAIGNS DURING THE WAR

Although the outbreak of the Second Sino-Japanese War in 1937 thwarted many of the Nationalist modernization programs, hygiene campaigns continued during the war. In 1941 the Executive Yuan of the puppet government in Nanjing proposed carrying out nationwide hygiene campaigns twice a year. In Shanghai, after a four-year hiatus, the wartime PHB administered its first hygiene campaign in May of 1941. Between that time and the summer of 1945, the city organized a total of five hygiene campaigns. Three were held in the summer, and two were held in the winter. These campaigns administered under the Japanese occupation were very similar in style and content to those before the occupation. The PHB organized a preparation team, selected members, and employed similar programs.[52]

Not only the programs themselves but also the logic and rationale for conducting the campaigns showed strong continuity from their initiation in the 1910s through the war years. Although the implied connotations for the "nation" were completely different from those of the prewar era, the familiar connection between personal health and national strength and prosperity remains a strong theme. Two excerpts of campaign proclamations from 1942 illustrate this point:

> We all know that the people are the components of a nation. We often say "Our country has a large population. It accounts for one quarter of the entire world." We say so as if we are satisfied with the quantity. In fact, even though a nation does need a population, weak and sick people do not help the nation's survival. On the contrary, they increase the nation's burden. Under current arduous circumstances, in which we want to satisfy

52. SMA R1-12-387.

and maintain our lives, yet our bodies are feeble, how can we struggle and strive? Therefore, if the economic situation is tough and the environment poor, we have to carry out a hygienic lifestyle even more [seriously]. We can find the way to national liberation only by doing this.[53]

Among methods of hygiene, cleanliness should be primary. If one's body and environment are clean, germs cannot live and reproduce. If we do not cultivate habits that appreciate cleanliness, but instead do not often change our clothing, do not comb our hair, and do not bathe frequently, then, it is easy to get lice and fleas. We will be infected with various diseases, such as plague, macula fever, typhoid, relapsing fever, and trench fever. Also, if one spits and urinates promiscuously, or dumps trash in a disorderly manner, such a person not only damages the city's appearance but also reveals bad, unsanitary habits, and represents a shame to the race and the nation. Moreover, one is spreading germs of tuberculosis, typhoid, and dysentery. This will jeopardize racial health and influence the national economy.

We hope each citizen will have a clear understanding of the significance and value of hygiene. Please be critical of yourself. Concerning personal hygiene, have you cultivated all the proper hygiene habits that you should? Have you improved your family's hygiene? Do you always follow the rules of public health? If each individual pays attention to these issues and implements them, only then can an individual be healthy, a family be happy, and a nation be strong and prosperous.[54]

These two passages include no indication of the Second Sino-Japanese War, and they are indistinguishable from prewar discourse on health and nation. The first passage underscores the connection between healthy people and national survival and calls for "national liberation" by way of good hygiene. The second passage addresses everyday hygiene practices and urges self-reflection of readers. It states that poor hygiene causes infectious diseases and shame and, in the end, weakens the nation. These themes commonly appeared in Republican-era literature on hygiene, and it is striking that these passages continued to be written during the war. In 1942, China and Japan were at war, and Shanghai was under Japanese military occupation. The city's public health bureau and hygiene campaigns

53.   "Wei benshi di-er jie xialing weisheng yundong gaoshiminshu."
54.   "Wei benshi di-yi jie dongji weisheng yundong gaoshiminshu."

were patronized by Japanese military forces and run by collaborators. While authors of these materials mention "national liberation," the very Chinese nation was in jeopardy. No mention is made about the poverty and damage inflicted by the war, and health and hygiene are handled as if they were completely nonpolitical and genuinely technical matters. Those who worked with occupiers were in an awkward predicament. Instead of protesting and lamenting the war, they found fault with individuals and addressed the "gospel of germs." They strove to live as normal life as possible and carry out campaigns in an ordinary and neutral manner.

Campaign Strategies

To achieve mass support, campaign organizers designed and adopted various programs and tactics with broad appeal. They emulated campaign methods from the West, borrowed publicity techniques from other activists, and used political symbols and rituals. A wide range of experiences and events in the city helped administrators design and organize hygiene campaigns and prepared the masses to participate in such programs. A more detailed discussion of the actual campaign strategies is now in order; below, I discuss five major campaign programs and place them within the dynamics of Shanghai's urban culture. Tracing connections and similarities between hygiene campaigns and other events can help explain the durability and effectiveness of hygiene campaigns.

EXHIBITIONS AND PERFORMANCES

Health exhibitions (*weisheng zhanlanhui*) were a significant component of hygiene campaigns. They served as a venue for the presentation of visual knowledge of hygienic modernity and provided a graphic way to assemble and present objects, panels, and data in a tangible manner. In fact, displaying and showing materials was a popular method of public health education. In the 1910s, the YMCA and other Christian institutions organized exhibitions, and the municipal government alone held thirty-six health exhibitions between 1928 and 1935.[55] Some medical schools in the city also displayed medical materials and instruments for viewing by the general public. Compared with these sporadic exhibitions, exhibitions connected to a hygiene campaign were larger, and they usually consisted of multiple events, including an opening ceremony, display of materials, entertainment programs, lectures, free physical and dental examinations, and various contests. All these events were held at the same site and were mostly free of charge. The entire program was designed to give audiences visual aids and live activities so that they could gain knowledge and have fun for free. Exhibitions were held at different places. The YMCA building, the Temple of the City God, schools, and an entertainment theater all served as exhibition sites. Sometimes more than one exhibition was held at multiple sites simultaneously. For example, during the 1934 campaign, exhibitions were held at five different locations around the city and in surrounding areas, including Pudong and Huxi.[56] Since no skill or fee was required to visit these exhibitions, the potential for running a very effective program that would attract a large number of people was high.

Health exhibitions were inaugurated in a formal manner, and the exhibition site was decorated like the site of a political assembly. A detailed description of an exhibition site of the Temple of the City God in the Nanshi area in 1934 illustrates this point. At the entrance gate stood a decorated archway, on the top of which was a sign that read "The City of Shanghai Thirteenth Hygiene Campaign Health Exhibition." In the auditorium, a platform was set up. Two scrolls hung to the left and right of the platform, and a portrait of the late Sun Yat-sen, a national flag, and a Party flag hung at the center. The commissioner of public health, the commissioner of education, the chairman of the Chamber of Commerce, and a movie actress attended the opening ceremony to give speeches.[57]

The display of materials was the core of the exhibition. A single exhibition might display a total of more than eight hundred items.[58] Visi-

55. *Shanghai Shi sinianlai weisheng gongzuo*, chap. 4.

56. Changwu weiyuanhui, "Shanghai Shi di-shisan jie weisheng yundong baogaoshu," 407.

57. "Weisheng zhanlanhui kaimuji."

58. Weisheng yundong choubeihui, "Benshi di-shiwu jie weisheng yundong baogaoshu (xu)," 393.

tors learned what *weisheng* looked like by seeing materials and displays set up for public viewing. Those in charge of the exhibition made elaborate preparation by collecting, classifying, and arranging the items from various organizations, including the municipal PHB, the Ministry of Public Health of the central government, medical schools in the city, and commercial firms. Collecting and transporting a large quantity of items and making the layout of the exhibition site took a considerable portion of the whole campaign expenditure. To subsidize the cost, the preparation team often linked up with an advertising company so that commercial firms could pay a fee for the advertisements of their merchandise.[59]

A detailed list of the items displayed in the 1935 exhibition survives. According to this list, four categories of items were displayed. First, there were educational materials on actual medical knowledge: Illustrated scrolls of emergency treatment, maternal care, and proper way of physical exercise; specimens of germs and pests; pictures showing the symptoms of diseases; and models and replicas of human bodies, skeletons, and internal organs were included in this category. In light of the goals of the health exhibition, these materials were the most important components. Spectators observed the structure of human body and gained a basic understanding of anatomy, physiology, and kinesiology. Also a picture of a patient suffering from cholera was shown, along with photographs of a magnified cholera bacillus and flies. Such images made the menace of microorganisms real and could generate lively interest among the spectators. These items brought medical science and bacteriology into focus and made them intelligible.

Second, the Shanghai PHB and its branch offices and attached clinics exhibited charts and illustrations of their activities. This category included charts of vital statistics, numbers of vaccinations given, numbers of children delivered, and results of school health examinations. They also displayed charts of the number of inspected livestock, the amount of trash removed, and the distribution of latrines in the city. The city's health stations and opium rehabilitation clinic also participated in the exhibition. They displayed photographs and diagrams to report their activities. These

---

59. Weisheng yundong choubeihui, "Benshi di-shisi jie weisheng yundong baogaoshu," 377.

data and charts were a living illustration of the good work of the public health bureau and other institutions, and they brought the concept of modern administration within the reach of the masses.

Third, pictures, slogans, and posters on hygiene practices were displayed at the exhibition site. These postings included not only those published by the campaign preparation team (PT) but also those contributed by city residents at large. The PT often solicited pictures and slogans from the general public. In 1935, the PT received 5,613 slogans and 362 pictures.[60] These submitted items were rated by the designated judges, and the items that received a high rating were awarded prizes.

Finally, commercial firms exhibited their merchandise. These firms included those that produced personal hygiene items, medical instruments, teaching materials, and pharmaceuticals. In 1935, for example, in addition to Commercial Press (Shangwu yinshuguan) and Chinese Institute of Scientific Instrument (Zhongguo kexue yiqiguan), more than twenty firms displayed their products.[61] Advertisement fees paid by participating businesses differed each year, but they were important source of income. In 1935, the total amount of the fees (1905.05 yuan) accounted for more than a half of the entire campaign budget (3153.05 yuan).[62]

The same exhibition site was used to provide free physical and dental examinations, entertainment, lectures, and various kinds of contests (such as a "healthy baby contest" and a "health slogan contest"). Among these events, performances by entertainers were perhaps the most popular part of the health exhibition programs. Professionals as well as nonprofessionals were invited to the exhibition site to give "performances on health and hygiene" (*weisheng biaoyan*), although no payment for performers was listed in the campaign budget. The offerings included Chinese opera, recitals, modern drama, dance, martial arts, farce, satirical talks, magic, and collective calisthenics. Unfortunately no hint of the actual content of these performances remains, but it is likely that they were at least loosely related to some aspect of health and hygiene. The health ex-

60. Ibid., 387.
61. Weisheng yundong choubeihui, "Benshi di-shiwu jie weisheng yundong baogaoshu (xu)," 393
62. Ibid., 404.

hibition held in the summer of 1935 boasted the most inclusive and extensive program, lasting for a period of ten days. Three or more performances were given each day, and the whole program lasted as long as nine hours a day.[63] In addition, slide shows and lectures by medical specialists were also popular programs.

Since a health exhibition consisted of various entertaining events, it could potentially make for a very appealing program. The wealth of activities associated with health exhibitions, however, was not without problems. The variety of events and displayed items may well have given visitors a somewhat jumbled overall impression. In fact, a member of a campaign's preparation team commented that "a shortcoming of the previous health exhibitions was that they tended to pursue only quantities of items. They did not care about the overlap of materials. Moreover, displays were not well organized. As a result, visitors could not concentrate, and an exhibition might not leave a profound impression on them."[64]

In spite of these problems, health exhibitions attracted a considerable number of visitors, and campaign records often included remarks like "visitors were enthusiastic" and "the site was full of excitement." According to the 1934 report, approximately sixty thousand people came to the Temple of the City God over a period of three days. In the same year, health exhibitions were also held at Pudong and Huxi for six days, and forty thousand people attended lectures and performances there. Altogether 100,000 people came to the three exhibition sites.[65] In 1935, there were more than fifty thousand visitors each day. Over a period of the ten days, the number of visitors to the exhibition site reached 500,000.[66] In 1936, twenty thousand people came to the site each day.[67] In 1945, a total of 350,000 to 400,000 people visited the exhibition site over a period of

63. Weisheng yundong choubeihui, "Benshi di-shisi jie weisheng yundong baogaoshu," 386.

64. Weisheng yundong choubeihui, "Benshi di-shiwu jie weisheng yundong baogaoshu (xu)," 393.

65. Changwu weiyuanhui, "Shanghai Shi di-shisan jie weisheng yundong baogaoshu," 411.

66. Weisheng yundong choubeihui, "Benshi di-shisi jie weisheng yundong baogaoshu," 386.

67. Weisheng yundong choubeihui, "Benshi di-shiwu jie weisheng yundong baogaoshu (xu)," 393.

six days.[68] Assuming that these numbers are accurate, the exhibitions and other programs successfully attracted large numbers of city residents.

In organizing exhibitions, YMCA members imitated the forms and styles of health education in the West, and the Shanghai Public Health Bureau followed YMCA examples. However, collecting and showcasing objects had a long history in China, and after the mid-nineteenth century, Chinese also learned about exhibitions and displays from Japan and the West. China participated in international expositions that boasted the industrial and commercial development of nations, and the Qing supported exhibitions at home to display national arts and crafts. In Shanghai, French Jesuits built the Siccawei (Xujiahui) Museum in 1868, and the British built the Shanghai Museum in 1874, both of which were open to the public. Through these institutions, Chinese became familiar with "museums" that classified, labeled, and preserved cultural artifacts and natural objects and made them public.[69] Likewise the municipal government and the Chamber of Commerce both established exhibition halls and museums to exhibit China's national products.[70] These exhibitions and pageants helped the public identify themselves with the ideas and images of the nation. Moreover, department stores and marketplaces also displayed commercial items; professional and amateur artists held art and photo exhibitions and fashion shows for public viewing. By the 1920s, Shanghai people were surrounded by and familiar with a wide range of spectacles in the city; in short, health exhibitions came from and contributed to Shanghai's spectacular culture. They were a depository of things, knowledge, and performances, and also a vehicle for transmitting information and practices in a concrete and perceptible form to as many people as possible. Spectacles could present multiple meanings and aspects of medicine and health, including shapes of bacteria, the structure of human skeleton and viscera, vital statistics, the proper way of brushing teeth, and much more. Campaign organizers were also well aware of the power of spectacles to visualize abstract ideas, attract attention, and enhance people's understanding of germs and diseases.

68. SMA R1-12-389; SMA R50-731.
69. Claypool, "Zhang Jian and China's First Museum," 573–75.
70. Gerth, *China Made*, 203–81.

TEXTS AND CARTOONS

The circulation of printed materials was always the most common technique utilized by Shanghai's hygiene campaigns. Early on, the Council on Health Education and the YMCA produced various materials, and since the 1890s, Public Health Department of the International Settlement created posters, handbills, and brochures for education.[71] During the Nationalist period, campaign organizers spent large portions of their budgets on printing.[72]

A wide range of printed materials was published for the hygiene campaigns, though the kind and amount differed from time to time. Usually five to ten different posters with a featured slogan were printed for each event. These posters were displayed around the city on public billboards, walls, and electric poles, and at ceremonial sites, exhibition sites, and amusement and entertainment venues.[73] Others were posted in public transportation vehicles, such as streetcars, buses, boats, and rickshaws.[74] In addition, five to ten different kinds of handbills were also printed and distributed.[75] In 1935 and 1936, the preparation team even rented an airplane from the China National Aviation Corporation to distribute handbills at opening-ceremony sites.[76] The wide range of materials used in the 1934 campaign demonstrates the variety of the printed media employed. Items included one hundred thousand copies of posters (five kinds altogether); five thousand copies of handbills titled "Notification of the Hygiene

71. Ma Changlin, *Shanghai de zujie*, 118–19.
72. For example, in 1928, 822.89 yuan was spent on printing, out of total expenditures of 2,313.59 yuan. See "Dahui jishi," 67. Likewise in the final financial report from the 1934 campaign, 645.18 yuan out of 2,007.05 yuan was spent for publicity, most of which was spent on printing fees and paper expenses. SMA U1-16-298, 45–46. Also, in estimating the whole budget for the 1942 campaign, 2,400 yuan out of 4,000 yuan was allotted to publicity, and 1,800 yuan out of 2,400 yuan was allotted to the printing of slogans and handbills. See SMA R1-12-388, 40.
73. "Second Health Campaign Mass Meeting."
74. Weisheng yundong choubeihui, "Benshi di-shisi jie weisheng yundong baogaoshu," 378; SMA U1-16-300, 15. For pictures of posters, see *Weisheng yuekan* (*WY*) 2, no. 12 (1929), and *WY* 5, no. 7 (1935). Also see SMA U1-16-299.
75. "Di-shier jie weisheng yundong baogao," 88.
76. Weisheng yundong choubeihui, "Benshi di-shisi jie weisheng yundong baogaoshu," 381; Weisheng yundong choubeihui, "Benshi di-shiwu jie weisheng yundong baogaoshu," 361. For a picture of the airplane, see *WY* 5, no. 6 (1935).

Emergency Law"; ten thousand copies of handbills titled "A Hygiene-Campaign Manifesto"; four thousand copies of handbills titled "Notice to the Citizens"; twenty thousand copies of other miscellaneous handbills; five thousand copies of cartoon books; one thousand copies of pamphlets titled "How to Protect Your Teeth"; and five thousand copies of pamphlets titled "The Song of Brushing Teeth." In addition to these, the Public Health Department of the International Settlement also published twenty thousand copies of pamphlets in English and Chinese.[77]

Because printed media commanded a considerable presence in Shanghai's urban culture, the variety and quantity of printed materials used in hygiene campaigns is hardly surprising. From the late nineteenth century onward, Shanghai had emerged as the national center for printing and publishing. Shanghai's machine shop proprietors and technicians quickly mastered Western-style printing machinery. Thanks to the development of new printing technology, newspapers and periodicals enjoyed wide distribution, and their readership among residents of the city and outlying communities was considerable.[78] In 1935 Shanghai was home to 260 publishing companies,[79] and 1,200 Chinese newspapers started publication in the city in the 1920s and 1930s.[80] Various forms of print materials and their readers were omnipresent in Shanghai. Government officials, merchants, Confucian educators, and religious preachers all extensively used handbills, pamphlets, posters, and newspapers to broadcast messages, instructions, and information across the city. Mass media based on written language also played a significant role in shaping public opinion. Hygiene campaign organizers were also familiar with the widespread presence of print materials and their potential to communicate with the masses. Most of the written materials that targeted the masses were short and simple so that those with limited literacy could understand them. Instead of complex texts, these materials adopted easy catch phrases,

---

77. Changwu weiyuanhui, "Shanghai Shi di-shisan jie weisheng yundong baogaoshu," 411–12.

78. On the printing industry and technology in Shanghai, see Reed, *Gutenberg in Shanghai*.

79. Of these companies, 164 were very small with assets of less than 5,000 yuan. Xiong Yuezhi, ed., *Shanghai tongshi*, vol. 10, *Minguo wenhua*, 106.

80. Ibid., 224.

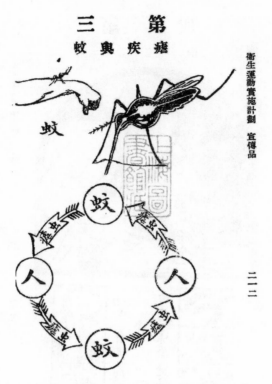

FIGURE 3.1 Malaria and mosquitoes. Lou, *Weisheng yundong*, 212.

colloquial expressions, and lyrics that could be recited. Cartoons and other visuals were also commonly used.

Germ theory was a popular subject of campaigns, and authors of campaign literature used plain language and visuals to teach basic ideas about germs and infection. Figures 3.1 and 3.2 illustrate educational materials carried in a book edited by a YMCA leader in 1928. Figure 3.1, "malaria and mosquitoes," describes how malaria parasites are transmitted by mosquitoes; figure 3.2, "microorganisms," shows drawings of the distinctive shapes of a roundworm, scabies worm, malaria parasite, rod-shaped bacillus, coccus, and chain coccus as seen through a microscope. These figures present what specific germs and parasites look like, how they are transmitted, and how to use a microscope.

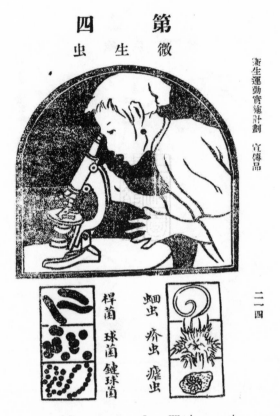

FIGURE 3.2 Microorganisms. Lou, *Weisheng yundong*, 214.

Whereas early YMCA materials were mostly informative and educational, those from the 1930s often conveyed messages that were not centered on germs per se but rather on personal habits and consciousness. Although these materials might mention that germs caused infectious diseases, they make it clear that the individuals who behaved in an unsanitary manner were the real source of disease. In other words, the responsibility for eliminating germs and preventing disease was deemed to lie mostly with individuals—not with city administrators or medical personnel. Whereas the printed media did not usually give a detailed explanation of germ theory, these materials explicitly described the connection between bad habits and diseases as if the cause-and-effect relationship was clear-cut. Such materials made the point that unsanitary habits not only caused diseases but also were injurious to a person's pride and public image. In short, poor hygiene habits were disgraceful and uncivilized. The presence of germs, personal behavior, and social etiquette were mutually related.

Cartoons (*lianhuanhua*) and posters (*biaoyu*) used in the 1934 campaign illuminate these points. In figure 3.3, the top frame shows a tubercular man coughing and spitting in the street; the middle frame portrays a man of science who studies the tuberculosis germs under a microscope; and the bottom frame shows the germs spreading in the air to be inhaled by another man. The cartoon describes the presence of germs, and they are clearly associated with what was then already a well-known disease. Importantly, it is not the germ but the unhygienic and unseemly behavior of the spitting man that really matters. What should one do to prevent disease? Figure 3.4 instructs, "When you need to spit, spit in appropriate places, such as into spittoons or a handkerchief." This poster highlights good personal habits. Knowledge of bacteriology and a lesson on proper conduct are nicely combined in these examples: the germs cause the disease, but as long as they stay in a spittoon or handkerchief they do not infect other people. It is noteworthy that these materials make no mention of the ventilation of residences or workplaces, or discuss general nutrition in the prevention of tuberculosis.

In other materials, germs are not even mentioned. For example, figures 3.5 and 3.6 both criticize a man who urinates in the street. The caption of figure 3.5 reads, "He urgently needs to urinate. But if he walks a few more steps, isn't there a public toilet?" In figure 3.6, the man urinating is compared with a dog that has neither medical knowledge nor a sense of shame; in the bottom frame, the man is caught by the police and ridiculed by passers-by. The message here is loud and clear: public urination is bad not only because it is unsanitary; it is also uncivilized and shows bad manners.

These cartoons and slogans do not convey complex theories on bacteriology or statistics of Chinese mortality or morbidity rates. But these visual images were more useful and compelling than lengthy essays in bringing admonition and lessons. Hygiene campaigns aimed at not

吐痰　（一）他
害着癆病，面黃飢
瘦，咳嗽不止，隨
地吐痰。（二）用
顯微鏡照照看，一
條條，活繞繞，心
驚膽怕！（三）塵
土飛天，毒菌飛在
空中，吸入走路人
鼻孔，為他捏着一
把汗。

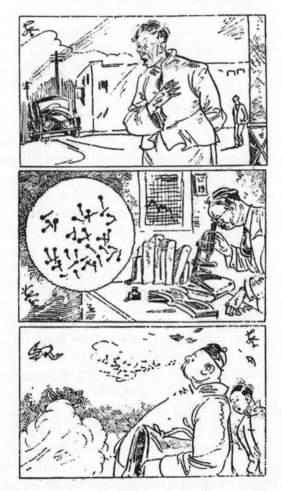

FIGURE 3.3 Expectoration (cartoon). *Weisheng yuekan* 4, no. 7 (1934), 290. This cartoon is titled "Expectoration." The text reads (1) He suffers from tuberculosis, and he is sallow and emancipated. He cannot stop coughing and spits everywhere. (2) Let us use a microscope and look at it carefully. We find something long. They are alive and moving around—make me tremble with fear! (3) Dust swirls, and poisonous germs also fly in the air. A passer-by inhales them through his nostrils. This make me feel very worried about him.

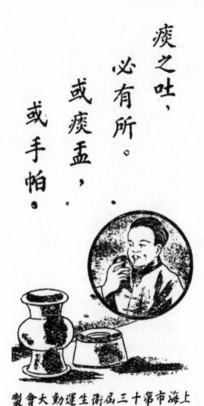

痰之吐，必有所。或痰盂，或手帕。

上海市第三十屆衛生運動大會製

FIGURE 3.4 Expectoration (poster). *Wei-sheng yuekan* 4, no. 7 (1934), 294.

only teaching about germs but also at cultivating modern civility and gentility.

LECTURES AND TALKS

In addition to printed materials, hygiene campaign programs drew significantly on a variety of spoken-language media, which was also abundant in the city. Shanghai people were exposed to lectures, speeches, and storytelling. Nationalist leaders, student activists, religious preachers, and entertainers all gave various kinds of speeches to draw the attention of the audience.[81] Hygiene campaign organizers were familiar with these

81. Wasserstrom, *Student Protests*, 214–16. Also see Smith, *Like Cattle and Horses*.

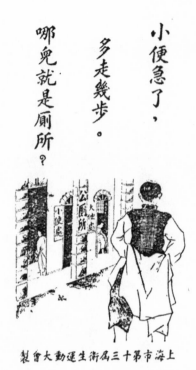

小便急了，
多走幾步。
哪兒就是廁所？

上海市第三十屆衛生運動大會製

FIGURE 3.5 Promiscuous urination (poster).
Weisheng yuekan 4, no. 7 (1934), 294.

methods and techniques and readily adopted them to spread their agenda.

During the hygiene campaign, medical doctors, city celebrities, and laypeople gave talks and lectures on medicine and hygiene. Whereas a substantial amount of money was spent on printed materials, a relatively small budget was allotted to spoken-language publicity; this was possible, in part, because laypersons often gave the lectures with very little monetary compensation or none at all.[82] The preparation team selected schoolteachers, youth, and factory workers and assigned them to give standardized lectures to their colleagues and neighbors. Schools were the primary sites for lectures, and schoolteachers were often appointed as

82. Weisheng yundong choubeihui, "Benshi di-shiwu jie weisheng yundong baogaoshu"; Chen Gao, "Shanghai Shi di-shiwu jie weisheng yundong choubei jingguo." The expenses of spoken-language publicity were often omitted from campaign budget plan. They were sometimes included in "miscellaneous expenses."

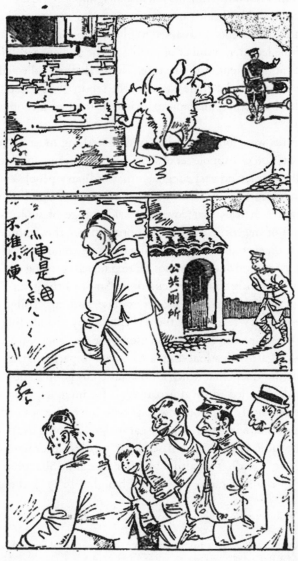

FIGURE 3.6 Promiscuous urination (cartoon). *Weisheng yuekan* 4, no. 7 (1934), 290. This cartoon is titled "urination." The text reads (1) A dog lacks knowledge and does not have a sense of honor. Thus he urinates promiscuously. (2) Isn't there a toilet over there? Why doesn't he walk a few more steps? Doesn't that make him equal to the dog that urinates anywhere? (3) A policeman has arrived. He is dragged into the police office. Why is he causing such trouble for himself?

lecturers. The publicity section of the preparation team designated reference books and issued "outlines" for the lectures.[83] These standardized materials were distributed to schoolteachers, and teachers gave their own lectures based on the "outline." School lectures were usually open to the public so that not only students but also neighbors could attend. In 1942, the wartime public health bureau instituted a report card system for the lectures. Each school was asked to fill out the card, reporting the date, name of the lecturer, number of people in the audience, response of the audience, and content of the lecture. The PHB then collected the cards and gave each school a grade based on the report.[84] As a result, some 110 schools held a lecture, and approximately thirty-seven thousand people attended.[85]

Lectures were longer and involved something more elaborate than the presentation of a simple set of short slogans and catchphrases. Yet they were still in clear and easy language that ordinary people could understand. The lecture outline for the 1942 summer campaign survives; it contained twelve articles that covered a wide range of subjects. (For the translation of the entire outline, see appendix 2.) The "outline" lists dos and don'ts on everyday life, suggesting that one could stay well by avoiding unsanitary food and drink, not sharing towels, keeping one's residence clean, and receiving cholera vaccinations. Some of the items, such as the benefits of sunlight, fresh air, proper exercise, and early rising, concurred with the ordinary regimen of the day that many already followed.[86] By heeding these tips and recommendations, the audience learned that they could avoid gastrointestinal diseases, cholera in particular, as well as tuberculosis and trachoma, which are all caused by germs. The outline does not provide detailed medical explanation for infection, but it gives the audience practical advice on how to prevent such diseases and stay fit.

In addition to lectures, hygiene campaigns adopted the new technology of the radio broadcast to disseminate medical information in a spoken language. Radio was also a popular media in Shanghai. After the opening of the first radio station in Shanghai in 1923, the number of

83.   Changwu weiyuanhui, "Shanghai Shi di-shisan jie weisheng yundong baogaoshu," 408–11.

84.   Reports with a grade from eighty-nine schools are filed in SMA R50-738.

85.   SMA R1-12-388.

86.   For the entire outline, see SMA R50-736, 45–48.

stations increased steadily, numbering fifty-four by 1934.[87] It is estimated that by 1937 Shanghai residents owned one hundred thousand receiving sets.[88] Because many of these sets were placed in stores so that customers as well as store clerks would listen, the actual number of radio listeners was much larger than one hundred thousand. The radio held a unique potential for the dissemination of ideas. Listening to the radio did not demand reading ability or physical presence at a specific site.[89] Just like commercial entrepreneurs and advertising companies, hygiene campaign organizers promptly made use of this media. As a part of the educational programs, the public health bureau sponsored 151 radio broadcasts between 1934 and 1936.[90] Moreover, a considerable number of commercial radio stations in Shanghai presented programs on health and hygiene. During the campaign period, the preparation team organized special radio programs broadcast from multiple radio stations. The team appointed medical experts, city commissioners, and other celebrities to give talks on the radio; typically each of them had a thirty-minute program. Two or three programs were broadcast from different stations every day.[91] Even Du Yuesheng, a well-known Green Gang boss-cum-businessman, gave a broadcast lecture during the health campaign of 1936.[92]

Exhibitions, written materials, and spoken-language media were all significant components of Shanghai's hygiene campaigns. They were also omnipresent in Shanghai's urban life; hygiene campaigns were not the only event that adopted them. Various groups in the city all used these methods and strategies to reach the masses and disseminate their messages. With the multitude of contemporary and historical examples of mass communication techniques, campaign organizers did not have to resort to new methods. They followed tried-and-true methods with which

87. Xiong Yuezhi, ed., *Shanghai tongshi*, vol. 10, *Minguo wenhua*, 243–244; Benson, "Manipulation of Tanci," 119–21.

88. Lee and Nathan, "Beginning of Mass Culture," 374–75.

89. Benson, "Manipulation of Tanci," 121–27.

90. *Shanghai Shi sinianlai weisheng gongzuo gaiyao*, chap. 4.

91. Changwu weiyuanhui, "Shanghai Shi di-shisan jie weisheng yundong baogaoshu," 412.

92. Weisheng yundong choubeihui, "Benshi di-shiwu jie weisheng yundong baogaoshu (xu)," 394–95.

Shanghai residents were already familiar; through these conventional methods, they introduced new concepts about germs, civility, and public health to the general populace. During the hygiene campaign, Shanghai people viewed, read, and listened to what germs and parasites looked like, how they were transmitted, and how people became infected. At the same time, they also learned that public health depended on their personal behavior and that they were responsible for avoiding and eliminating germs. The main subjects of the popular media were quotidian practices—what to eat and drink, where to spit and urinate, and when to wake up and go to bed. But such personal behavior was not only personal, and public health was not only public. Shanghai's hygiene campaigns presented a set of standards of civilized behavior in public and private through familiar forms of mass media. This familiarity bridged the gap between intellectual discourse and commoners' lives, as well as between bacteriology and everyday habits, and helped a large number of people take part in campaigns. Eventually hygiene campaigns became a common feature of the urban life. Moreover, promotion of good manners was a significant part of China's effort to challenge Western racism and to build a strong nation.[93] The connection between personal practices and the state came to the fore in ceremonies and rituals related to hygiene campaigns.

OPENING CEREMONIES AND STREET SWEEPING

Hygiene campaigns were an occasion in which organizers took full advantage of the city's mass media to communicate with Shanghai's general populace. At the same time, campaigns involved ceremonial performances with rituals, rites, and symbols. Ceremonies and rituals bestowed legitimacy and authority on those who organized campaigns and united those who participated in the events. After 1928, and after 1934 in particular, hygiene campaigns transformed from educational programs organized by medical elites to official events overseen by the Nationalist state. In this process, they were carried out in an increasingly ritualistic and standardized manner and put allegiance to the party in the spotlight.

93.   Zhiwei Xiao, "Movie House Etiquette Reform"; Yamin Xu, "Policing Civility."

Formal opening ceremonies were a case in point. Each campaign kicked off with an opening ceremony.[94] Campaign organizers would rent a public space or theater for the ceremony so that a large number of people could assemble. The ceremony sites included the Public Recreation Grounds, the Municipal Educational Institute, the Confucian Temple of the City, and the Nanjing Grand Theater.[95] The ceremony was held at a different site every year, but the site was always decorated in a similar way. Following are descriptions of the decoration in 1934 and 1936, respectively: the 1934 ceremony was held at the Public Recreation Grounds, and the 1936 ceremony was held inside the building of the Shanghai Popular Citizens' Educational Institute.

> After more than a month of preparation, at 10:30 in the morning on June 19, an opening ceremony was held at the Public Recreation Grounds. Fine rain was pattering down, and many people had begun to gather. Two slogans written on cloth, "Heed order" (*zhuyi zhixu*) and "Neat and clean" (*zhengqi qingjie*) were posted all around the site. Other colorful posters were also put up. They were beautiful and eye catching. The wordings of these slogans were rhymed, lively, and could be recited. Above the platform, a big horizontal scroll read: "The Shanghai Municipality Thirteenth Hygiene Campaign Mass Meeting." To the left and right, hung a couplet. The left one said "Rejuvenate our nation, and promote health" (*fuxing wuminzu er tichang weisheng*), and the right one said "Practice New Life, and carry out the campaign" (*shijian xinshenghuo er juxing yundong*). The last two characters of each scroll, *weisheng* and *yundong* thus cleverly inserted the words "hygiene" and "campaign" [into these slogans].[96]

> At the front gate of the Shanghai Popular Citizens' Educational Institute, a national flag and a Party flag were displayed, in a crossed fashion. Above them, hung a horizontal inscription board that read "The Shanghai Municipality Fifteenth Hygiene Campaign." Below the flags hung a large

94. Sometimes the opening ceremony of the campaign and that of the health exhibition took place simultaneously.

95. For example, see "Weisheng yundong kaimuji," 295; Weisheng yundong choubeihui, "Benshi di-shiwu jie weisheng yundong baogaoshu (xu)," 392; SMA R1-12-388; SMA R1-12-389, 14; SMA R50-736, 34.

96. "Weisheng yundong kaimuji," 295. Also see *Shenbao* June 19, 1934, 15–16; June 20, 1934, 9.

shield made of cardboard, on which appeared two artistically stylized characters, "wei" (for *weisheng*) and "yun" (for *yundong*) were written. The ceremony took place in a lecture hall of this Institute. Around the hall stood policemen on point duty, and Boy Scouts were dispatched to maintain order. At the hall entrance hung a horizontal cloth streamer bearing a slogan written in red ink: "Shanghai New Life Movement Promotion Association, Public Health Bureau, Public Health Department of the International Settlement, and forty-some other organizations jointly administer this Fifteenth Hygiene Campaign." The hallways of the Institute were hung with various kinds of health-related posters.[97]

As these accounts demonstrate, ceremony sites were typically loaded with political symbols: the national flag, the party flag, and a portrait of Sun Yat-sen commonly adorned opening-ceremony venues. The wartime public health bureau employed a similar style, using the national flag of the puppet government and the portrait of Dr. Sun as if claiming they were Sun's legitimate successors.[98] The opening ceremony was not open to the public. Attendees were delegates of selected social organizations in the city, including schools and factories, the New Life Guidance Squad, the police, the public security squad, the YMCA, the YWCA, and the Boy Scouts. They arrived to the ceremony site in groups, and altogether, they represented the entire city. In addition, city celebrities, such as the mayor, the chairman of the local branch of the party, municipal commissioners, the chairman of the Chamber of Commerce, delegates of the two foreign settlements, and delegates of the medical and dental associations in the city also attended the ceremony as guests. After 1941, those who were associated with Japanese organizations also attended the ceremony. For example, delegates from a detachment from the Japanese military forces, the Shanghai Special Agency (Tewu jiguan/Tokumu kikan), and the medical department of the Japanese Embassy, among others, were invited to the opening ceremony of the 1942 winter campaign.[99]

97. Weisheng yundong choubeihui, "Benshi di-shiwu jie weisheng yundong baogaoshu (xu)," 392.
98. SMA R50-731.
99. SMA R50-732.

Participants of the opening ceremony performed a series of civic rituals. The ceremony was formally inaugurated with a salute and an overture. The attendees bowed toward the party flag and Sun's portrait, then sang a party song. Sometimes they recited Sun's last words and observed a moment of silence. Then the commissioner of public health delivered a report, followed by speeches by the mayor, other city celebrities, and medical experts. To conclude, attendees sang a "hygiene song" (*weishengge*) and made a final salute. One small but revealing example of the ritualization of opening ceremonies is the "oath of hygiene" (*weisheng xuanshi*) given by Boy Scout members in 1935. Following the speeches by celebrities, selected Boy Scout members and students stepped forward and took the following oath, right hands raised: "On my honor, I will do my best, to help other people and obey the following five creeds. One: I will receive preventive injections. Two: I will only drink boiled water. Three: I will not eat unsanitary food. Four: I will not spit. Five: I will eradicate flies."[100]

Oath-taking is a highly ritualistic act often used to create a solid alliance or pseudo-kinship. It frequently appeared in popular novels, dramas, and theatrical performances about rebels and revolutionaries. People from many different backgrounds took oaths during the Republican period. For example, Shanghai's student protesters in the May Fourth Movement swore a solemn oath to demonstrate their solidarity and to preserve their determination.[101] The Green Gang bosses also took an oath of pseudo-brotherhood.[102] Most interesting and reminiscent of the Boy Scout hygiene oath is the oath taken by Blue Shirts members when they inaugurated their organization. In February of 1932 Chiang Kai-shek called his close disciples from the Whampoa Military Academy to come to his villa in Nanjing. There, they held a meeting to establish the Lixingshe (Society for Vigorous Practice), the core organization of the Blue Shirts Society. At the end of the four-day meeting, Chiang and his students assembled in a classroom. The students raised their hands and pledged, in front of the chairman, to practice the Three Principles of the People.[103] In fact,

100. Weisheng yundong choubeihui, "Benshi di-shisi jie weisheng yundong baogaoshu," 380–81. For a picture of oath-taking, see *WY* 5.6 (1935).
101. Wasserstrom, *Student Protests*, 78–79.
102. Martin, *Shanghai Green Gang*, 20–21.
103. Wakeman, "Revisionist View," 405–9.

the Chinese Boy Scouts in the 1930s were closely associated with the Blue Shirts. The Boy Scouts organization in Shanghai had been created under the guidance of foreigners in 1913,[104] but by the 1930s it had been reformulated as a "satellite" organization of the Blue Shirts. Blue Shirts members infiltrated the Boy Scout organization as officers and instructors so that the youth would be trained as militaristic and revolutionary patriots.[105] Just as Blue Shirts members swore loyalty to Chiang Kai-shek, the youth trained by these Blue Shirts members pledged to follow official hygiene instructions before the city administrators and celebrities at the campaign ceremony. The posture, attitudes, and clothing of these youths embodied the ideal of the healthy strong citizen of a modern nation.[106] The actual content of the oath was not political or complex; rather it was about everyday practices. Here, the language of the Boy Scouts not only conveyed information but also was meant to have an emotional and psychological effect on the audience that would inspire and mobilize them. Symbolic references and practical advice were combined together and evoked emotional engagement among the attendees. National symbols, solemn rituals, allegiance to the Nationalist Party, and personal practices were placed side by side.

After the speeches, oath, and song, a final musical performance concluded the assembly. Each attendee then took a broom and left the ceremony site to march through the city sweeping the streets. In some years, nurses, police, and musicians also joined the procession. At a certain point, the celebrities would gather for a memorial photo and depart. This was the official end of the ceremony. The other attendees continued their sweeping until the afternoon.[107] The marching and street sweeping were an important part of the hygiene campaign demonstration. Even in 1933, when there had been no opening ceremony, the city's street sweepers performed a street-sweeping procession. The PHB dispatched forty-some vehicles, including trash collecting cars, sprinkling cars, and others, and the Police Bureau also dispatched some ten motorbikes.

104. Xin Ping, Hu Zhenghao, and Li Xuechang, *Minguo shehui daguan*, 642–48.
105. Wakeman, "Revisionist View," 418–19.
106. On Chinese Boy Scouts and scout training, see Culp, *Articulating*, 178–97.
107. "Weisheng yundong kaimuji," 296.

The vehicles and street sweepers were divided into two groups: one group marched in the Zhabei area, and other marched into Nanshi. Slogans were tied to the vehicles, and the street sweepers carried brooms and shovels on their shoulders. They wore yellow jackets on which two characters, *qingdao* (cleaning streets), were inlayed. They also held aloft banners with slogans. As they marched, they shouted slogans and distributed handbills.[108] Those who participated in these marches made a public and conspicuous presentation of hygienic modernity, implying that their experience should be shared by all Shanghai people.

The subject matter of these activities was health and hygiene, but the activities incorporated many common features that paralleled other events in the city. Except for the speeches made by medical and public health experts, opening-ceremony procedures bear a striking resemblance to other civic and political gatherings held in the Republican period. One example is National Day celebrations on October 10 that commemorated the founding of the republic. On that day, Shanghai people decorated schools and offices with flags, posters, and archways and held ceremonies that included a musical overture, bowing before the national flag, and celebrity speeches. Not only festivals but also the rallies of the May Fourth and other protest movements followed a similar structure and used similar symbols. Street processions were also copious in Shanghai's public life, and a wide range of religious and secular events took the form of parade.[109] Shanghai people observed annual parades held by native-place organizations to celebrate folk cults and deities and a parade on the Jubilee of Queen Victoria, staged in the International Settlement. Funeral processions and protest demonstration marches were also common in the city.[110] These parades transformed the city into a venue of imaginary journeys of spirits, pageants of power, and theatrical performances. Together, Shanghai people experienced various examples and precedents of mass gathering and street marches. In particular, after the Nationalist takeover of the city, the party designated national holidays and organized

108. "Di-shier jie weisheng yundong baogao," 89.

109. For a fascinating study on street culture in Chengdu, see Di Wang, *Street Culture in Chengdu*.

110. Goodman, "Improvisations on a Semicolonial Theme"; Qiliang He, "Spectacular Death."

memorial ceremonies.[111] As the party sought to capture and exploit these ceremonies to impose its legitimacy, the ceremonies became increasingly standardized and routinized.

The opening ceremony and street-sweeping march in hygiene campaigns were variations of these existing events, and they were more symbolic and demonstrative than practical. To understand the function of the ceremony and procession, we must pay attention to the significance of rituals in Republican Shanghai. Drawing on Clifford Geertz, Wasserstrom argues that power holders depended on ceremonies, popular images, and rituals to justify their authority and legitimacy. Conversely, such rituals and ceremonies can be also used to challenge and undermine authority. Rituals often expressed and evoked emotion and created solidarity among participants. During assemblies and parades, flags, songs, oaths, cheers, and shouts symbolically united participants and audiences to the broader community and nation.[112]

Campaign organizers recognized the power and importance of rituals and gatherings to link hygiene practices, public decorum, and the nation. As campaigns became official, they also provided an opportunity for the Nationalist government to demonstrate, at least symbolically, its concern for the people's well-being, as well as its command of modern medical knowledge. Ceremonies and political objects used in hygiene campaigns symbolized not only the Chinese nation but also the Nationalist state; they connected state authority with personal habits. With a national flag, anthem, and Sun's portrait, the opening ceremony portrayed the party and the state as the legitimate ruler and protector of the people. The wartime government under the Japanese occupation used the same rhetoric and symbols. At the same time, by attending and observing ceremonies and processions, Shanghai residents took part in the campaigns and identified themselves with the ideal of a "healthy citizen." They internalized the behavioral norms presented by the state authority and accepted the idea of the hygienic life defined by the state.

111.   Henrietta Harrison, *Making of the Republican Citizen.*
112.   Wasserstrom, *Student Protests,* 283–93.

MONITORING AND POLICING

During the hygiene campaigns, Shanghai residents gained information and instructions on how to practice good hygiene through written and spoken media, exhibitions, and entertainments. They also observed and participated in ceremonies and street marches so that they could physically take part in particular campaigns. At the same time, hygiene campaigns provided an opportunity for administrators to watch and directly intrude into people's bodies, residences, and everyday lives. To keep an eye on people's behavior, campaign organizers created a monitoring (*jiucha*) section that consisted of Boy Scouts, the police, and the Peace Maintenance Corps (*bao'andui*). They supervised city residents and ordered, and sometimes even forced, rather than instructed, them to behave properly. With help from the police, the purview of monitors was considerably expanded from the 1930s through the 1940s.

Originally, monitors were brought in to keep order at exhibition and ceremony sites.[113] Since these events involved gatherings of large numbers of people, maintaining order was a concern for campaign organizers. Monitors were stationed around the exhibition and ceremony sites to maintain overall order, assist evacuation in case of emergency, and make sure the displays and posters were kept in an orderly manner. They also supervised the entrance of visitors to the exhibition. When the numbers of the visitors exceeded the capacity of the site, the monitors blocked further entrance. Anyone in untidy dress was refused entrance as well. In case of fire, fire extinguishers were prepared, and the monitors were in charge of them.[114]

Keeping order of public sites was probably the monitors' easiest job. They also supervised and reviewed the sweeping and cleaning of the city. During the campaign periods, the campaign headquarters urged people of the city to clean public, residential, and commercial areas, and they monitored their activities. The city's street sweepers became the first target of inspection. They were instructed to keep streets tidy and re-

113.　SMA U1-16-298, 47, 64; SMA R1-12-387, 39; SMA R1-12-406; "Weisheng yundong choubei jingguo baogao," 284; Changwu weiyuanhui, "Shanghai Shi di-shisan jie weisheng yundong baogaoshu," 413–14.

114.　Weisheng yundong choubeihui, "Benshi di-shiwu jie weisheng yundong baogaoshu," 364.

move trash from their assigned areas. The campaign preparation team sent inspectors to supervise their work and make sure their sweeping was done in a satisfactory manner. Inspectors scrutinized not only their work but also their dress, work ethic, and attitudes.[115] The Education Bureau and Social Affairs Bureau, respectively, issued orders that schools and shops should carry out cleaning.[116] The sanitation of certain shops, including restaurants, food shops, barbershops, bathhouses, and hotels, was most carefully supervised. The preparation team and the Public Security Bureau ordered all the food store owners in the Chinese sector of the city to clean out their stores, sweep the stores' environs, and wash the walls with lime powder.[117] In 1936 and 1937, the preparation team offered training courses on occupational hygiene to the staff of these shops. In 1936, 11,194 people from thirteen different occupations took the training.[118] City residents at large were also advised to clean their homes, nearby alleys, and places of work during the campaigns.[119] Policemen on duty were sent to each household to advise residents about cleaning and to examine the state of their houses. In addition to the policemen, the *baojia* system was also used under the Japanese occupation to monitor household cleaning. Staff from the PHB provided notices and instructions to *baojia* chiefs, and these chiefs were responsible for contacting and instructing each resident.[120] Monitors demonstrated the proper way to clean and examined the way in which city residents performed their cleaning duties.[121]

Moreover, monitors patrolled the city and watched people's behavior. Monitoring culminated in the promulgation of the Hygiene Emergency Law (*weisheng jieyanling*) announced in the 1934 hygiene campaign. The

115.   SMA U1-16-298; SMA U1-16-301; SMA R1-12-388; "Di-shier jie weisheng yun-dong baogao," 88; Changwu weiyuanhui, "Shanghai Shi di-shisan jie weisheng yun-dong baogaoshu," 408, 413.

116.   SMA R1-12-387; SMA R50-735; "Di-shier jie weisheng yundong baogao," 88.

117.   "Di-shier jie weisheng yundong baogao," 88.

118.   SMA U1-16-301, 17–18; Weisheng yundong choubeihui, "Benshi di-shiwu jie weisheng yundong baogaoshu (xu)," 400–402.

119.   SMA R1-12-388, 39; "Di-shier jie weisheng yundong baogao," 88.

120.   SMA R1-12-389.

121.   Weisheng yundong choubeihui, "Benshi di-shiwu jie weisheng yundong baogaoshu (xu)," 396–99.

Emergency Law consisted of five articles: (1) Do not spit in public; (2) Do not urinate in public; (3) Always drink boiled water; (4) Always dump refuse in trash boxes; and (5) Seek out anti-epidemic vaccinations. Although this set of articles was called an "emergency law," its contents in fact pertained to mundane personal practices.[122] In addition to the police force and the Boy Scouts, the New Life Advisory Corps (Quandaodui) also joined the monitoring section to carry out the Emergency Law of 1934. With the campaign kickoff, monitors were sent to patrol the city.[123] According to the plan for this campaign, when a policeman discovered any resident spitting in public, he should order the offender to wipe up the spittle with a piece of paper or a handkerchief. If the offender refused, he or she could be arrested. Likewise, a policeman could arrest anyone who urinated in public and punish them accordingly.[124]

In implementing the Hygiene Emergency Law, monitors and policemen were directly involved in people's everyday behavior and imposed penalties on unseemly practices. The use of laws and penalties to maintain a clean environment was not unique to hygiene campaigns. In fact, the city had a bylaw that prohibited anyone from spitting in public, and enforcement of that law and imposing fines on offenders had been a topic of debate among Shanghai's public health administrators for some time. In this regard, a discussion in the Public Health Department of the International Settlement in 1942 deserves special attention. The topic of the discussion concerned the enforcement of the bylaw that prescribed a five-dollar fine for those who spat in public spaces. The inspectors agreed that the bylaw had been applied reasonably well in licensed premises, such as food shops, restaurants, and laundries. However, it was almost impossible to enforce it in the streets, on public vehicles, and in other public areas. The inspectors were understaffed, and, with a large number of offenders, they were afraid that the imposition of a fine might antagonize the whole community. They believed that many, though not all, of the offenders were "uneducated" Chinese who lacked knowledge of or consciousness

122.   "Dahui biaoyu ji jieyanling"; SMA U1-16-298.
123.   "Weisheng yundong kaimuji," 297; Changwu weiyuanhui, "Shanghai Shi di-shisan jie weisheng yundong baogaoshu," 414.
124.   "Public Health Movement."

about hygiene. Thus, they concluded that an educational campaign on the harm of spitting was necessary. Yet, they also doubted the effectiveness of conventional campaign methods. They pointed out that even though civic organizations had held anti-spitting campaigns for three years, and even though the city was filled with anti-spitting posters and streamers, public spitting had not decreased that much. Some thought a penalty against offenders could be more effective in preventing spitting than posters and notices, but they also realized the imposition of a penalty could be very difficult. The discussion went round and round, and did not reach a conclusion.[125]

The Emergency Law also raised the issue of penalty and law enforcement in the context of public health. But since it was the 1934 campaign preparation team—an agency with no law-enforcement power—that created and implemented the Emergency Law, and the measure was only temporary, the actual effectiveness of the measure was uncertain. Again, the "law" was symbolic rather than practical. Nevertheless, the use of law enforcement was a considerable departure from the YMCA's educational campaigns. It meant the city residents were now closely watched and expected to behave properly and conform to the hygiene regulations.

Most closely monitored was the anti-epidemic vaccination drives carried out as part of campaign programs.[126] Of all the campaign programs, the anti-epidemic injection drive stood out, because unlike other campaign activities, it was a medical program aimed at preventing specific diseases. Medical knowledge and expertise were required to produce the vaccine and give the injections, and physicians and nurses had to have direct physical contact with the people to administer injections.

The cholera vaccination program in the 1934 hygiene campaign is well documented, and the records suggest that the delivery of vaccinations betrayed a degree of social discrimination. The vaccination programs were conducted in three ways. First, anyone in the city could receive a free vaccination at designated hospitals and clinics on a voluntary basis. City

125. SMA U1-16-2192 contains the accounts of the anti-spitting campaign of 1942.
126. The vaccine used combined anti-cholera, anti-typhoid, and anti-dysentery agents, but it was usually referred to as either an "anti-epidemic vaccine" or an "anti-cholera vaccine."

residents were strongly encouraged to receive a vaccination, but they were not forced to do so. Second, the PHB sent doctors to schools, factories, and shops so that students and workers could receive an injection without going to a hospital. Finally, rickshaw pullers and shantytown dwellers were slated to receive compulsory injections. They were considered malnourished and not able to care about the quality of their drinking water. Only the poorest of the working poor were subjected to compulsory injections. To deliver vaccinations to Shanghai's rickshaw pullers, campaign organizers set up nineteen "injection stations" across the city. They enlisted forty doctors, seventy nurses, eighty-two Boy Scouts, forty-six staff persons, and fifteen detective inspectors from all three sectors of Shanghai to administer the vaccinations. When the hygiene campaign got under way, staff persons and Boy Scouts were sent into the streets, where, in cooperation with the police, they stopped rickshaw pullers to determine whether or not they had been vaccinated. Unless a rickshaw puller could show a valid certificate of vaccination, he was taken to a nearby injection station to receive a shot. If he refused the vaccination, he would either be arrested or have his rickshaw license confiscated.[127] Those who lived in Shanghai's shantytowns were another target of compulsory injections. In 1934 the anti-epidemic section of the hygiene campaign designated five areas in which compulsory vaccinations should be implemented. An inspector or a detective, a doctor, and a nurse made up a team. These teams were sent into shantytown areas and paid house visits. The inspector explained to the residents the significance of the vaccination and supervised the injection, while doctor and nurse administered it.[128] The PHB reported that the anti-epidemic section vaccinated tens of thousands of rickshaw pullers and shantytown residents on the first day of the campaign.[129]

Compared with other campaign programs, these cholera vaccination drives were more pragmatic and could have a direct effect on the prevention of diseases and the improvement of the city's public health. In spite of the intrusive nature of injections, the vaccination programs did not

127. "Public Health Movement."
128. Ibid.
129. "Weisheng yundong kaimuji," 297.

meet much resistance. In fact, one *Shenbao* writer complained about the shortage of free injection stations.[130] Not everyone might have received injections willingly, but many did so voluntarily.

Indeed, injection was one of the most popular medical programs in Republican Shanghai. The injection drive remained a standard campaign program during the Japanese occupation period.[131] This popularity grew not only from the medical efficacy of the vaccine but also from the popular belief in effectiveness of injection and the use of syringes. As Frank Dikötter has pointed out, the syringe was omnipresent in Republican Shanghai's medical culture. Injections were regarded as an effective method to nourish the body, as well as to cure and prevent many diseases.[132] As we have seen in previous chapters, doctors in summer-disease hospitals boasted about saline injections for cholera patients, and the PHB frequently organized injection drives. Since injections were an important technique of Western biomedicine, and only qualified doctors were allowed to administer them, the syringe helped establish the medical authority of doctors. In the 1920s and 1930s, the common use of syringes and the popularity of vaccination went hand in hand. Hygiene campaign organizers took full advantage of the popular belief in the efficacy of injections. Medical knowledge and technique became an instrument of the municipal authority to discipline and control people's bodies and obtain people's consent.

Health and hygiene remained the responsibility of individuals. However, as the municipal government became the sponsor of the campaigns, with its capacity to deploy law enforcement and command of medical knowledge, the state became actively involved in people's lives and bodies. The belief in modern medical science superseded the fear of intrusive injections and supported hygiene campaigns.

130. Mengruo, "Tanyan."
131. For the Japanese accounts on cholera in Shanghai, see GK I-3-2-0-6, 7, 8, 9, 10, 11, and 12. On the injections in Manchuria under the Japanese rule, Rogaski, "Vampires in Plagueland."
132. Dikötter, "Cultural History of the Syringe."

Conclusion

Overall, how effective were these hygiene campaigns to educate people? Did they improve Shanghai's public health and attain their goals? Several scholars have argued that, in spite of the persistence of sanitary problems, the overall standards of public health improved in Republican China; such scholars have given Nationalists high marks.[133] Christian Henriot, in particular, has concluded that, in Shanghai, given the limited resources and time constraints, the public health policies of the Nationalists were mostly successful.[134] Demographers have also discussed the relationship between mortality and changes in public health and personal hygiene habits. In his study of Beijing, Cameron Campbell has pointed out that China's death rate had begun falling in the early twentieth century without substantial improvements in living standards. He has suggested that public health work in the 1920s and 1930s, including health education, contributed to the decrease in mortality.[135] In early twentieth-century Shanghai, the fear and danger of germs and infection were real. As a greater number of people moved to the city and lived in close proximity to one another, and the city lacked proper sewage systems, infectious diseases posed serious threat. Although hygiene campaigns taught only rudimentary knowledge of pathology and bacteriology (and medical science alone did not solve problems of public health), they induced Shanghai people to change their behavior. Shanghai residents heard practical and useful information and admonition through campaign programs. The focus of many of the teachings of the campaigns, including washing hands, drinking boiled water, and not sharing cups and towels, are still regarded and promoted as effective ways to avoid germs. These personal habits prevented dangerous encounters with diseases and likely contributed to helping Shanghai people stay well.

At the same time, hygiene campaigns were a sociopolitical event. Their subjects were health and hygiene, but they served other needs as well: to teach people moral lessons, unite them under the national flag,

---

133. Yip, *Health and National Reconstruction*.
134. Henriot, *Shanghai, 1928–1937*.
135. Campbell, "Public Health Efforts in China"; Campbell, "Mortality Change."

and strengthen the nation. Various scholars have discussed how the concern for national survival helped the expansion of state power and how state authorities controlled and supervised the quotidian lives of people in Republican China.[136] In this chapter I have also suggested that hygiene campaigns promoted the links among personal bodies, social manner and etiquette, and national strength. Believing that they were helping Shanghai people learn how to stay well, the city's elites initiated hygiene campaigns. The Nationalist government's involvement in campaigns and the advent of the New Life Movement made these campaigns state-sponsored events, and it became clear that the health of the nation depended on personal hygiene practice and the Nationalist state should guide the masses. Hygiene campaigns began as educational programs organized by progressive elites, but, as campaigns became official and grew larger, their goal shifted from achieving individual well-being to national salvation. Hoping that the state could bring order and discipline and save the Chinese people and Chinese nation, Chinese elites designed campaign programs and closely worked with the Nationalist state to monitor and even force people to follow prescribed norms by using the police forces. The bodies and behavior of Shanghai people served as a primary site and target of the exercise of power. In the end, hygiene campaigns fostered docility among the population. Being healthy and hygienic was a citizen's duty—not a right.

However, overseeing and supervising were only an aspect of the campaign programs. Campaigns adopted many other methods that evolved from the city's urban culture. Power operated not only between the Nationalist state and Shanghai people; it could be interactive and flowed among individual citizens through social and cultural networks. In addition to monitors and the police force, various types of people were involved in campaigns. They included YMCA members who published campaign materials, schoolteachers who gave public lectures on hygiene, workers and students who attended opening ceremonies and sweeping marches, Boy Scouts who performed the "oath of hygiene," and doctors and nurses who gave compulsory injections on the street. These individuals and groups worked as agents of the state to promote the ideals of a

136.   Glosser, *Chinese Visions of Family and State*, 19; Zhiwei Xiao, "Movie House Etiquette Reform"; Yamin Xu, "Policing Civility."

hygienic life and a healthy body, and their goals and interests also shaped the meanings and practices of hygiene campaigns. In the hygiene campaign, coercion, policing, publicity, education, and rituals all coexisted and complemented each other. The city's mass media promoted germ theory and supported compulsory injections, while campaign ceremonies and processions helped attendees and spectators identify themselves with the nation.

Henrietta Harrison has discussed the emergence of a new sense of Republican citizenship and nationhood in early twentieth-century China. She argues that this new sense was not simply imposed by political elites on the people; it developed through daily customs and objects that symbolized the new Republic, and its creators, disseminators, and recipients were all involved in the process of its development.[137] Harrison's points are relevant here. Hygiene campaigns offered occasions in which the abstract concepts of national strength and hygienic modernity interacted with and penetrated into the everyday lives of Shanghai Chinese through various programs, and many Shanghai people voluntarily joined together in these programs. Campaign programs created a readiness among the population to accept such opportunities and eventually became part of the city's culture.

In this regard, the Republican-era hygiene campaigns influenced the patriotic hygiene campaigns of the Communist period. As Campbell has noted, the Communist state also identified health-related work with modernity. Patriotic sentiment motivated individuals to voluntarily perform unpaid labor and made society receptive and willing to cooperate with state policies. In her discussion of the Patriotic Hygiene Campaign in Tianjin in 1952, Rogaski also notes that the Communists adopted campaign methods similar to those of the Nationalists, and the Communist Patriotic Hygiene Campaign was both a "continuation and culmination" of the pursuit of public health since the Republican period.[138]

Finally, hygiene campaigns were related to the efforts of Shanghai elites to create a national identity and social unity among the city's

---

137. Henrietta Harrison, *Making of the Republican Citizen.*
138. Patriotic hygiene campaigns in the Communist period also adopted methods similar to the Republican campaigns. See *SWZ*, 217–231; Campbell, "Mortality Change," 224–25; Rogaski, "Nature, Annihilation, and Modernity."

populace. Although some campaign programs targeted working-class people and the poor, the campaigns did not emphasize class or gender distinctions. Campaign organizers and their agents differentiated those who were healthy and hygienic from those who were not, but they did not attempt to eliminate or exclude the "unfit" or "unclean." Rather, the campaigns attempted to unify everyone in Shanghai. They even provided a marketing opportunity for the city's merchants, which is the subject of the next chapter.

CHAPTER 4

Selling Hygiene, Supporting Nation

Health, Hygiene, and Commercial Culture

In this chapter I examine the issues of health and hygiene from the angle of business and commerce, and focus on industrialists, merchants, and entrepreneurs—another important group in the city that contributed to the creation and development of the discourse of health, cleanliness, and nationalism. People of Shanghai had many concerns about and insights into physical well-being and environmental sanitation. But the focus and nature of particular concerns and insights were framed differently by diverse elements of Shanghai's population. Whereas Chinese reformers, medical elites, and Nationalist administrators believed that a healthy people and a clean environment were signifiers of a modern nation, Shanghai's businessmen realized that "being healthful" could add market value to their merchandise. They made the most of this potential with advertising that emphasized how their goods would make consumers healthy and clean. They also diligently searched for the best gimmicks and schemes to reduce prime costs and attract price-conscious clientele. Through an examination of commercial strategies and pitches employed by a group of Shanghai businessmen, we learn how the idea of health became integral to Shanghai's commercial culture and how Shanghai's merchants and manufacturers affected consumers' awareness and understanding of health and hygiene.

In the early twentieth century, Shanghai's entrepreneurs established a variety of businesses that manufactured and retailed products that were directly or indirectly related to personal health and hygiene. In their commercial activities, these businesses also helped promote the ideal of physical well-being and bodily cleanliness and connected personal hygiene to national health and the act of buying. The commercial rendering of hygiene practices had as much, if not more, influence in shaping people's perceptions of the body, society, and nation as did the efforts of administrators and intellectuals. Shanghai's businessmen sold more than just "things." In their commercial promotions, they gave symbolic meanings and values to their goods, and manipulated these meanings to generate greater demand for their merchandise. At the same time, consumers had the freedom to select particular products. Their choices reflected not only their financial means but also their attitudes toward hygiene, appreciation of science, and loyalty for the nation. In sum, selling and buying were not only personal: both actions had larger social and cultural implications.

The scholarship on Chinese entrepreneurs is broad and diverse. Some studies focus on power relations between the urban capitalist class and the state,[1] while others pay close attention to the culture created by and developed through commercial activities. I have been profoundly influenced by a number of historians of business, consumerism, and culture in China, such as Sherman Cochran, Parks Coble, Wen-hsin Yeh, and Weipin Tsai. These scholars have pointed out that China's local businesses skillfully emulated and appropriated Western ideas, products, and business styles. Moreover, Chinese merchants cleverly invented their own marketing strategies by exploiting native-place ties and family connections. They were able to overcome political constraints and successfully create commercial networks that extended across regional and national boundaries, and in the end, they outdid their foreign counterparts.[2] At the same time, the very acts of sales and purchase could be overtly political. In his study of the National Products Movement (Guohuo yundong), Karl Gerth observes the close connection between the consumption of commodities and nationalism. He argues that Chinese entrepreneurs and consumers contributed to the formation of modern nationalism by making

    1.   Coble, *Shanghai Capitalists*; Fewsmith, *Party, State, and Local Elite*.
    2.   Cochran, ed., *Inventing Nanjing Road*; Cochran, "Marketing Medicine"; Cochran, *Chinese Medicine Men*; Yeh, *Shanghai Splendor*; Tsai, *Reading Shenbao*; Coble, *Chinese Capitalists*.

a point of buying and selling China's "national" products.[3] Using various methods and approaches, all of these scholars illustrate how commercial activities and entrepreneurship fashioned not only the economy but also Chinese politics, social values, and national identity.

Building on this scholarship, I demonstrate that Shanghai entrepreneurs materialized, commodified, and popularized various connotations and conceptualizations of health and hygiene. Over the first three decades of the twentieth century, a number of Chinese entrepreneurs opened light industries to manufacture various consumer goods related to personal health and bodily cleanliness. Unlike social reformers, philanthropists, and public health officers, the primary motivation for these entrepreneurs was profit. Precisely because they were doing business, they had every incentive to present the "hygienic effects" of their merchandise in an easily understandable manner and to place their "healthful goods" within easy reach of consumers. Their commercial activities significantly contributed to the creation of a national discourse on health and hygiene.

Sherman Cochran has done extensive research on the development of Chinese-owned Western-style drugstores and pharmaceutical industries in late nineteenth- and early twentieth-century Shanghai.[4] Cochran argues that, in selling Chinese brands of Western medicines and supplements, Chinese owners of these drugstores freely and rather arbitrarily used both Chinese and Western images in their ads. Disregarding academic and political struggles between the supporters of Western medicine and Chinese medicine, Shanghai's drugstore owners took advantage of the permeable boundary between Chinese and Western ideas on health and medicine in their sales strategies to promote various kinds of pseudo-Western drugs and supplements. Consequently, by the 1930s, these Chinese retailers commanded a considerable share of Shanghai's pharmaceutical market. Shanghai residents purchased Western drugs primarily from Chinese-owned stores and acquired firsthand knowledge and images of Western drugs through their advertisements and store displays.

3. Gerth, *China Made*.

4. On the development of new-style drugstores in Shanghai, see Cochran, "Marketing Medicine"; Shanghai shehui kexueyuan jingji yanjiusuo, ed., *Shanghai jindai xiyao hangyeshi*.

Cochran's study made a significant contribution to our understanding of China's commercial culture. However, drugstore owners were not the only ones to publicize the healthful effects of their goods. A quick review of popular magazines and newspapers from the 1920s and 1930s reveals that many different businesses used the terms "hygienic" (*weisheng*), "healthful" (*jiankang*), and "clean" (*qingjie*) to describe a wide range of merchandise. Toiletries, cosmetics, clothes, bedding, home appliances, shoes, food, beverage, and even tobacco were products described with such terms.[5] Of the many Shanghai businesses that advocated the healthful effects of their products, this chapter focuses on "everyday use chemical product industries" (*riyong huaxue gongye*), which, under the aegis of germ theory and sanitary science, introduced and sold personal-hygiene items, including soap, toothpaste and toothpowder, and other toiletries, as well as pesticides and disinfectants for domestic use.[6] Supposedly having the capacity to neutralize harmful objects, all these items were intended for direct use on individual bodies or in personal residences. They were also "chemical" products: chemically manufactured, composed of chemical compounds, and chemically, rather than mechanically, eliminating germs, dirt, and other filthy materials. Owners of these businesses generally had some background in chemistry and applied their knowledge to the manufacturing of their merchandise. These products all harnessed chemical means for practical use—removing dirt and tartar and killing germs and pests. In sum, these personal-hygiene items had the potential to evoke clear and powerful images of clean bodies and a hygienic lifestyle based on modern science. They helped define standards of cleanliness and the proper appearance of the body, as well as promote the "common sense" of hygiene and social etiquette among ordinary Shanghai residents.

These personal-hygiene items were promoted on the back of China's nation-building discourse from the late nineteenth and early twentieth centuries. As discussed in previous chapters, under pressure from the West and Japan, Chinese elites of all political stripes were convinced that a healthy people was the foundation of a strong nation and that a hygienic

5.   For a range of *weisheng* items, see Juanjuan Peng, "Selling a Healthy Lifestyle."
6.   This term "chemical products for everyday use" (*riyong huaxuepin*) is still used today. See, for example, Wang Shenmin, ed., *Riyong huaxuepin*; Zhou Xueliang, ed., *Riyong huaxuepin*.

lifestyle was a mark of civilization. During the Republican period, owners of industries that sold personal-hygiene items were well aware of these ideas and their broad appeal. They were quick to seize on such ideas to produce effective rhetoric to sell their products and gain comparative advantage over foreign competitors. In doing so, they actively participated in and responded to the city's mass movements. They cooperated with the municipal government and took part in hygiene campaigns; they supported the New Life Movement; and they strongly endorsed the National Products Movement. By advocating these mass movements, Shanghai's everyday-chemical industrialists worked closely with the Nationalist state. Their efforts indirectly and inadvertently aided in the expansion of state authority; state and business interests in promoting hygiene practices and cultivating modern civility converged. At the same time, however, these mass movements were not always conducted in a top-down manner. In fact, Shanghai's entrepreneurs exercised considerable discretion in how to participate in these movements and used them for their advantage. They provided the new everyday-chemical industries with opportunities to promote their products and gave them a certain prestige. In their efforts to expand their markets, Shanghai's businessmen manipulated and exploited patriotic rhetoric presented by the state, and invented new representation of their products.

Zwia Lipkin wrote that the Nationalists "created a myth of a unified China and a Chinese nation that was stronger than reality."[7] She has argued that in its efforts to make a new society, the Nationalist state discovered "undesirable" social elements and attempted to correct them so that they would be fit for the ideals of the "myth." Shanghai's businessmen also contributed to this myth-making and used the language of national strengthening in their sales talks. They established their patriotic credentials, and their ads invoked a sense of community and nation that included and united all Chinese. In doing so, however, they also added new twists and nuance to the patriotic discourse in order to stimulate consumers' desire and build a larger customer base for their products. Unlike the state, they did not identify or label people as "undesirable" or "unwanted." Rather they encouraged and invited Shanghai people of all social strata to participate in the myth-making process by buying

7. Lipkin, *Useless to the State*, 203.

their merchandise. Anyone could buy and use their soap, toothpaste, and other items. Together, all Chinese people could defend their society and nation from dirt, disease, and foreign capitalism.

Below we examine the close and complex relations between hygiene practices, state-sponsored mass movements, and private businesses.

Development of Light Industries and Interest in Chemistry

Westerners first brought mass quantities of personal-hygiene items to China after the opening of treaty ports following the Opium War. Of these goods, soap quickly became popular; individually wrapped bars of Western soap (*yangjian*) were among the first items to attract the attention of Chinese consumers.[8] As early as 1859, Chinese literati regarded Western soap as a suitable gift for friends, and by the 1860s, specialty shops in Shanghai were selling Western goods, including soap.[9] Western soap even became a subject of *zhuzhici*, Shanghai's popular verse, during the Guangxu era (1875–1908). One author described laundry soap (*xiyi feizao*) as "beautiful and inexpensive" (*wumei lianjia*) and "widely recognized" (*ming yuanbo*). Another author wrote that toilet soap (*xiangyi*) was "nicely packaged" (*zhuangxiamei*) and had a "sweet smell" (*fenfang qiwei*).[10]

As soap became popular and demand increased, Western and Japanese soap companies opened factories in Chinese coastal cities.[11] The

8. Before the introduction of Western soap, Chinese commonly used ashes from plants or clams, which contain potassium compounds, and native soap (*tujian* or *tuzao*) made of lime as laundry detergents. They also used pig pancreas (*zhuyi*), which contains enzymes that dissolve fat and protein, and pods of Chinese honey locust (*zaojia*), which contain saponin, to wash their bodies and clothing. See Yang Dajin, ed., *Xiandai Zhongguo shiyezhi*, 472; Chen Xinwen, *Zhongguo jindai huaxue gongyeshi*, 122–23; Liu Shanling, *Xiyang feng*, 187–88.

9. Li Changli, *WanQing Shanghai*, 54, 127.

10. For some *zhuzhici* about Western soap, see Gu Bingquan, ed., *Shanghai yangchang zhuzhici*, 154.

11. Yin Wei and Ren Mei, *Zhongguo muyu wenhua*, 170; Liu Shanling, *Xiyang feng*, 188–89; Yang Dajin, ed., *Xiandai Zhongguo shiyezhi*, 472, 493.

earliest soap factories in Shanghai were opened by small Japanese entrepreneurs. Virtue Accumulating Company (Sekizen yōkō) opened the first factory around 1900, and by 1913 at least seven Japanese factories operated in the city. The Japanese continued to open soap factories throughout the 1920s and 1930s. Except for Shanghai Oil and Fat Corporation (Shanghai yushi kabushiki gaisha), most of these companies were small and obscure, and many of them did not endure very long. But they introduced basic soap-making techniques to China and provided an example for the Chinese to follow.[12]

In addition to these small Japanese makers, Lever Brothers in China (LBC), a British corporation, entered China. LBC opened its headquarters in Shanghai in 1911 to take charge of distribution of British soap exports. In 1923, under the name China Soap Company (Zhongguo zhizaochang), LBC built its own factory in Shanghai for manufacturing several well-known brands of British soap, including Lux and Sunlight. In 1930 LBC merged with a Dutch margarine company to form the Unilever Corporation. Unilever evolved into the largest supplier of Western soap in China.[13] Taking advantage of China's low tariffs and lack of legal restrictions, and viewing China as an important prospective market, Western and Japanese businesses became active in China.

Encouraged by the evident profitability of these companies, Chinese entrepreneurs soon mastered the basic chemical techniques for producing soap and launched their own businesses. Xu Huafeng (1858–1928) opened Broadening Skills Company (Guangyi gongsi) in 1889 in Shanghai to produce soap and candles.[14] Song Zejiu (1867–1956) opened Tianjin Soap Manufacturing Company (Tianjin zhiyi gongsi) in 1905 to produce soap and toothpowder.[15] Following their lead, other Chinese

12. On Shanghai's Japanese soap makers, see Xu Jinsheng, *Jindai Shanghai Rizi gongyeshi*, 78–84.

13. On Unilever in China, see Zurndorfer, "Imperialism, Globalization, and the Soap/Suds Industry"; *Shanghai zhizaochang changzhi* bianshen weiyuanhui, ed., *Shanghai zhizaochang changzhi*; Wang Daren, "Yingshang Zhongguo feizao gongsi"; Xiang Zenan, "Yingshang Zhonguo feizao gongsi."

14. Xu Huafeng is the third son of Xu Shou. Chen Xinwen, *Zhongguo jindai huaxue gongyeshi*, 342–45.

15. Guo Hongxiao, "Song Zejiu," 426.

entrepreneurs began opening factories to produce soap and other toiletries in the early decades of the twentieth century.

Many of these enterprises began their operations in the 1910s and 1920s, with Shanghai at the center of their business activities, and the sector continued growing until the outbreak of the Second Sino-Japanese War in 1937. Following the opening of Nanyang Candle and Soap Manufacturer (Nanyang zhuzaochang) in the late years of the Guangxu era, many soap factories were built in the city.[16] Between 1912 and 1924, more than sixteen Chinese soap factories had opened.[17] On the eve of the war, some sixty to seventy soap makers operated in the city.[18] Among the city's Chinese soap makers, Five Continents-Guben (Koopun) Soap Manufacturer (Wuzhou Guben zaochang) was the largest.[19]

Contemporary accounts of the toothpowder and toothpaste industry are scarce. Like soap, toothpowder was first introduced to China by foreign companies, Japanese and American in particular. But Chinese industrialists lost no time in entering this business. In 1890, Zhang Jinqing opened a "powder shop" and sold Tiger toothpowder, the first Chinese brand.[20] Because toothpowder production was simple and easy, the industry developed rapidly.[21] In the late nineteenth century, some twenty-eight kinds of foreign toothpowder were sold in the Chinese market, and by 1910, dental-care products were widely available in China.[22] In the 1910s, several well-known Chinese brands of toothpowder appeared on the market. These included Three Stars (Sanxing), made by China Chemical

16. Yang Dajin, ed., *Xiandai Zhongguo shiyezhi*, 473; Chen Xinwen, *Zhongguo jindai huaxue gongyeshi*, 125.

17. Chen Xinwen, *Zhongguo jindai huaxue gongyeshi*, 126.

18. Yang Dehui and Dong Wenzhong, *Shanghai zhi gongshangye*, 39; Shanghai Shi shehuiju, ed., *Shanghai zhi jizhi gongye*, 109–112; Shanghai tebieshi shehuiju, ed., *Shanghai zhi gongye*, 57–59.

19. In 1921, Five Continents Drugstore (Wuzhou yaofang) purchased a German soap plant in Shanghai and reorganized it into Five Continents-Guben Soap Manufacturer. Five Continents Drugstore had been opened some years earlier by Huang Chujiu. Xiang Songmao replaced Huang to become the store's owner in 1916. On Huang Chujiu and Xiang Songmao, see Cochran, *Chinese Medicine Man*, chap. 3; Tan Yulin, "Huang Chujiu"; Tan Yulin, "Xiang Songmao, Xiang Shengwu."

20. Huang Zhiwei and Huang Ying, eds., *Wei shiji daiyan*, 237.

21. Yang Dajin, ed., *Xiandai Zhongguo shiyezhi*, 540, 547.

22. Huang Zhiwei and Huang Ying, eds., *Wei shiji daiyan*, 237; Dikötter, *Exotic Commodities*, 209–11.

Industries Company (Zhongguo huaxue gongyeshe); Invincible (Wudi), made by Household Industries Company (Jiating gongyeshe); and Girl in Moon (Yueli chang'e), a product of Yonghe Enterprises Corporation (Yonghe shiye gongsi). Before long these companies began producing and marketing toothpaste, though toothpaste did not completely replace toothpowder.[23] In the 1930s, numerous small workshops still manufactured toothpowder, and by the 1940s there were at least seventy-eight dental-care enterprises in Shanghai.[24]

Although they differed with respect to age and social background, many of the owners of these early twentieth-century businesses shared certain similarities. Unlike the supporters of the self-strengthening movement, who worked closely with late-Qing officials to initiate new industries, these entrepreneurs did not enjoy government connections or backing; unlike the compradors, who acted as crucial middlemen for Western businesses, none had strong ties with Western companies; unlike medical doctors, with some exceptions, they had not received advanced educations in science at a university. Since these businesses required only small amounts of capital and simple equipment, many started out as cottage industries. Unlike classically trained literati, these entrepreneurs were more interested in hands-on work and practical experiments than book learning. Few had much training in the classics, but many of them had some knowledge of elementary science, in particular basic chemistry. Among these entrepreneurs, the educational background of Chen Diexian, the founder of Household Industries Company, was exceptional. Chen's literati training, work as the chief editor of *Jiating changshi huibian* (*JCHB*) (Collection of Household Common Knowledge), and activities in the National Products Movement will be discussed later in this chapter.[25]

---

23. Toothpowder and toothpaste were often classified in the same category as cosmetics. Yang Dajin, ed., *Xiandai Zhongguo shiyezhi*, 540.

24. Ibid., 540–41, 547; Yang Dehui and Dong Wenzhong, *Shanghai zhi gongshangye*, 38; *Shanghai riyong gongyepin shangyezhi* bianzuan weiyuanhui, ed., *Shanghai riyong gongyepin shangyezhi*, 82; Shanghai Shi shehuiju, ed., *Shanghai zhi jizhi gongye*, 113–18; Shanghai tebieshi shehuiju, ed., *Shanghai zhi gongye*, 52–57.

25. On Chen Diexian and Household Industries, see, for example, Zhang Huimin, "Chen Diexian"; Zhang Huimin, "Chen Diexian yu Jiating gongyeshe"; Meng Yuan, "Zhongqing riyong huagong."

Soap, toothpaste, and other personal-hygiene items were categorized as "chemical products" (*huaxue yongpin*) produced by "chemical industry" (*huaxue gongye*). For the early twentieth-century Chinese, these items embodied modern Western chemistry and its efficacy, and this status contributed to their popularity.[26] Western chemistry was first introduced to China in the late nineteenth century through translations of foreign texts.[27] Following the loss of two Opium Wars and the devastating Taiping Civil War, Chinese reformers realized the necessity of learning and promoting Western military technology and science. They opened arsenals, shipyards, and new schools; they also sponsored the translation and publication of scientific works. Jiangnan Arsenal Translation Bureau was an important center for the translation of various works on science and technology, including treatises for specialists as well as introductory textbooks targeting lay readers.[28] Although official support for science was marginal in the Qing government, the popularity of science books and magazines among the reading public steadily increased from the 1870s through the early twentieth century. Lay readers of these magazines could acquire basic knowledge of chemistry, and some of them applied that knowledge to simple experiments, such as making soap and toothpowder.

The earliest recipe for making soap appeared in *Gezhi huibian* (*GZHB*) (The Chinese Scientific Magazine) in 1876.[29] The goal of *GZHB*, edited by John Fryer (1839–1928), Xu Shou (1818–84), and other members of the Chinese staff of the Jiangnan Arsenal Translation Bureau, was to spread scientific knowledge to a wide audience.[30] Altogether sixty issues of *GZHB* were published between 1876 and 1892, with some interruptions. It is estimated that three thousand copies of this magazine were printed

26.   For an overview of the history of light industries and entrepreneurs in modern Shanghai, see Xu Xinwu and Huang Hanmin, eds., *Shanghai jindai gongyeshi*; *Shanghai riyong gongyepin shangyezhi* bianzuan weiyuanhui, ed., *Shanghai riyong gongyepin shangyezhi*; Huang Hanmin and Lu Xinglong, *Jindai Shanghai gongye qiye fazhanshilun*. Also see Yang Dajin, ed., *Xiandai Zhongguo shiyezhi*; Yang Dehui and Dong Wenzhong, *Shanghai zhi gongshangye*.

27.   On the history of chemistry in China, see Reardon-Anderson, *Study of Change*.

28.   On scientific translation in late-Qing China, see Wright, *Translating Science*.

29.   Liu Shanling, *Xiyang feng*.

30.   On Fryer and Xu Shou, see Bennett, *John Fryer*. On *GZHB*, see Elman, *On Their Own Terms*, 314–19.

at the start of the publication, and four thousand copies circulated monthly in the 1880s. Issues were distributed in Shanghai and other treaty port cities.[31] The magazine exclusively covered science, technology, and engineering. In addition to translations of English articles and original Chinese articles, the magazine also contained letters and inquiries from readers, many of which concerned practical matters and technical issues.

The September 1876 issue of *GZHB* carries an exemplary inquiry from a reader in Fuzhou who asked about the ingredients and recipe for making soap. The editors responded to his inquiry by providing the following instructions. First, prepare pig lard (*zhuyou*) or olive oil. Then, melt it in an iron or lead pan; cow or sheep lard (*niuyangyou*) could be used as substitutes. Use a cloth of tight texture to filter it, then, add six *liang* of refined salt (*jingyan*) and three *liang* of white vitriol (*baifan*) per one hundred *jin* of lard. Mix well and keep it still for a while. Heat it again and gradually add caustic soda (sodium hydroxide) (*jianshui*). Mix it well with a wooden spoon, add coloring and perfume if desired, pour it in wooden molds, and let it sit for twelve hours until it coagulates. The editors also explained how to produce caustic soda: to obtain one hundred *jin* of caustic soda, mix twenty-five *liang* of quicklime with water; after the white solid precipitates, use the top clean layer. Finally the editor commented that "since soap making does not require particularly high heat, soap can be conveniently made at home. This home-made soap is a bit costly but of good quality."[32]

Two years later, a certain Mr. Yang from Guangzhou also wrote to ask about the proper kind of caustic soda to make soap. He had used potassium hydroxide (KOH), but the final product was too soft to sell. He asked where he could obtain sodium hydroxide (NaOH) to make harder soap. The editors responded that sodium hydroxide could be purchased in Hong Kong and also advised that it was easily produced by blending water and sodium oxide.[33]

Before the twentieth century, scientific knowledge did not have much pull in China's mainstream political system or within its intellectual

31. Britton, *Chinese Periodical Press*, 60–61. Also see Wright, *Translating Science*, 181.
32. "Huxiang wenda" (1876), 10–11.
33. "Huxiang wenda" (1880), 16.

framework. Nevertheless, interest in science was clearly growing. These accounts in *GZHB* suggest that by the late 1870s there was a readership for popular science that was sufficiently familiar with new chemical nomenclature to understand the basic process of saponification—turning fat or oil into soap by a reaction with alkali—in scientific terms. As the letter from Mr. Yang suggests, amateur scientists also considered selling their soap. China's defeat in the First Sino-Japanese War and the collapse of the Qing dynasty had opened the way for scientific development, and science would be wholeheartedly embraced by May Fourth intellectuals as a way forward for the nation.

Increasing numbers of Chinese became interested in industrial chemistry and chemical manufacturing in the twentieth century. Chinese universities opened chemistry departments, and university graduates went abroad to pursue higher degrees. Interest in chemistry was not limited to elites and those in the academic community. Popular interest in chemical manufacturing continued to grow among the reading public as well. Pieces that appeared in *JCHB* illustrate this point. In the 1910s, *Shenbao ziyoutan* (Shenbao Free Talks), a popular supplement to *Shenbao*, featured the column "Household Common Knowledge" (*jiating changshi*), which included contributions from readers. Chen Diexian, the chief editor, and his assistants compiled these contributions together with other subjects in the book series *JCHB*.[34] First published in 1918, the series included eight volumes and had gone through twenty editions by 1941.

JCHB was divided into several sections, such as *fuyong* (clothing and articles), *yinshi* (food and drink), *renti* (human body), *dongwu* (animals), and *gongyi* (technology or craft). It covered a wide range of topics and tips on housekeeping, including how to properly wash hats, how to polish silverware, how to recycle ashes, how to make fruit preserves, how to prepare home remedies for headache, and so on. According to Chen, when he received submissions from readers, the editorial team conducted follow-up experiments to check and confirm their accuracy.[35]

The *gongyi* section is the most relevant to our discussion of popular chemistry and chemical manufacturing. In the preface to this section, Chen Diexian reported that quite a few Chinese were studying industrial

34.   On Chen Diexian and *Free Talks*, see Tsai, *Reading Shenbao*, 85–91.
35.   Chen Diexian, ed., *Jiating changshi huibian* (*JCHB*), vol. 1, 3–4.

technology through translated foreign texts. However, many of the available translations were rambling and made simple matters too complex. When he reviewed a number of contributions from readers, he found them plain and straightforward. Thus Chen decided to use them to create the *gongyi* section. In this section, he tried to spread industrial technologies in an easily accessible language, and he hoped it would be "a good teacher and friend" (*lianghao shiyou*) to the industrial community (*gongyejie*).[36] Though this book was about housekeeping, Chen seemed to be confident that some of his readers were actually engaged in light industries. The *gongyi* section covered how to manufacture simple industrial goods, such as artificial cotton, camphor, cosmetics, candles, and alcohol. Soap making was an especially popular topic, and a couple of the contributors also wrote about recipes for toothpowder.

A *JCHB* contributor by the name of Ye Zeting described how to make "top-quality hygienic toothpowder" (*shangdeng weisheng yafen*). The ingredients of this toothpowder are one *liang* of magnesium carbonate (*tansuanmei*), one *liang* of calcium carbonate (*tansuangai*), five *li* of menthol peppermint, a few drops of rose oil, one *fen* of salicylic acid, and a small amount of camphor (*zhangnao*). Making toothpowder involved grinding the ingredients into a fine powder with a mortar and pestle. According to Ye, commercial toothpowder often contained glass fiber (*bozhi*), which might hurt the gums, and carmine, which is poisonous. Ye's recipe for toothpowder contained neither of these harmful ingredients. He also described an easier process for making "ordinary toothpowder" (*putong yafen*) by grinding oyster shells or cuttlefish bones into fine powders and drying them well.[37]

These accounts in *GZHB* and *JCHB* indicate that by the 1910s the Chinese reading public was in a position to understand the basic processes of making soap and toothpowder, and that some had experience in producing these items. Although the manufacturing techniques introduced in these accounts are neither complex nor difficult, they are still based on chemical formulae. The readers and contributors might not have had college degrees, but they were educated enough to read scientific magazines and understand basic chemical reactions. They might not have had

36. Chen Diexian, ed., *JCHB*, vol. 1, 121.
37. Chen Diexian, ed., *JCHB*, vol. 2, 124–125.

technical expertise or sufficient funds to open full-blown factories, but they could afford to purchase the ingredients to make soap and tooth-powder and perform a few experiments at home. Some of them would go on to open cottage industries and engage in mass production and the sale of personal-hygiene items.

In fact, some Republican-era entrepreneurs started their everyday-chemical operations with little formal training in science. For example, Xue Kunming (1885–1945), the founder of Pacific Soap Manufacturer (Taipingyang feizaochang), learned basic soap making as an apprentice working in a Japanese factory in Wuhan. Because the recipe was kept con-fidential by the Japanese, Xue memorized the names of various ingredients written on pails and carefully observed the activities of Japanese engi-neers. He purchased alkaline materials, different kinds of oil, and neces-sary instruments, and performed experiments at home after work. By mimicking Japanese methods, he eventually mastered soap making and opened his own factory in 1914.[38] Zhang Meixuan (1883–?), a cofounder of Nanyang Candle and Soap Factory (Nanyang zhuzaochang), worked at a silver shop before he began his soap-making business.[39] Xue and Zhang were both self-taught amateur scientists who launched their busi-nesses with relatively little capital.

As a rudimentary knowledge of chemistry spread among the reading public, a new appreciation of business and industry also developed. In fact, from the late Ming through the Qing, scholar-officials had gradu-ally come to evaluate merchants in a more positive light and to accept the pursuit of wealth as legitimate.[40] In the Republican period, commerce and industry gained increased respectability. In Wen-hsin Yeh's words, "economic affairs gained growing prominence in the state's agenda." In-stead of traditional literati, merchants and industrialists, with their ability to compete with foreigners, became recognized agents of modernization and national strengthening. When the Nationalists took power, they ac-tively encouraged economic enterprise.[41]

38. Xue Ziren, "Xue Kunming yu Taipingyang feizaochang," 197–209.
39. Xiandai shiyejia, 523.
40. On the commercial developments of the Ming-Qing period, see Brook, Confu-sions of Pleasure; Myers and Yeh-chien Wang, "Economic Developments, 1644–1800."
41. Yeh, Shanghai Splendor.

Mastery of chemical knowledge and entrepreneurship were necessary but not sufficient conditions for success in business. To promote their brand-name products, Chinese businessmen asserted their sociocultural value. Soap, toothpowder, and other goods were not simply chemical compounds; they were effective products for cultivating a clean body and good hygiene.

Ideals of Clean Bodies, Public Health, and a Strong Nation

When Westerners first introduced personal-hygiene items to China, their products did not meet significant resistance. The Chinese were by no means xenophobic. Though they often associated Western things with strangeness, extravagance, and imperialism, they had a practical attitude toward foreign goods. Li Changli points out that by the 1870s, many stores in Shanghai sold a wide range of Western commodities, including both daily necessities (e.g., matches, needles, soap, and socks), and nonessential items (e.g., sunglasses, jewelry, and perfume).[42] Dikötter further elaborates on Li's points in his discussion of foreign commodities and material culture in China. Taking issue with the conventional view, Dikötter argues that the Chinese people, both elites and non-elites, were very open and receptive to Western goods. By the end of the nineteenth century, ordinary Chinese people were using various Western commodities in their everyday lives, and China had become a part of the global circulation of goods. The Chinese creatively appropriated Western commodities and often marketed them very differently by representing them in ways that would be meaningful to their Chinese customers. They were also quick to imitate and copy foreign designs and to offer similar items at a less expensive price. According to Dikötter, the Chinese did

42. Li Changli, *WanQing Shanghai*, 127–28. Various Western institutions and goods became subjects of Shanghai's *zhuzhici* during the Guangxu era. For examples of *zhuzhici* describing Western goods, see Gu Bingquan, ed., *Shanghai yangchang zhuzhici*, 93–182.

not adapt to Western goods; rather, they adapted Western goods for their own use.[43]

Li and Dikötter's points are relevant here. When Chinese entrepreneurs opened industries to produce soap, toothpowder, and other cosmetics, local consumers already familiar with such products did not see them as "foreign" or "alien." Still, the Chinese merchants did have to create marketing for local brands that would be relevant to their Chinese customers. To differentiate their products from foreign brands and to promote sales, they endowed their commodities with new meaning. They labeled them "healthful goods" and identified them as "national products." By bestowing their products with these meanings, they connected their use to bodily cleanliness, good health, and beautiful appearance. They also affirmed that the use and purchase of their products could contribute to building the Chinese nation.

Owners of everyday-chemical industries promoted products that would clean both the body and the home. The revelation that mouths, hands, and bodies harbored germs and that house dust and dirt was a serious health menace heightened anxiety about cleanliness. Cleanliness became an indicator of an individual's physical well-being. Personal-hygiene items not only directly defended skin, teeth, and residences from germs but also invoked lessons of chemistry that justified the sale of such products. Promotional literature promised consumers that using particular personal and home-care products would make their bodies and residences clean, germ- and odor-free, and resistant to diseases. Removing dirt, tartar, and odor from one's body and residence was an important goal of hygiene practices. Carrying this out was a means to achieve physical health. To make personal-hygiene items even more appealing, consumers were assured that products were manufactured according to scientific procedures. To endorse the cleansing effects of their products, marketers drew on rudimentary knowledge of science. Along with syringes, microscopes, and X-ray machines, personal-hygiene items also embodied modern science and components of medical culture for the early twentieth-century Chinese. Yet, unlike medical instruments, anyone could easily purchase and use personal-hygiene items, providing

43. Dikötter, *Exotic Commodities*.

laypeople with an easy way to experience and benefit from "medical science."

In their marketing efforts, Chinese manufacturers placed their merchandise in a larger nationalist context. In the 1920s and 1930s, most, if not all, industry owners participated in the National Products Movement. As Gerth has discussed, the National Products Movement had many phases and various components, but Shanghai's businesses played a significant role in the movement. Shanghai's industrialists joined the Chinese National Products Preservation Association (Zhonghua guohuo weichihui) and later established the Shanghai Union of Machine-Made National Products Manufacturers (Shanghai jizhi guohuo gongchang lianhehui, or Jilian) as an independent organization of manufacturers. Jilian actively organized exhibitions and opened markets that exclusively displayed and sold Chinese-made products. Among the participants were Xiang Songmao (1880–1932), the owner of Five Continents-Guben Soap Manufacturer; Fang Yexian, the founder of China Chemical Industries Company; Chen Diexian; the Ye brothers (founders of Yonghe Enterprises Corporation); and Zhang Meixuan.[44] These entrepreneurs sold Western goods, promoted Western-driven hygiene practices, and mimicked (and sometimes stole) foreign technologies and designs. Yet in their commercial promotions, they often ignored or concealed the Western origins of their products. Instead, these industrialists positioned their goods as China's "national" products, and they urged Chinese consumers to purchase their products as a way to support the country's businesses and economy. The products were both "healthful" and "national," and their manufacturers and marketers straddled the two common slogans of Republican China: "Business rescues the nation (*shiye jiuguo*)"[45] and "Health rescues the nation (*kangjian jiuguo*)."[46]

The Nationalist state also connected cleanliness and hygiene to national strength by organizing several mass movements in Shanghai. As discussed in chapter 3, beginning in 1928, the Nationalists sponsored city-

44. The National Products Movement had many phases and various components, but Shanghai's businesses always played a significant role. Gerth, *China Made;* Guohuo shiye chubanshe bianjibu, *Zhongguo guohuo gongchang shilüe;* Pan Junxiang, *Jindai Zhongguo guohuo yundong yanjiu.*

45. Wang Yansong, "Xu."

46. Song Guobin, "Fakanci"; Lu Yipei, "Jiankang yu jiuguo."

wide hygiene campaigns twice a year.[47] Public health administrators employed various methods and programs, both prescriptive and coercive, including verbal and visual propaganda, rallies, and marches. In 1936, the Shanghai New Life Movement and hygiene campaign essentially merged.[48] In this concerted form they successfully mobilized various grassroots organizations.[49] During mass events, administrators instructed the entire Shanghai populace to live a disciplined life and practice good hygiene.[50]

These Nationalist mass-mobilization programs helped the expansion of state power, while also providing an opportunity for Shanghai's industrialists and merchants to promote various products, including food, drugs, and supplements. But the everyday-chemical industries really made the most of these events, and their for-profit marketing benefited from the interplay with state-sponsored compulsory initiatives and private desires. During the periods of these mass movements, industrialists advertised their products in newspapers and magazines. Their ads stood out from others by providing specific, product-based solutions to public and personal health problems. They also participated in "health exhibitions" (*weisheng zhanlanhui*) and displayed their merchandise as "healthful goods" alongside replicas of germs and pests and specimens of the human body.[51] These public displays were meant to be educational, but they were also effective in creating desire and demand for specific brands. The mass movements helped the spread of knowledge and information about personal-hygiene items and hygiene practices. While the city's administrators were busy distributing handbills and posters about hygienic lifestyles and lecturing about the harmfulness of flies and bugs, Shanghai's industrialists were encouraging city residents to use soap to wash their bodies and clothing, to use toothpowder and toothpaste to clean their teeth, and to use insecticides and antiseptics to kill pests and germs.

47. For the Nationalist guidelines for the campaigns, see Zhongguo Guomindang zhongyang zhixing weiyuanhui xuanchuanbu, ed., *Weisheng yundong xuanchuan gangyao*.

48. SMA U1-16-300.

49. Ferlanti, "New Life Movement."

50. Van de Ven, *War and Nationalism*, 163–68.

51. For more on public health exhibitions, see various issues of *Weisheng yuekan*, 1934–1936; *Shanghai Shi sinianlai weisheng gongzuo gaiyao*, 1932–1936, chap. 4.

Personal-hygiene products best responded to and supported the themes and goals of the Nationalist mass movements; indeed, the strong symbiotic relationship between the Nationalist discourse on health and hygiene and product marketing is unmistakable.

Personal Hygiene Items in Commercial Advertisements

Developments in early twentieth-century Shanghai fueled a dramatic increase in advertising.[52] Taking advantage of the city's various mass media and advancement in graphic technologies, manufacturers of personal hygiene items used advertisements extensively to communicate with consumers. These ads became a powerful medium for diffusing images about germs, dirt, and cleanliness, and illustrate the social and cultural values that Chinese industrialists attached to their products through visual and verbal depictions.

One commonly used strategy was to highlight the medico-scientific effects of hygiene products. Nancy Tomes has discussed how American entrepreneurs incorporated scientific lessons and precepts into their businesses, and how their advertisements invoked bacteriology and chemistry, even though they sometimes misrepresented scientific knowledge.[53] Likewise, Chinese manufacturers often associated their products with popular science. For example, an ad for Invincible brand toothpaste, a successful product of Chen Diexian's Household Industries, identifies germs as responsible for tooth decay and depicts toothpaste as if it were a kind of medical sterilizer, which removes tartar, controls lactobacillus, and kills germs (fig. 4.1).

Household Industries also published a short commercial text, "Ten Great Functions of Invincible Brand Scrubbing Toothpowder" (Wudipai

52. Yeh, *Shanghai Splendor*, 51–78. On the new printing technology that contributed to the creation of the new visual culture, see Reed, *Gutenberg in Shanghai*.

53. Tomes, *Gospel of Germs*, 68–87.

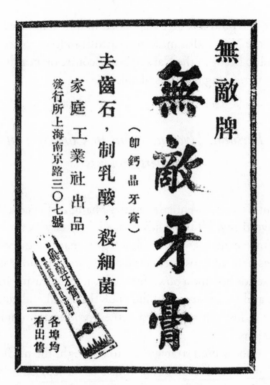

FIGURE 4.1 Invincible brand toothpaste. Shanghai shizhengfu, *Shanghai Shi chengli shizhounian gongye zhanlanhui tekan*, n.p. This ad explains that Wudi toothpaste is a "calcium grain toothpaste" that has various medical effects.

camian yafen de shida gongyong).[54] This text states that the toothpowder's main ingredient—magnesium carbonate—prevents halitosis, tooth decay, and throat inflammation. But, according to this ad, Invincible toothpowder had other, non-oral uses as well: applied to the face, the powder could remove greasy spots and freckles; applied to the body, it could prevent heat rash and kill body odor; applied to clothing, it could remove stains and whiten fabric; and applied to razor rash, it could stop the bleeding. Although we do not know how many Chinese consumers actually applied Invincible toothpowder to their faces and bodies, this text promotes the powder as a handy and convenient item for cleaning up just

54.   This ad appears on the back cover of Bao Xiang'ao and Mei Qizhao, *Meishi yanfang xinbian*.

about anything. Thus, this ad pulls together medico-scientific knowledge, cleanliness in a general sense, and usefulness for everyday household life.

Yuhua Chemical Industries, Ltd. (Yuhua huaxue gongye gufen youxian gongsi) adopted the similar logic to promote their soap. Consider for example the ad shown in figure 4.2. Here Yuhua presents the various benefits of Tiger brand medical soap. According to this ad, Tiger brand medical soap, which is made in China, can safeguard a family's health and has four great merits (*sida youdian*): (1) kills ticks and other insects (*shachong*); (2) prevents epidemics (*fangyi*); (3) eliminates germs, viruses, and other poisons (*qudu*); and (4) refreshes the skin (*shengji*). Not only could this soap kill germs and pests and clean the body; it could also defend one's family from diseases and contributes to the welfare of society by preventing epidemics (fig. 4.2).

Personal-hygiene-item advertising often featured beautiful women. In an advertisement for Pure and White (Jiebai) toothpaste, created by Household Industries (fig. 4.3), the image of the smiling young woman in the ad suggests that the toothpaste will give consumers both an attractive appearance and clean, germ-free teeth. At once, this ad promotes the aesthetics of white teeth (an attractive appearance) as well as the medical effects of toothpaste (a clean mouth). Dental hygiene and halitosis appeared regularly in popular medical magazines in the 1930s. These ads reflected rising concerns about dental health among ordinary Chinese. Whereas the number of qualified dentists was still small, even in Shanghai,[55] toothpaste was an inexpensive and readily available commodity for keeping one's teeth clean, healthy, and charming (fig. 4.3).

With the proliferation of ads for tooth-care products focused on female beauty, some Shanghai soap companies followed suit.[56] Adopting what Juliann Sivulka calls the "emulation formula,"[57] they used portraits and photographs of female movie stars along with their testimonials in ads to connect beauty with the consumption of their soap. Yuhua Chemical manufactured "movie star toilet soap" (*yinxing xiangzao*) and its ads featured the endorsement of nineteen Chinese female movie stars,

55. Yip, *Health and National Reconstruction*, 63.
56. For more examples of tooth-care product advertisements, see Huang Zhiwei and Huang Ying, *Wei shiji daiyan*, 237–38
57. Sivulka, *Stronger Than Dirt*, 192–201.

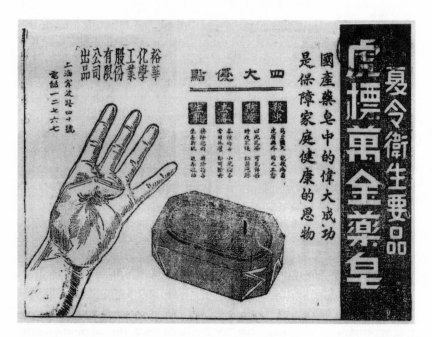

FIGURE 4.2 Tiger brand medical soap. Shanghai shizhengfu, *Shanghai Shi chengli shizhounian gongye zhanlanhui tekan*, n.p. The right two vertical lines read, "A necessity for summer hygiene, Tiger brand medical soap for everything." The ad continues, "This Chinese-made medical soap achieves great success in ensuring the blessing of family health."

with the catch phrase "the favorite of nineteen stars" (*mingxing shijiu aiyong*).[58]

These ads targeted women as potential customers and enticed readers into believing that they, too, could have the romantic life and beautiful appearance of movie stars. Images of young and progressive women were also a popular icon among international corporations' advertising in China. Unilever, Kotex, and other Western companies engaged fashionable women to promote their products.[59] Such women

58. Yuhua Chemical was founded in Shanghai by Liang Songling in 1933. Huang Zhiwei and Huang Ying, *Wei shiji daiyan*, 234–35. Household Industries adopted a similar strategy and employed twelve female movie stars in their ads. See Yi Bin, Liu Youming, and Gan Zhenhu, eds., *Lao Shanghai guanggao*, 44–45.

59. For Unilever's soap advertisements featuring female movie stars, see Huang Zhiwei and Huang Ying, *Wei shiji daiyan*, 230–32. For Kotex's ads, see Barlow, "Wanting Some."

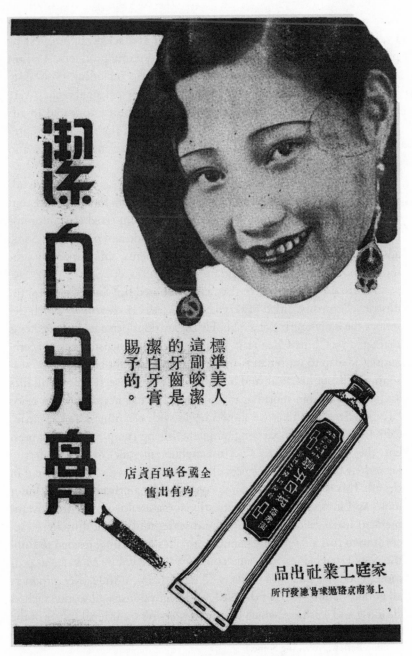

FIGURE 4.3 Pure and White toothpaste. *Xiandai shiyejia*, n.p. The text reads, "This is a standard beauty. Her clean teeth are a gift from Pure and White brand toothpaste."

were tastemakers, set the standard for "modern beauty" and "modern hygiene," and contributed to China's social and scientific progress by practicing good hygiene and by using brand-name products. As Tani Barlow has pointed out, female life practices, including grooming, bathing, and even menstruation, were not purely personal—they were also scientific and public. Virtually the same women appeared in ads for both Chinese and Western corporations, and their pictures represented and reinforced transnational values of science, beauty, and cleanliness.[60]

At the same time, however, Chinese industrialists also devised advertising strategies to differentiate their products from foreign brands and appeal to the entire Chinese population. They connected the consumption of personal hygiene items with national pride and patriotism. Some ads explicitly refer to Nationalist mass movements, simultaneously promoting both the movements and products.

Figure 4.4 shows an advertisement composed by China Chemical Industries Company, titled "Everyday Life" (*Mei ri shenghuo*), which describes the daily routine of a man. He uses various personal hygiene items marketed by China Chemical. These included toothpaste to clean teeth, antiseptic soap to wash hands and face, toilet water for bathing, food seasoning to flavor his meal, and mosquito coils and insecticides to kill flies and bedbugs, from morning to bedtime. The top horizontal line reads "To practice New Life, we should begin with cleanliness and hygiene" (Shixing xinshenghuo xu cong qingjie weisheng zuoqi), and the ad presents the "New Life Pledges" (Xinshenghuo gongyue) to urge readers to keep their bodies and residences clean and hygienic just like the man in the ad. This is a commercial pitch composed by a private business, but it looks as if it were taken from educational material issued by the government to teach readers how to avoid diseases and live healthy lives. According to this ad, China Chemical provides everything needed to fulfil the New Life Pledges. This ad champions the New Life Movement, promotes good hygiene, and markets China' Chemical Industries' products all at once. Some items of the pledges concern household works, such as cleaning and washing, which belong to women's traditional sphere of the

60. Barlow, "Wanting Some."

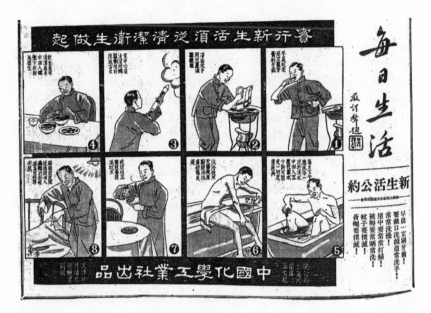

FIGURE 4.4 "Everyday Life." *Shenbao*, June 19, 1934, 15. On the right, under the heading "New Life Pledges," seven admonitions are listed:

You must always brush your teeth in the morning!

You must rinse your mouth, wash your hair, and frequently wash your hands!

You must bathe often!

You must clean your room often!

You must dry your bedding in the sun and wash it often!

Mosquitoes must be eradicated!

Flies must be eradicated!

home. Yet this ad does not show a stylish woman. Instead, it features a man in traditional dress. The New Life Movement also encouraged austerity, frugality, and discipline, and these features of the New Life gainsay commercial marketing. Yet, the fact that the authors of this ad simply concentrated on hygiene practices underscores the company's contributions and commitment to the pledges. In the end, this focus seamlessly integrates the New Life Pledges into marketing. Here, official slogans and commercial promotions are nicely combined. The personal-hygiene items in this ad were vehicles to practice New Life and contribute to revive the Chinese nation.

Figure 4.5, an advertisement for Nanyang Candle and Soap, also promotes its product by aligning it with the New Life Movement and the National Products Movement.[61] With the rise of these two movements, medical concern about personal hygiene, state concern about personal discipline, and patriotic concern about personal consumption merged. This ad calls out the scarcity of washing and bathing as damaging to China's reputation. In the second and third lines of this ad, the copywriter repeatedly uses the word *shao*, meaning "not enough" or "deficient."[62] This word also calls attention to the discourse of "Chinese deficiency."[63] High mortality and morbidity rates, dirty streets, contaminated water, and the poor hygiene standards of bakeries and slaughterhouses were all marks of Chinese deficiency. But here Chinese deficiency is reduced to a simple matter of inadequate consumption of soap—an easily corrected problem.[64] While Shanghai administrators were working hard to make the city cleaner and healthier on a limited budget, Chinese merchants offered an easy way to overcome the deficiency and relieve national shame at the personal level.

Purchasing and using soap were simple private actions, but they were not independent from social and national concerns. Consumers could contribute to the public good while performing these actions. With soap, they could clean their bodies and clothing, eradicate the stigma of being unclean, and improve China's international image all at once. They could also support a homegrown industry and thus participate in the National Products Movement. Even though soap was originally brought from the West, Chinese consumers could use soap to improve China's international status.

Figure 4.6 promotes various products from Yonghe Enterprises[65] in an advertisement run in conjunction with a Shanghai hygiene campaign.

61.   Nanyang was founded by Zhang Changfa and Zhang Meixuan in 1904 in Shanghai. It was the earliest Chinese soap manufacturer. Huang Zhiwei and Huang Ying, *Wei shiji daiyan*, 234; Yang Dehui and Dong Wenzhong, *Shanghai zhi gongshangye*, 39.

62.   My thanks to Professor Ruth Rogaski for pointing this out.

63.   On Chinese deficiency, see Rogaski, *Hygienic Modernity*, 4–9.

64.   This ad concurs with descriptions found in popular science books published during the Republican period. These books remark that the degree of a nation's civility can be measured by the amount of the soap the nation consumes. For example, see Li Zongfa, *Feizao*.

65.   Yonghe Business Corporation was founded by Ye Zhongting, Ye Jiting, and Ye Xiangting. On the Ye brothers, see *Xiandai shiyejia*, 67.

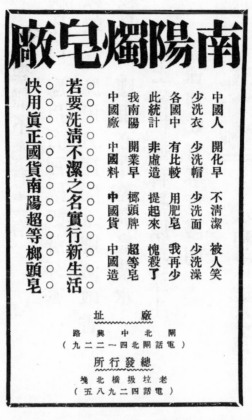

FIGURE 4.5 Hammer brand soap of Nanyang. *Xiandai shiyejia*, n.p. The left two lines of text read, "If you want to wash away the stigma of being unsanitary and to practice New Life, now [is the time to] use Nanyang's Hammer brand soap. This is a genuine national product of supreme quality." The main text in the right block is written in rhyme:

The Chinese people have an old civilization.

But we are not clean, and are laughed at by other peoples.

We do not do laundry often.

We do not wash our hats often.

We do not wash our faces often.

We do not bathe often.

Compared to other nations, we use the least amount of soap.

We do not fabricate these statistics.

It is very embarrassing to speak about this.

Our Nanyang factory is an old company.

Our Hammer brand soap is of supreme quality.

We are a Chinese factory.

Ours are China's national products made of Chinese ingredients and made in China.

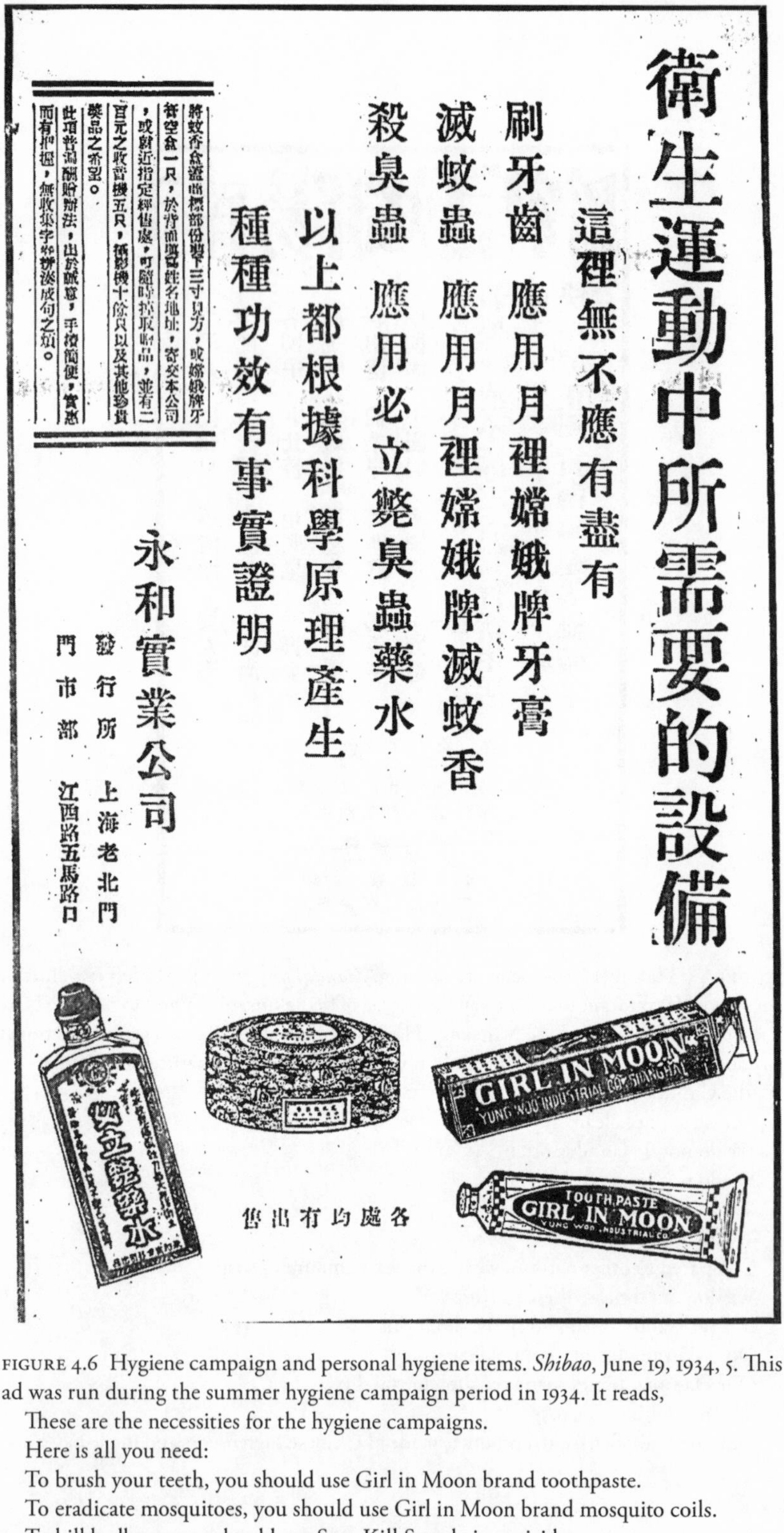

FIGURE 4.6 Hygiene campaign and personal hygiene items. *Shibao*, June 19, 1934, 5. This ad was run during the summer hygiene campaign period in 1934. It reads,

These are the necessities for the hygiene campaigns.

Here is all you need:

To brush your teeth, you should use Girl in Moon brand toothpaste.

To eradicate mosquitoes, you should use Girl in Moon brand mosquito coils.

To kill bedbugs, you should use Sure Kill Speedy insecticides.

These items are all manufactured according to scientific principles.

Facts prove these various products to be effective.

Here hygiene practices such as brushing teeth and eradicating vermin are taken for granted. The focus of the ad is not on these practices per se, but on the particular brand to be used. It is also noteworthy that the copywriter chose the word *ying*, meaning "should" or "ought to," instead of *shao*, "deficient," to urge consumers to purchase Yonghe brand products. Consumers "should" use these products as part of their participation in the hygiene campaign because they were all scientifically manufactured. This ad proudly announces the effectiveness of Chinese brand items and promotes the hygiene campaign. The Chinese might still be "deficient" in their use of personal-hygiene items, but they were capable of taking advantage of modern science and becoming better. With these Yonghe products, it was relatively easy and affordable to live up the ideal of a "modern citizen."

The Sociocultural Significance of Commodities

The ads shown here are but a few examples of the advertisements for personal-hygiene items abundant in Republican Shanghai. These ads used popular conceptions of Western science as the basis for touting the efficacy of Chinese brands and urged Chinese consumers to use their products to be more attractive, more hygienic, cleaner, and healthier. They also presented commodity purchases as an affordable way to support native industries and improve China's national prestige.

Though it was not always explicitly expressed, such advertising addressed a modern Chinese desire to meet global—that is, Western—standards of health and hygiene; however, Western standards could claim only a relatively short history. Notions of cleanliness and filth being variable, norms of a hygienic body were not well consolidated in the West until the early twentieth century. Historians have discussed the changes in the use of water and the custom of bathing in the West. Georges Vigarello has argued that although the scientific concept of cleanliness came to prevail among the French bourgeoisies in the mid-nineteenth century, premodern images of corporeal composition and physical sensibility did not disappear. He has pointed out that the habit of bathing with soap and hot water still met resistance in late nineteenth-century France because it was believed that a hot bath might cause moistness and weakness of the body and awaken sexual desire.[66] Bushman and Bushman have also illustrated that the usual method of everyday cleaning in eighteenth-century America was "a basin of water and towel"—even in well-off families. In the nineteenth century, the religious link between moral purity and physical cleanliness, aspirations of gentility, and the new view of the function of skin all promoted the new practice of bathing in hot water with soap.[67] The use of toothpaste in the West was also relatively new. The first toothpaste in America was sold in the late nineteenth century, and Colgate distributed toothpaste and toothbrushes to schools to promote the practice of tooth brushing among school children in 1911.[68] As the Western bourgeoisie promoted physical cleanliness to indicate strength, vigor, and energy, and as their sanitation standards became increasingly accepted, hygiene practices and bodily cleanliness began to differentiate social classes at home and distinguish different races in the colonies. Cleanliness became a marker of social and racial hierarchy, and public health reforms in the metropoles and colonies often went hand in hand.[69]

When Chinese industrialists sold their products, they were not necessarily aware of the ambiguity and variability of Western concepts of cleanliness. Nor did they question the validity or efficacy of hygiene practices. Chinese manufacturers took the Western origins of their products for granted and presented their commodities as a means to correct Chinese deficiencies. They were optimistic that their products would improve China's hygiene practices and render Chinese bodies clean;[70] they were also careful not to offend prospective consumers. Although advertisements admitted that Chinese people were not as clean as they should be,[71] local

66. Vigarello, *Concepts of Cleanliness*.

67. In the eighteenth century, many American physicians came to understand that skin perspired and thus removed certain bodily wastes. Bushman and Bushman, "Early History of Cleanliness."

68. http://www.colgate.com/app/Colgate/US/Corp/History/1806.cvsp.

69. Stepan, *Idea of Race*; Kupinse, "Indian Subject of Colonial Hygiene"; Anderson, *Colonial Pathologies*.

70. On the demand for cleanliness in China, see Dikötter, *Exotic Commodities*, 205–13.

71. In fact, the Chinese in Republican Shanghai did bathe often. In 1936, more than two thousand hot water shops providing small bathing spaces at a budgeted cost

industrialists insisted that their products could easily help consumers improve. Some illustrations of these ads depicted middle-class people as their subjects, but their creators assumed that their audience and prospective buyers included the entire socioeconomic range of the Chinese people. Rather than differentiating social classes, gender roles, or ethnic groups, personal-hygiene products were a means to unite and safeguard the entire family and population from germs and disease and to create national pride. Soap, toothpaste, and other personal-hygiene items may have come from the West, but Chinese industrialists and merchants successfully domesticated them.

Some of the advertising bears a striking similarity to the posters and slogans used in the mass movements in Republican Shanghai. Seemingly mundane practices, such as bathing and washing, took on social meaning and became the focus of mass movements and ceremonies.[72] By selling and promoting their merchandise, Shanghai's merchants and industrialists certainly cooperated with the Nationalist state in connecting the private body to the nation. Unlike the state, they possessed neither political authority nor legal power. Instead of disciplining people's bodies and regulating their behavior, they pursued business; their primary goal was to persuade consumers that their products were worth purchasing.

This discussion of personal-hygiene items and their promotion calls to mind the issue of commodity fetishism. Scholars ranging from Marx to contemporary anthropologists and economic historians have assessed the sociocultural significance of commodities. In Igor Kopytoff's words, commodities are "not only produced materially as things, but also culturally marked as being a certain kind of thing."[73] Marxian historians have suggested that the ability to create desire and demand often depends more on the sociocultural values associated with particular things than with their actual utility. They also assert that the power of modern capitalism lies in its ability to create and manipulate the sociocultural values

---

operated in Shanghai. Larger bathhouses were also common. They had large tubs with hot water and offered various services, including back washing, massage, and pedicure. On hot water shops and bathhouses, see Hanchao Lu, *Behind the Neon Lights*, 263–68; Yao Fei, "Jindai Shanghai gonggong yushi yu shimin jieceng."

72. For posters and slogans used in the Shanghai hygiene campaigns, see, for example, *Weishang Yuekan* 5, no. 7 (1935).

73. Kopytoff, "Cultural Biography of Things."

of goods. Big capitalists are neither the only nor the most powerful agents engaged in this process: local traders, brokers, and consumers can also play important roles.[74] Moreover, sociocultural values are not fixed: they are related to the practical use of materials, but they are also created as a result of specific social and historical conditions.[75] As Chinese industrialists domesticated personal-hygiene items, they also expanded the social and cultural significance of these products; personal-hygiene items not only cleaned teeth, bodies, and clothing, but also helped remove a national stigma and create a public health citizenship that was neutral and open to everyone. Consumer products could also be useful devices in the fight against foreign economic imperialism. For Chinese industrialists, creating new meanings for products constituted a significant part of their business activities.

Largely because of the efforts of merchants and industrialists, using soap and toothpowder had become standard practice for Shanghai residents by the 1920s, as social surveys conducted in the 1920s and 1930s illustrate. From November 1927 to October 1928, Yang Ximeng (1900–?) surveyed 230 Caojiadu working-class families having an average monthly income of 32.89 yuan.[76] On average, each household had 4.77 people, including children, elders, and other relatives,[77] and a monthly expenditure of 32.50 yuan.[78] Out of these households, 225 owned soap.[79] The amount of money spent on soap varied each month, ranging from 0.08 yuan (March and April) to 0.15 yuan (July and September). In total, each household consumed 27.2 pieces of soap and spent 1.36 yuan on soap annually.[80] Likewise each household purchased 4.3 packages of toothpowder and spent 0.08 yuan on toothpowder annually.[81] The Shanghai Social Affairs Bureau (Shehuiju) carried out a similar survey of 305 working-class families, whose average annual income was 416.51 yuan, from

74.   Ibid.; Burke, *Lifebuoy Men, Lux Women*; Cochran, *Chinese Medicine Man*.
75.   Bayly, "Origins of Swadeshi."
76.   Yang Ximeng, *Shanghai gongren*, Part 1, 31.
77.   Ibid., 19.
78.   Ibid., 35.
79.   Ibid., 83.
80.   Ibid., Part 2, 26.
81.   Ibid., 27.

April 1929 to March 1930.[82] In this survey, each household had 4.62 people,[83] with an average monthly expenditure of 37.86 yuan.[84] All these families had purchased soap during the year surveyed. Each family had consumed on average 50.827 pieces of soap and had spent 2.592 yuan. Also, 299 families out of the 305 spent on average 0.511 yuan on toothpowder.[85] These accounts indicate that soap and toothpowder were common household items. The amount of money spent on these items may seem small, but their retail prices were also low. Around 1935, the most expensive toothpowder cost 0.75 yuan per bottle; cheaper brands cost less than 0.02 yuan per package. Inexpensive toilet soap cost 0.18 yuan per bar,[86] and laundry soap was even less costly. The modest price of these Chinese products contributed to the rapid spread of new hygiene customs among Shanghai's populace.

Although not all Chinese manufacturers of personal-hygiene items endured, some outdid foreign rivals and their brands became quite popular. Chinese producers of tooth-care products fared especially well. By the 1930s Chinese toothpowders dominated the market. Toothpaste production also developed quickly in Shanghai. During the 1930s, sixteen Chinese companies in Shanghai produced twenty-four brands of toothpaste; by the 1940s, seventy-eight makers produced a total of 43.2 million tubes in 110 brands. Three Stars, Invincible, Girl in Moon, White Jade (Baiyu), and Darkie (Heiren) were among the best-known and most popular Chinese brands.[87] In the soap market, Unilever and other foreign-owned factories were operating in Shanghai, and China was still importing a significant amount of the soap it consumed in the 1930s. However, in spite of its size and access to capital, Unilever did not dominate the soap market. Out of thirty-three soap makers in Shanghai listed by Yang Dajin, thirty were Chinese.[88] Chinese brands, Five Continent-Guben's

82. Shanghai shizhengfu shehuiju, ed., *Shanghaishi gongren shenghuo chengdu*, 15, 99.

83. Ibid., 7, 91.

84. Ibid., 17, 101.

85. Ibid., 73, 157.

86. Yang Dajin, ed., *Xiandai Zhongguo shiyezhi*, 564, 576–79.

87. Ibid., 540–42; *Shanghai riyong gongyepin shangyezhi* bianzuan weiyuanhui, ed., *Shanghai riyong gongyepin shangyezhi*, 82; Shanghai tongzhi bianzhuan weiyuanhui, ed., *Gongye*.

88. Yang Dajin, ed., *Xiandai Zhongguo shiyezhi*, 491–96.

Guben and China Chemical's Arrow and Sword (Jiandao) in particular, outsold Unilever products.[89] Clearly, the strategy of connecting hygiene practices with nationalism used by Chinese businessmen garnered them a significant advantage in China's growing soap market.

Doing Business in Shanghai: Fang Yexian and Chen Diexian

Some Chinese manufacturers that started in the early twentieth century developed into large companies that still exist today. Among these successful entrepreneurs, Fang Yexian and Chen Diexian, both based in Shanghai, were the best known. Fang founded China Chemical Industries Company, the largest company to produce and sell toiletries and personal-hygiene products in pre-1949 China.[90] After 1949 it was reorganized as Shanghai Toothpaste Manufacturer (Shanghai yagaochang). It is now called Shanghai Maxam Company and remains a leading manufacturer of toothpaste in China today.[91] Chen Diexian was the founder of Household Industries Company, which also sold personal-hygiene items and cosmetics. Household Industries Company merged with Continental Chemical Products Plant (Dalu huaxue zhipinchang) and became Shanghai Daily Chemical Products Plant (Shanghai riyong huaxuepinchang) in 1958.[92] In the 1980s this company was once again reorganized into Shanghai Daily Chemical Fragrance Ltd. (Shanghai rihua fangfang youxian gongsi).[93] Examining the careers of these two businessmen illustrates how Chinese entrepreneurs learned elementary chemistry, opened and expanded their companies, and popularized personal-hygiene items among Chinese consumers.

89. Zurndorfer, "Imperialism, Globalization, and the Soap/Suds Industry"; Shanghai tongzhi bianzhuan weiyuanhui, ed., *Gongye*, chap. 5, sec. 3.

90. In 1948 all the directors of the Shanghai Everyday Chemical Industry Association were from either the China Chemical or Household Industries. See SMA S86-1-10.

91. For its official website, see http://www.stof.com/old/stf.html (English) or http://www.maxam-sh.com/about_overview.aspx (Chinese).

92. Xue Shunsheng and Lei Chenghao, eds., *Lao Shanghai*, 62.

93. For its official website, see fangfang.binzhuang.com.

In Chinese historiography, Fang Yexian is referred to with two epithets: "Ningbo merchant" (*Ningbo shangren*) and "patriotic businessman" (*aiguo qiyejia*).[94] Both his paternal and maternal families hailed from Ningbo and had been engaged in various businesses in Shanghai. Because of his family background, Fang is regarded as a Ningbo businessman even though he was born and grew up in Shanghai. From 1919 until his death in 1940, Fang, along with Chen Diexian, was a leading figure of the National Products Movement in Shanghai. With other businessmen in the city, Fang opened the United Market for National Products in Shanghai and organized the National Products Company, which sold Chinese-made goods exclusively. Throughout his business career, Fang was helped significantly both by his family ties and by the National Products Movement.

Although his parents wanted him to work in finance and banking, Fang Yexian was more interested in chemical experiments. He went to a missionary school in Shanghai and studied chemistry with L. W. Dupre, a German chemist who worked for the International Settlement. In 1912, at age nineteen, he founded China Chemical Industries with financial help from his mother. With a moderate capitalization of 10,000 yuan, his company started out as a domestic workshop. Soon Fang entered into partnership with Li Zuhan (1891–1964), his maternal cousin, and employed several workers and apprentices to make cosmetics such as vanishing cream, toilet water, perfumes, and hair lotion, as well as toothpowder. They were unable to match the quality of foreign brands, and business did not go well initially. Although Fang dispatched itinerant peddlers into the city and offered free samples of his merchandise to promote sales, he suffered losses every year. After burning through all his initial capital, Fang managed to raise more money, including 15,000 yuan from Li Yunshu (1867–1928), his maternal uncle. With this investment, he employed accountants and salespeople and expanded his workshop to produce other items. In 1915 he also began manufacturing Three Stars brand

94. There are many accounts of Fang Yexian and his China Chemical Industries Company. For example, see Fang Zhixiong, "Zhongguo riyong huaxuepin gongye de dianjiren"; Lin Rukang, "Zhongguo huaxue gongyeshe"; Lu Zhilian, "Fang Yexian"; Shen Yuwu, "Fang Yexian"; Guohuo shiye chubanshe bianjibu, *Zhongguo guohuo gongchang shilüe*, 63–64; SMA A38-2-242; Shanghai jilianhui, "Zhongguo huaxue gongyeshe."

mosquito coils to compete with Japanese imports. Still, business did not pick up, and the company was teetering on the brink of bankruptcy.

With the May Fourth Movement of 1919 and ensuing boycotts of foreign goods, China Chemical was able to launch a comeback. Fang became a vocal leader of the National Products Movement and emphasized that his goods were made in China. The boycott movement helped China Chemical's publicity and product sales. In the 1920s he successfully promoted his Three Stars brand as China's national brand. Three Stars cosmetics also enjoyed brisk sales, and soon the company began turning a profit. At this point Fang received financing of 50,000 yuan from Fang Jiyang, his paternal uncle. He used this money to reorganize the company into an unlimited liability enterprise. Fang Jiyang agreed to serve as company president, and Fang Yexian worked as general manager. Since Fang Jiyang was an influential figure among Shanghai's traditional bankers, his investment and involvement improved China Chemical's financial reputation. With its financial footing secure, the company built a new plant in West Shanghai and recruited technical staff with advanced degrees in chemistry and engineering.[95]

By the mid-1930s China Chemical had developed into the largest everyday-chemical-industry company in China and was producing a variety of personal-hygiene items (see fig. 4.2).[96] It possessed assets of two million yuan in 1938. As the company grew from the 1920s to the 1930s, its primary products shifted from cosmetics to other items. In 1923, in addition to its toothpowder, Fang Yexian promoted Three Stars toothpaste as China's first "national" toothpaste. He also opened a second plant to manufacture food seasonings. In 1928, he built a third plant to exclusively manufacture mosquito coils. In 1937, his fourth plant began to manufacture Arrow and Sword laundry soap.[97] Toothpowder and toothpaste, mos-

---

95.   SMA A38-2-242 and A38-2-255, 70–77, list technical staff of the company, some of whom had degrees from Chinese and Western colleges.

96.   Also see Yi Bin, Liu Youming, and Gan Zhenhu, *Lao Shanghai guanggao*, 44–45.

97.   Originally the brand name of the soap was "scissors" (*jiandao*). But "scissors" was already a registered trademark of Unilever. China Chemical changed the name to "arrow and sword," which is a homophony of "scissors." Li Zufan, "Yagao shengchan jianshi," 95.

quito coils, food seasoning, and laundry soap thus became the main products of China Chemical Industries.[98]

Fang Yexian promoted his commodities as "national" products—even though many of his products were imitations of foreign brands and their ingredients and recipes were based on those of foreign companies. When he began producing food seasoning, he visited Japan to study the manufacturing process of Ajinomoto, a brand of monosodium glutamate powder popular in Japan and China. He also brought some half-finished Ajinomoto products back to China and chemically analyzed their ingredients. Likewise when he began producing mosquito coils, he dispatched one of his employees to Japan to study the techniques used by his Japanese competitors for mechanically pressing the shape of the coil. For Three Stars brand toothpaste, Fang used the American Colgate brand as a model, imitating both its formula and package design.[99] When sales of toothpaste overtook those of toothpowder in the late 1920s through the 1930s, Three Stars toothpaste became one of China Chemical's most important products. To increase sales, Fang Yexian adopted various marketing strategies. Most importantly, he set a retail price much lower than that of foreign brands. To attract retailers, Fang offered a 10 percent discount off the wholesale price and 0.5 percent in rebates. In addition to these incentives, he also offered commissions of 3 to 8 percent, depending on total retail sales. Some retailers were even willing to sell the Three Star brand toothpaste at the wholesale price just to receive the commission. Fang also gave retailers a grace period for payment, delivering his products to shops in May and allowing them to pay in September. The profitability of toothpaste per unit sold was not as high as cosmetics or mosquito coils, but the production process was not complex, and toothpaste could be sold over the entire year. Fang therefore adopted a "low-margin, high-volume" strategy. His goal was to distribute Three Stars brand items across the market and make them widely known. Soon Three Stars toothpaste became popular, and in the 1930s Fang's company commanded the largest share of China's toothpaste market. As toothpaste production increased and his company accumulated wealth, Fang and Li Zufan (1897–1992), another

---

98. For lists of China Chemical's products, see SMA S59-1-39-146.
99. Meng Yuan, "Zhongqing riyong huagong," 397; Li Zufan, "Zhongguo huaxue gongyeshe jianshi," 218.

of his cousins, opened a separate plant to produce calcium carbonate, the key ingredient in the toothpaste formula. Then he used glycerin, a by-product of soap manufacturing, with the calcium carbonate to produce toothpaste. By creating a reliable, self-sufficient system, the company was able to reduce raw-material costs.

After the outbreak of the Second Sino-Japanese War, China Chemical moved its facilities into Shanghai's International Settlement and continued operation. When Fang Yexian refused to collaborate with Shanghai's Japanese occupiers, he was kidnapped and killed in 1940. After Fang's death, his family members took over the management of the company. Fang Jiyang, Li Zuhan, Li Zufan, Fang Yexian's wife and children, and Li Mingyue (1911–98), Fang Yexian's nephew, all joined the board of directors. They remained in charge of the company until the Communist takeover.[100]

Along with Fang Yexian, Chen Diexian was another important entrepreneur who sold personal-hygiene items. Like China Chemical, Chen's Household Industries made a modest start in 1918 as a small, family-run business producing toothpowder and simple toiletries. Ultimately, it developed into a major manufacturer of personal-hygiene items. Chen Diexian, a man of varied attainments, was born to a literati family in Hangzhou and received a traditional education in reading and writing. He grew up to be a prolific writer and composed a variety of texts. He joined the editorial boards of some journals, including *Libai liu* (Saturday) and *Youxi shijie* (Pastime world). As a member of the Mandarin Duck and Butterfly school, he published novels under the pseudonym Tianxu Wosheng. He also wrote scripts of *tanci* storytelling and translated Sherlock Holmes stories into Chinese. Even though he had no formal training in science or medicine, he was well versed in classical medical texts. Chen had become an established writer by his early twenties. His writing also included music scores, popular science books, cookbooks, and how-to manuals on housekeeping.[101]

---

100. SMA A38-2-255, 76; SMA A38-2-242, 24.

101. For biographies of Chen Diexian, see Zhang Huimin, "Chen Diexian"; Meng Yuan, "Zhongqing riyong huagong"; Shanghai jilianhui, "Jiating gongyeshe"; Hanan, "Introduction"; Chen Xinwen, *Zhongguo jindai huaxue gongyeshi*, 283–85. On Chen and the Mandarin Duck and Butterfly school, see Link, *Mandarin Ducks and Butterflies*.

In addition to writing and editing, Chen Diexian held a variety of positions. In 1898 he left Hangzhou for Wukang to serve as a secretary to the commissioner of customs. The following year, he resigned from the position and ran a tea and bamboo dealership in Wukang. In 1900 he went back to Hangzhou and opened a store that sold books and imported electric appliances, such as gramophones and radios. But this store earned a reputation as "strange" (*guai*), "supernatural" (*shen*), and "messy" (*luan*) and was not successful. From 1901 to 1908 Chen opened a publishing house and library and launched a new literary journal. At the same time, he continued writing and publishing his own novels and essays. From 1909 to 1913 he worked as a private adviser (*muliao*) to a number of governmental offices in Zhejiang and Jiangsu; it was during these years that Chen became interested in chemical manufacturing. He also studied Japanese and hired a Japanese chemist as a tutor. He built a small thatched hut as a laboratory and conducted public exhibitions of chemical experiments. His show of a chemical fire extinguisher was particularly popular. One day, he botched the performance and burned down the hut, but this failure did not stop his interests in experiments. When he was in Zhenhai, he came up with a plan to produce toothpowder by using cuttlefish bones that washed up on the beach. At the time, his brother was a director of a rehabilitation facility for criminals in Zhenhai. Together with his brother, he proposed making toothpowder at the facility and applied for a 2,000 yuan subsidy. When this proposal was rejected, Chen Diexian went to Shanghai.

In Shanghai, Chen Diexian decided to go into business on his own. He invited Wu Juemi, a graduate of the Science Department of Dongwu University, to become his partner, and they jointly collected 200 yuan. With this tiny amount of capital, Chen began producing chilblain ointment. Ointment production was technically easy and required only a small amount of capital. Without hiring workers, Chen mobilized his wife and children to make the ointment manually and sell it from their home. Because ointment did not cost much to produce, Chen accumulated a profit, though the amount produced was small. After the death of Wu Juemi, Chen brought in his friend Li Xinfu as a technical advisor, and they invested 2,000 yuan and 500 yuan, respectively; together, Chen and Li opened an unlimited liability company to begin toothpowder making in 1918. Because this company was run by Chen's family members and friends, he named the company Household Industries. Chen adopted Wudi (Invincible) as the brand name of the tooth-care products,[102] and this toothpowder and toothpaste became the key products produced by Household Industries.

At first Household Industries did not make much profit, and Chen had to use his writing royalties to support the company. He experimented with different raw materials and tried several production methods to help improve the operation of the business. His initial idea to use cuttlefish bones found on seashores as abrasive agents in the toothpowder proved harmful to teeth and gums. Chen wondered if there was some other way to cut down on raw-material costs, and he hit on the idea of utilizing alkaline earth halogens (*kulu*)[103] found in saltpans. He succeeded in producing magnesium carbonate from the halogens. Because these halogens were waste materials from salt making, he could obtain them cheaply. When salt pan owners required higher prices for alkaline earth halogens, Chen contacted individual salt workers and purchased the halogens he needed directly from them. His methods worked, and the company developed quickly. To expand the market for his toothpowder and familiarize consumers with his brand name, he offered Invincible-brand toothpowder free to retailers. Taking advantage of the National Products Movement, Chen extensively publicized his toothpowder as one of China's national products. In 1923, Household Industries was reorganized into a limited liability company. The company invited outside investors and accumulated total assets of 20,000 yuan. In 1926 the company raised capital by selling shares, and its assets reached 50,000 yuan. In addition to the main plant for toothpowder production, it opened a number of subplants for glasses, boxes, printing, and package papers. It also established two magnesium-production plants in Wuxi and Pudong and created a self-sufficient system for making toothpowder. In 1930 the share price of Household Industries rose significantly, and its total assets reached

---

102. Wudi literally means "invincible." Since this is a homophony of *hudie* (butterfly) in Shanghai dialect, the English brand name of the toothpaste was "Butterfly." Chen Xinwen, *Zhongguo jindai huaxue gongyeshi*, 283.

103. Alkaline earth halogens are by-products of salt production and are compounds of various chemical elements, such as chloride, potassium, magnesium, iodine, bromine, calcium, etc.

500,000 yuan. Around this time, Chen also began producing Butterfly brand vanishing cream (Dieshuang). From this time on, tooth-care products and vanishing cream became the major products of Household Industries. In 1935, Household Industries had a total of some two thousand employees, including some three hundred workers at the main toothpowder plant. Though pirated replicas and imitations damaged the sales of Invincible-brand items, the total sales of the company reached 1,400,000 yuan that year.[104]

Chen gave up writing novels after founding the company, but he kept on writing short essays, columns, and commercial advertisements. In particular, he fully implemented his talent as a writer in the National Products Movement. He was one of the founding members of Jilian, and the editor-in-chief of various periodicals published by Jilian. He published numerous articles calling for patriotic consumption.

Household Industries was prospering, and Invincible became a well-known brand of toothpowder, but Chen Diexian did not stop. He had a wide range of interests and carried out extensive business ventures in various areas until he died of pneumonia in 1940. He studied the process of peppermint-essence production and opened a factory in Taicang to produce it. He also studied different botanical strains of peppermint plants and encouraged Taicang peasants to grow peppermint. Though the peppermint factory was soon closed, a lasting knowledge of peppermint-plant cultivation was spread among the peasants in the Taicang area. Chen also opened paper mills in Wuxi and Hangzhou to produce toothpowder packages, and a number of plants for aerated water and glass bottles and Invincible-brand mosquito coils. His interests in manufacturing were not limited to chemical products. He gamely attempted to manufacture small Western appliances, including chemical fire extinguishers, portable duplicators, and offset printers. Not all of these attempts were successful, and many of his smaller plants were short-lived. But Chen Diexian became famous as a vocal leader of the National Products Movement, and Household Industries thrived.

104. Shanghai jilianhui, "Jiating gongyeshe," 115–16.

Conclusion

Chinese businessmen took every opportunity to attract consumers and expand their businesses. Karl Gerth and Frank Dikötter offer different opinions regarding how Chinese consumers made their choices: whereas Gerth concludes that the National Products Movement was successful in creating "patriotic consumption," Dikötter argues that pragmatism, not economic nationalism, ruled China's market.[105] Yet the accounts of Fang Yexian and Chen Diexian suggest that both forces played a role. These men were flexible about marketing strategies and took whatever actions were needed to sell their products. By definition, a business should be expansive, efficient, and profitable. To achieve these goals, Fang and Chen studied basic chemistry and conducted experiments; they set up workshops and factories, sought new sources of inexpensive raw materials, and created a self-sufficient production system to help keep prices low. They exploited family and friend connections. They did not hesitate to make cheaper imitations of foreign brands. They offered monetary incentives to retailers. And they actively participated in and took advantage of New Life and other mass movements, appealing to consumers' patriotism when needed. Through various business strategies, Fang, Chen, and other Chinese manufacturers were able to expand their businesses and promote their "healthful goods." Westerners introduced soap, tooth-powder, and other personal-hygiene items to China, and Chinese intellectuals championed personal cleanliness. But it was the small Chinese manufacturers who first popularized personal-hygiene items and spread hygiene practices among the Shanghai populace.

Fang and Chen bear some resemblance to Huang Chujiu and other Chinese sellers of Western drugs. Sherman Cochran uses the concepts of "poaching" and "popularizing" to explain the significant role that Huang played in spreading Western ideas and values through his commercial activities. In Cochran's words, "Huang co-opted some of the Chinese intellectual elite's most cherished causes—advocacy of Western medicine, economic nationalism, and women's liberation—and commodified

105. Gerth, *China Made*; Dikötter, *Exotic Commodities*, 36–47.

them to promote his products."[106] Like Huang, small manufacturers of personal-hygiene items referred to the ideas of modern science, a healthy body, hygiene practices, and national salvation in their promotions. They also succeeded in linking their products to the idea of *weisheng*. *Weisheng*, an abbreviation of *baowei shengming*, was a term that "achieved an unprecedented status of power and prestige"[107] in early twentieth-century China. During the Republican period, it became the subject of various writings (both academic and popular), education programs, and urban reforms. But the meaning of the term was by no means fixed, and different people used it in different contexts. *Weisheng* can be translated into numerous English words and phrases: it connotes health, hygiene, sanitation, public health, hygiene practice, cleanliness, self-cultivation, nutrition, proper diet, and so forth.[108] Shanghai's hospitals aimed at "protecting lives" (*baowei shengming*) of patients from sickness and other misfortunes, administrators opened a public health bureau (*weishengju*), and reformers organized hygiene campaigns (*weisheng yundong*). Not only intellectuals but also Shanghai's general populace adopted the term to describe a variety of items, actions, and conditions in a very casual manner. Some obscure authors of *zhuzhici* sarcastically commented on the strange and indiscriminate use of this term. It could be used to describe soy sauce and vegetarianism and was even employed as a name of a brothel.[109] Shanghai industrialists and merchants were aware of these various discourses on *weisheng* and added a new dimension. *Weisheng* meant being clean and germ-free, and cleanliness resulted from using personal-hygiene items. Anyone could achieve *weisheng* by purchasing and using their goods.

This discussion of personal-hygiene items offers us a new perspective on state-society relations in twentieth-century China. In her discussion of family reforms, Susan Glosser points out close connections among the

106. Cochran, "Marketing Medicine," 91.
107. Dikötter, *Sex, Culture, and Modernity*, 23; Dikötter, *Exotic Commodities*, 206.
108. Rogaski, *Hygienic Modernity*; Lei Hsiang-lin, "Weisheng weihe bu shi baowei shengming?"; Furth, "Introduction: Hygienic Modernity in Chinese East Asia," 7. Historians have observed that the development of modern nationalism in different societies created new ideas about the body and promoted state control over the individual's body. See Parker et al., eds., *Nationalisms and Sexualities*.
109. Gu Bingquan, ed., *Shanghai yangchang zhuzhici*, 235.

nation, state, and society. She contends that during the Republican and early Communist period, most Chinese intellectuals did not make a clear distinction between the nation (the community to which people belong) and the state (the bureaucratic governmental apparatus). Because they believed that the Chinese nation would collapse without a strong state, they accepted and facilitated invasive policies by the state and the expansion of state power over the society. Glosser writes that "given certain desperate circumstances, societies may prostrate themselves to authoritarian states in hopes of saving the nation. Reformers and revolutionaries of all political stripes welcomed state intervention and willingly subordinated individual rights to the demands of the state in return for its promise to save China."[110] Glosser's points are relevant here. The threat to China's sovereignty solidified the alliance between the Nationalist state and society. China's medical elites hoped to restore the nation's strength and independence by creating a healthy and hygienic population, and there was a growing acceptance of the concept that the state was responsible for protecting and guiding the people. Shanghai's entrepreneurs' rush to produce and sell hygiene items is a testament to how successful administrators were in awakening consciousness about hygiene practices among the populace, and some commercial pitches drew heavily on patriotic versions of hygiene. The rise of nationalism and the development of everyday-chemical industries occurred in tandem. Shanghai's industrialists agreed with the Nationalist agenda based on state authority and national strengthening. National-salvation discourse was prominent in their advertisements, and their rationale for selling and advocating "healthful goods" drew on the currency of the link between healthy individuals and a strong nation. Shanghai's entrepreneurs actively participated in Nationalist-sponsored mass movements and encouraged consumers to practice hygiene as the state prescribed it.

However, the main interest of Shanghai's entrepreneurs still lay in sales of their commodities—not in supporting national salvation or spreading medical knowledge. Their vision of hygienic modernity remained a personal matter. Instead of looking to the state to construct medical facilities or improve urban sanitation, entrepreneurs focused on the everyday customs of individual people. Each individual was obliged to clean

110. Glosser, *Chinese Visions of Family and State,* 19.

his or her body and surroundings and to contribute to the nation; personal-hygiene items promised a means for fulfilling these obligations. Most such items were inexpensive and readily available, and they provided a small but effective material foundation for achieving personal hygiene. Administrators used hygiene practices as a vehicle for disciplining and educating citizens, while Shanghai's businessmen used it as a channel to sell their merchandise. They welcomed the detailed instructions the state provided about private practices of grooming and washing because state intervention helped promote and even legitimate the use of their products. They did not really prostrate themselves to the Nationalist state; rather, they recognized a marketing opportunity in the state's public health policies.

CONCLUSION

B y considering what it meant to be healthy and hygienic for various people in late nineteenth- and early twentieth-century Shanghai, I have aimed to show how global public health became an inherent aspect of Shanghai's domestic life. Under pressure from Western and Japanese imperialism, Shanghai's pursuit of good health was accompanied by a strong desire to participate in global modernity and an increasing awareness of Chinese inferiority. Yet, this pursuit took various forms. People followed different strategies and methods to stay well and clean, and these strategies and methods were embedded in local culture and particular environments. Physical health and hygiene were personal matters, but they were not independent from Shanghai society and the Chinese nation. I have attempted to link issues associated with health and hygiene to Shanghai's local settings, such as traditions of philanthropy and social networks of Shanghai elites, the presence of the West in the city and the city's semi-colonial status, the prevalence of mass media, the repertoire of collective actions and civic rituals, and the development of commerce and industry. Through a discussion of these issues and links, I have tried to illuminate how Shanghai's urban culture and concerns for national survival interacted with people's perceptions of their own bodies.

From the late Qing through the Republican period, Shanghai's social and medical elites were primarily responsible for introducing Western science and medical systems and for promoting ideas about public health among the general populace. The city's medical doctors opened hospitals to protect people's lives from diseases and other troubles and to help them conform to social norms. As biomedicine gained confidence among the Chinese populace, hospitals transformed from charitable institutions for the poor to venues for research and education. In this process, hospitals also became vibrant centers for medical elites to raise and assert their prestige and authority. Creating a healthy population was also a state project. After Chiang Kai-shek and the Nationalist Party consolidated their power, the Ministry of Public Health took steps to build a nationwide public health system. Nationalist leaders and elites believed that public health should serve the interest of the state, and the state required a sturdy and hardworking citizenry. Shanghai's Public Health Bureau (PHB) was part of this Nationalist scheme, and recovering Chinese sovereignty was one of its mandates. At the same time, however, the Shanghai PHB had local origins, and its work was significantly augmented by nongovernmental hospitals and other social organizations in the city. Administrators strove to provide necessary services, while also implementing public health policies through inspection, policing, and compulsion. In particular, during the Japanese occupation, Chinese health officers and Japanese military forces worked together to carry out systematic anticholera injection drives. The idea of protecting people from cholera by means of modern medicine provided a basis for Chinese collaboration and was used to justify coercive measures in public health work.

At the same time, Shanghai's elites and administrators did not maintain exclusive control over the discourse on health and hygiene. Public health involved not only discipline and coercion but also an "internalization of desire for health on the part of each citizen."[1] Administrators extended education and spread information. By doing so, they invited "individuals voluntarily to conform to their objective [and] to discipline themselves."[2] We have seen that, during citywide hygiene campaigns, campaign organizers were able to leverage the city's cultural capital and familiar rituals to persuade and mobilize a broad spectrum of society. We have also seen that not only administrators participated in these campaigns; merchants also participated in them and took advantage of opportunities to promote their businesses. Through a discussion of institutions, practices,

1. Bashford, *Imperial Hygiene*, 11.
2. Lupton, *Imperative of Health*, 11.

and products related to health and hygiene, I have addressed reciprocal interactions among Western medicine, state authorities, colonial powers, and Shanghai's local culture.

Health and Hygiene in post-1949 China

The Communist victory in the civil war in 1949 brought considerable change to Shanghai and to the lives of Shanghai's residents. Once the new regime was in power, Communists strove to remake Shanghai from a semi-colonial city to a revolutionary city that was free from imperialism, capitalist exploitation, and various urban vices and decadences. They expelled foreigners and confiscated their properties; collectivized private businesses and attacked "reactionaries" and "unpatriotic" bourgeois; balanced budgets and controlled inflation; and rehabilitated prostitutes, opium addicts, and gangsters. Early Communist writings are full of descriptions of "liberation from the feudal past" and the "renewal of the city."[3]

Like Republican elites and Nationalists, Chinese Communists also regarded a healthy people as the foundation of national strength. They reestablished the nation's public health administration and resumed medical services. At the same time, they prioritized economic development and political correctness over social welfare. A case in point is the set of four "principles" established by the Communists as directives for China's public health work. Communist leaders convened public health conferences in 1950 and adopted three primary principles: medicine should serve workers, peasants, and soldiers (*gong-nong-bing*); priority should be placed on preventive medicine; and Western medicine and Chinese medicine should be integrated. In 1952, after the alleged American germ attack during the Korean War, Communist leaders added the fourth principle: health work and mass mobilization should be combined.[4]

---

3. For posters that feature "socialist transformation" of Shanghai, see http://chineseposters.net/themes/shanghai.php.
4. Sidel and Sidel, *Serve the People*, 21; Huang Shuze and Lin Shixiao, eds., *Contemporary China*, 3–4; Scheid and Lei, "Institutionalization of Chinese Medicine," 249.

These principles are an interesting mixture of multiple elements. The first two, the socialist ideals of "for the people" and emphasis on prophylactic measures rather than clinical studies, derived from the Soviet Union. In the early years of the PRC, medical policies of the Soviet Union served as a model. Even after China-Soviet relations cracked apart and Russian experts and advisers left China in 1960, the Soviet legacy remained, and Marxist-Leninist ideology continued to feature China's medical education. The third principle displayed Communist efforts to rejuvenate and make sense of Chinese tradition within a framework of a new revolutionary culture. Finally, the fourth principle directly responded to the recent international crisis. These principles were open to multiple interpretations and applications; overall, they reflected political and ideological considerations to a greater degree than the medical or therapeutic efficacy of specific programs. Instead of allocating large resources or making a high investment, the new Chinese state relied on individual efforts and commitment. The principles served as the general guideline for China's public health and medical professionals for most of the twentieth century.

In this context, Communists restructured national and local public health administration and centralized and standardized medical education. They turned hospitals and other medical facilities into public institutions and trained not only doctors but also various kinds of medical workers, including midwives, pharmacists, and assistants. To give medical aid to people in rural and suburban areas, the Party dispatched "barefoot doctors," local paramedics who had received short-term training in primary care. Under state patronage and funding, traditional Chinese medicine regained official recognition and national prestige. The Communists introduced the work unit (*danwei*) system and provided medical care and health insurance through this system. Under the new socialist regime, basic medical care became widely available, general sanitation significantly improved, and various infectious and parasitic diseases were largely eliminated by the late 1970s. Except during the Great Leap Forward, China's life expectancy increased and its infant mortality rate decreased to a considerable degree. Progress in Shanghai's public health was particularly impressive. Authors of *Shanghai weisheng* proclaim that the city's health made "significant achievements." As of 1983, the entire city had a total of 6,451 medical facilities, including hospitals, workplace clinics, and health stations.[5] The average life expectancy of Shanghai residents was 74.90 in 1990 and 78.14 in 2000, significantly higher than measures of the national average (68.55 and 71.04).[6] Yet, in spite of these images of a complete transformation during the Communist era, 1949 was not a clear dividing line. Many of the changes, reforms, and innovations Communists introduced were, in fact, already in place during the Nationalist era. As Hanchao Lu has written, "the changes brought by the 'Liberation' may not be as thorough and fundamental as people have previously thought."[7] Moreover, these changes were not always the intended outcome of Communist plans for the revolutionary society, nor did they always reflect positive medical progress. Rather, they were slow and gradual processes that involved contingencies, compromises, and political consideration.

Post-Mao economic reforms that began in 1978 brought about dramatic social changes to the direction of profit-making, and health care was one of the key sites for building a market economy. A great deal of governmental control and support was withdrawn from hospitals and clinics, and global capitalism entered China's medical market. Although capitalism provided a broader range of health-care products and services, it also altered and, in fact, deteriorated the state-subsidized medical system. Rather than relying on paramedics and district nurses to provide community health care, doctors and specialists who conducted hospital-based clinical work came to play major roles. The rapidly burgeoning presence in Chinese cities of pharmaceutical industries and other health-related businesses have directly exposed citizens to new goods, practices, and ideas to protect and promote their physical and mental well-being. With the expansion of commercialism and the dismantling of the state-run insurance system and workplace benefits, the search for good health required money and connection. Commercialization has created disparities between the rich and poor, and cities and the countryside. The Communist state is still pervasive, but it is not the only or predominant power to

5. *Shanghai weisheng gongzuo congshu* bianweihui, *Shanghai weisheng, 1949–1983* (*SW*), 3–4.
6. Wang Shucheng., eds., *Zhongguo weisheng shiye fazhan*, 40.
7. Hanchao Lu, *Beyond the Neon Lights*, 316.

provide health care and regulate or control the medical market. Shanghai has always been the center of the Chinese economy; state power, commercial interests, and medical concerns have continued to interact with each other in the city throughout the reform-era to this day.

Physical well-being has always been an individual, a social, and a national concern. As such, exploring changes and continuities in Chinese perceptions of body and health from the Republican era to the Communist era, and tracing the trajectory from the radical Maoist era to the more recent reform era, could offer a promising way to sharpen our understanding of nationhood and citizenship in modern China. Yet, it would require another volume to thoroughly examine Shanghai's public health since 1949. Thus, rather than providing a comprehensive account, I concentrate on two relevant topics to conclude this book.

First, in this conclusion, we trace the transformation of hospitals and other health-care-providing institutions after 1949. We explore how Communists reorganized medical institutions and recruited medical workers so that they would conform to socialist norms and could meet the needs of the local populace. In doing so, Communists exploited and capitalized on preexisting institutions and resources and trained and fostered grassroots-level health-care workers in particular neighborhoods. This chapter also shows how medical care has increasingly diverged from early ideals based on Marx-Lenin ideology to help the masses, and has become more and more commercialized since the 1980s. As Nancy Chen notes, with the development of a market economy, China's health care transformed "from socialist communal care to individual consumption."[8] Such a transformation is particularly evident in Shanghai. Discussing changes in medical facilities and services connects this conclusion to chapter 1, which traces the history of hospitals, and to chapter 4, which focuses on commercial culture.

Second, following chapters 2 and 3, we discuss how the Communist state dictated power and incorporated individual and national health into mass movements. Once Mao Zedong and the Communists took over the country, they repeatedly carried out political campaigns to involve the masses and to attack class enemies. Through these campaigns, they strove to construct "revolutionary citizenship" to create legitimate members of a

8.   Nancy Chen, "Health, Wealth, and the Good Life," 165.

new China.[9] The Patriotic Hygiene Campaigns, which launched in 1952 in the middle of the Korean War to fight against American germ attacks, were one of these campaigns. Mao applied the concept of "people's war" to the campaigns and required the people, instead of experts and scientists, to participate in this war. In Shanghai, too, local cadres organized patriotic hygiene campaign committees and carried out citywide movements to mobilize the masses. Connections between physical well-being, environmental sanitation, patriotism, political correctness, commitment to the revolution, and medical knowledge were featured more strongly and prominently than ever in these campaigns. After 1952, patriotic hygiene campaigns became regular events, and these have been carried out throughout the twentieth century. However, hygiene campaigns were not a Communist invention. Communists carried them out in a similar manner to Nationalist-era events, and campaign programs and methods were deeply embedded in China's cultural repertoire. Yet, since the late twentieth century, along with economic, social, and cultural changes, campaigns have been increasingly losing their centripetal force. Examining Communist hygiene campaigns and looking into what has changed and what has not will highlight the significance of public health in China's social and political life.

Reorganizing Medical-Care Facilities

When Communists arrived in Shanghai, they sorted out, adjusted, and reorganized the city's medical-care institutions. First, they seized and expropriated existing hospitals operated by the Nationalist government, foreigners, and social organizations (such as native-place associations, schools, and churches). They also took over health stations under the Nationalist government. Concurrently, they assumed tighter control over private institutions. The new Public Health Bureau set up a unified price schedule for medical treatments, drugs, and tests and imposed it on all private hospitals in the city. Then, in the early 1950s, Communists gradually rearranged and reorganized private institutions. Under party directives,

9.   On revolutionary citizenship, see Perry, *Patrolling the Revolution*.

some were merged with others, some ceased operation, and those that remained were turned into public institutions. Eventually, by 1956, all the hospitals in the city were placed under governmental jurisdiction. The Communists also opened new hospitals and new departments that practiced Chinese medicine and Chinese-Western combined medicine (*zhongxiyi jiehe*).[10] At the same time, with guidance and financial help from the new government, the city's smaller clinics and private practitioners, including those who did not have a medical degree but had relevant experiences, were grouped into joint factory health stations (*gongchang lianhe baojianzhan*), joint clinics (*lianhe zhensuo*), and joint health stations for women and children (*lianhe fuyou baojianzhan*). These small institutions were collectively called "joint-medical-care institutions" (*lianhe yiliao jigou*) and included those that practiced Chinese medicine.[11]

Using these institutions as the starting point, the new public health bureau under the Communist regime classified the city's medical facilities into three levels and eventually created a three-layered health-care network. The institutions at the most basic level were "lane" or "block" hospitals (*jiedao yiyuan* or *diduan yiyuan*) in the city proper, township health stations (*xiang weishengyuan* or *zhen weishengyuan*) in the suburbs, and public health stations (*baojianzhan*) at workplaces. Second-level institutions included district hospitals (*qu yiyuan*) in the city proper and county hospitals (*xian yiyuan*) in the suburbs. Third-level institutions, also called municipal-level hospitals (*shiji yiyuan*), included large general hospitals, university hospitals, and large hospitals that practiced Chinese medicine. With this hierarchy, Communists introduced a division of labor among medical institutions. Whereas basic-level institutions offered primary care and easy access, second- and third-level institutions examined more complex cases. In particular, top-level hospitals were also engaged in advanced research and teaching. These institutions were connected and supplemented each other's work. Lower-level institutions referred and sent patients to upper-level ones, and upper-level ones gave advice and offered training to those who worked at lower-level institutions.[12] With subsidies

---

10. Scheid, "The People's Republic of China," 239–83.
11. *SW*, 18–19.
12. *SW*, 18–30; *SWZ*, 84–90.

from the central government, the costs for basic medical services were kept very low.

Of all these medical institutions, lane hospitals, which had direct contact with local residents, best represented the socialist ideal of community health. These institutions developed from the various joint medical-care institutions discussed above and were small operations, located throughout the city. As cooperative organizations of medical workers, they served as the foundation of grassroots health care. In 1951, Shanghai PHB held a conference to which they invited the city's medical professionals. At this conference, professionals decided that establishing "joint institutions" was one of their significant tasks. Then, in 1956, the PHB convened "The City of Shanghai Joint Medical Care Institution Professionals Meeting." Attendees agreed that "joint institutions" were the foundation of socialist medicine and that the development of these institutions should be promoted. As a result, the number of "joint institutions" continued to increase. As of 1957, there were a total of 417 "joint institutions" in the city proper. Around 1958, when the Great Leap Forward launched, these institutions were collectivized within a particular lane so that they could share medical facilities, equipment, and personnel and eventually reorganized into lane hospitals. Lane hospitals were collectively owned and operated by medical workers and served those who lived and worked in the lane. By 1965, the Municipal Public Health Bureau had issued laws and regulations about the duties, operation, and management of lane hospitals, defining them as the primary component of China's socialist public welfare.[13] Lane hospitals were supposed to be self-supporting, but in practice they received financial subsidies from the state.

In general, lane hospitals offered both Chinese and Western medical treatment and had multiple departments, including internal medicine, surgery, gynecology, Chinese medicine, acupuncture, and the five sensory organs (*wuguan*) (eyes, ears, nose, mouth, and tongue). They examined mostly outpatients, but some had inpatient facilities. Some also administered a "family-care hospital bed" (*jiating bingchuang*) system and made house calls. In addition to providing clinical care and treating emergency cases, lane hospitals also supervised and inspected food safety and took charge of the occupational and school health of small businesses and

13. *SW*, 18–21.

schools in the lane. As of 1983, there were a total of 103 lane hospitals in Shanghai proper.[14]

The lane hospital was significantly supported and augmented by residents' committees (*jumin weiyuanhui*) (RC). Organizationally, the RCs were located at the intersection between the vertical administrative hierarchy and horizontal interpersonal network. Next to municipal-, district-, and lane-level institutions, they were the "fourth-level" administration to govern, monitor, and serve the neighborhoods; they also represented the interest of the specific locale. An RC consisted of delegates of "cells." A cell, in turn, consisted of residents of an apartment complex or a block. RC members comprised mostly "retirees in good health and housewives who are popular in the neighborhood, who have the time and desire to serve the public interest wholeheartedly"[15] and many of them were women. The function of the RC was reminiscent of that of the prewar *baojia* system, but when the Communists enacted regulations on the RCs in 1954, RCs were given greater responsibility and assigned more duties.[16] Most relevant to this discussion, the RCs operated residents' committee health stations (*juwei weishengzhan*). RC health stations first emerged around 1956 out of the enthusiasm for the patriotic hygiene campaigns. In some cases, they were run by the Red Cross Society. These health stations provided the most basic site for environmental hygiene and medical services for a neighborhood. Station staff were called "red medical workers": local residents who had received basic training in primary care, an urban equivalent to barefoot doctors in the countryside. Like their rural counterparts, they gave advice on birth control and maternal care; carried out simple physical tests, such as measuring blood pressure; administered various vaccinations and immunizations; circulated information and reports on infectious diseases; organized sanitation efforts, such as catching flies and eradicating larvae; supervised people's hygiene practices and fitness activities; and tended to those with chronic illnesses and

---

14. *SW*, 20; *SWZ*, 88.
15. Cheng Gang, "Neighborhood Committee," 31.
16. On residents' committees, see Read, *Roots of the State*; Chen, Cooper, and Sun, "Spontaneous or Constructed?" For a personal account of an RC member in Shanghai, see Frolic, ed., *Mao's People*, 224–41.

mental disabilities. They also practiced acupuncture and prescribed herbal drugs.[17]

Communist experiences in the 1930s and 1940s, earlier precedents from the Nationalist era, and local adjustments and cooperation all helped the new government apply socialist ideals to local health care and make these arrangements. When they were at war against the Nationalists and Japanese, Communists developed their medical programs in base areas. In addition to field and rear hospitals, they set up small clinics and medical and pharmaceutical cooperatives for civilians. They also recruited Chinese-style practitioners and herbalists and trained medical aides. In this process, Communists learned how to optimize available resources and connect medicine with the revolution. In the Communist scheme, hospitals and other institutions were operated by and for the "masses," and the community medical care was a marker of "socialist superiority." Medicine should serve the common good and the revolution. In addition to fighting the Nationalist army and Japanese invaders, medical workers were "white-coat warriors" who fought against not only diseases and pathogens but also superstitions and ignorance. As such, they were discouraged from pursuing personal profit.[18] When Communists brought their programs to post-1949 Shanghai, they did not create a new system from scratch. They took over existing institutions and personnel and converted and adjusted them to accord with their vision. The majority of the hospitals and clinics in the city had been opened before 1949, and small medical institutions and health stations and offices were also in operation. The RCs and RC health stations, the most basic element of Communist health care, were staffed by local "grannies" and "aunties" who were familiar with neighborhood affairs. The Communist medical system was neither a complete break from the past nor a simple copy of early examples. Rather it was a combination of various elements.

With the introduction and the development of the market economy, the entire social structure that supported the Communist health-care system has changed. The new economic reforms that began in the early 1980s improved China's living standard. At the same time, reforms also

17. *SW*, 22; *SWZ*, 84; For detailed reports on lane hospitals and health stations in China in 1971 and 1972, see Sidel and Sidel, *Serve the People*, 68–74.
18. Watt, *Saving Lives in Wartime China*.

resulted in the withdrawal of the state from various service sectors, including health and medicine, which caused problems. As state-owned enterprises became privatized, and the communes were dissolved, they were no longer able to fund the medical or health insurance costs of employees and members. Although China's GDP and government revenue has continued to increase from the 1980s through the twenty-first century, the proportion of health-care spending from government expenditure has not increased. State subsidies for hospitals also decreased, and hospitals have had to be financially independent. To this end, the government launched the reorganization and deregulation of medical institutions, and accordingly, hospitals and clinics transformed from being providers of socialist welfare to self-supporting businesses. The Communists introduced the "responsibility system" (*chengbao zerenzhi*) to hospital management. Under this new system, hospitals were still owned by the state, but hospital directors were given greater discretion and responsibility over management.[19] The state policy still required hospitals to keep prices for basic medical care low, but allowed them to charge higher prices for drug prescriptions and complex procedures and examinations. As a result, hospitals have tended to overprescribe expensive drugs, overprovide high-tech tests to generate more revenue, and overlook less lucrative primary care.[20] The government also legalized medical practice by private doctors. After 1949, as most medical institutions were placed under governmental control and supervision, the number of private practitioners significantly decreased. In particular, during the Cultural Revolution, those who had received advanced education became targets of political persecution. However, economic reforms have encouraged the reemergence and growth of private practices. Not only doctors of biomedicine but also those who practice Chinese and Chinese-Western medicine as well as former barefoot doctors have opened private offices. These private doctors were entrepreneurs interested in turning a profit rather than in being the servants of the people.[21] In addition to medical practitioners, pharmaceutical companies and other health-related industries have been flourishing since

19. Yoshida, *Chūgoku shin iryō eisei taisei no keisei*, 50–53.
20. Saich, *Providing Public Goods*, 83.
21. Yoshida, *Chūgoku shin iryō eisei taisei no keisei*, 43–46, 53–55. On private practitioners of Chinese medicine in a county town in Shandong, see Farquhar, "Market Magic."

the 1980s. With the increased use of prescribed medicine and a greater number of people willing and able to afford to purchase over-the-counter drugs and supplements, foreign and Chinese pharmaceutical companies have opened and expanded operations in China. Nancy Chen has observed the window displays and storefront clinics of fancy drugstores as well as colorful advertisements for drugs on television and in magazines.[22] These medical businesses and entrepreneurs offer more options and choices for consumer-patients and create a different ambience from that of the state-run hospitals.

Economic development has brought diverse medical services and advanced curative measures to the Chinese people. However, as the overall quality of health care has improved, it has become more expensive. A big question is, who should pay the bill? The total health expenditure per year in China was 14.3 billion yuan in 1980, 74.7 in 1990, 458.7 in 2000, and 759 in 2004. Accordingly, per capita health expenditure per year also increased rapidly. It was 14.5 yuan in 1980, 65.37 in 1990, and 361.9 in 2000.[23] In spite of soaring medical and health-related costs, in relation to the total health expenditure, the proportion of the expenditure covered by the government, state-owned-enterprises, and communes has decreased. This means that individuals have had to take more responsibility for their own bills. Personal spending made up less than 30 percent of total health expenditure in the 1980s; it reached 40 percent in the 1990s, and was over 50 percent by the early 2000s.[24] These figures indicate that medical costs have squeezed family budgets and caused financial problems for some individuals and families. Because of high medical fees, those without health insurance, such as retirees and migrant workers, have had trouble receiving proper health care.[25] Cities have more hospitals, doctors, and beds per capita than are found in the countryside; in spite of this, medical care has become less affordable and less accessible for the urban poor.

22. Nancy Chen, "Health, Wealth, and the Good Life," 174–80.
23. Yoshida, *Chūgoku shin iryō eisei taisei no keisei,* 89–90; Saich, *Providing Public Goods,* 79.
24. Yoshida, *Chūgoku shin iryō eisei taisei no keisei,* 103–4; Saich, *Providing Public Goods,* 77.
25. Saich, *Providing Public Goods,* 82.

Shanghai provides an illuminating example of health disparity within a city. Beginning in the 1980s, and after the 1990s in particular, Shanghai's urban planners have been striving to physically transform the city into a modern megalopolis by building highways and skyscrapers. At the same time, by retaining and renovating historical monuments and architecture, they also have been working hard to preserve and uphold the city's cultural heritage from the pre-1949 era. This grand project—creating a cosmopolitan city with tradition—does not evenly benefit Shanghai's entire population. While the city is rising as the business and financial center of the nation and East Asia, state-owned factories are being downsized and closed. Factory workers, who once were the vanguard of the revolution, are being laid off without monetary compensation or health insurance. Even though Shanghai offers various medical services, these services are not within the financial means of laid-off workers. These people tend to live in the city's "lower quarters," which used to feature graveyards and shantytowns. As Pan Tianshu's study demonstrates, neither the Communist Revolution nor the post-socialist renovation completely eliminated the "spatial dichotomy" between the poor and well-off sectors in the city.[26] This dichotomy also reflects social and economic inequalities and disparities in terms of available medical care. The ideals of providing public health to protect the corporeal and mental life of all men and women have not yet been attained.

In the twenty-first century, the Chinese state seems to have reentered the market for a cure to alleviate these problems and to improve the health of the nation. The government has organized a series of meetings, issued statements on health-care reforms, and announced that their objectives are to provide "equal access of all Chinese residents to basic medical care and health services" and "to establish fundamental medical and health care system covering both urban and rural areas by 2020."[27] China is now facing a challenge to balance governmental involvement and effective marketization in the field of public health. Liberalization of the economy and competition should allow private doctors and entrepreneurs to enter the medical market and offer affordable services. At the same time, medical care is a part of social welfare, and the government

26. Pan Tianshu, "Place Attachment."
27. State Council Information Office, *Health Care in China*, 2–3.

needs to take more responsibility and invest in public funding. These issues have larger implications not only for Shanghai and China but also for every country in the world. Further studies are needed to understand how professionals and administrators of other countries are attempting to solve similar problems.

Organizing Hygiene Campaigns

Along with community-based health care, mass campaigns have been a significant feature of Communist public health programs. Following the precedents of the Nationalist-era campaigns, Communists resumed hygiene campaigns to involve the city residents almost immediately after they arrived in the city. In June 1949, they convened a conference and decided to conduct mass campaigns to improve citizens' health and urban sanitation. Accordingly, they organized injection teams to administer anti-cholera injections. They also mobilized some 3,600 people to dispose of debris and corpses. In January 1950, the People's Government of Shanghai issued a notice on sanitation and hygiene campaigns (*qingjie weisheng yundong*), and mayor Chen Yi (1901–72) wrote an epigraph: "Let us promote and develop sanitation and hygiene campaigns, preserve citizens' health, and hope all citizens will contribute to the joint effort." Responding to this call, Shanghai people created sanitation and hygiene campaign committees in districts and lanes. They also organized more than twenty thousand neighborhood hygiene groups (*jumin weisheng xiaozu*). Beginning on January 8, some 200,000 people undertook a range of activities for a month, aiming at cleaning the war-torn city: they removed trash and waste, disposed of abandoned coffins, and cleaned and drained ditches.[28] Also, some 183,000 people joined "propaganda troops" (*xuanchuan duiwu*) to teach people how to avoid epidemics. Then, in May, the city carried out a summer anti-epidemic campaign. Schools and other units organized demonstration marches and gave various performances, including folk dances, waist-drum concerts, and masquerades, to promote knowledge about summer infectious diseases. They also used posters, pic-

28. *SW,* 43–44; *SWZ,* 217–18.

tures, radio programs, and films.[29] Following these efforts, the city organized similar cleanup campaigns and injection drives several times in 1950 and 1951.[30]

Shanghai's hygiene campaigns entered a new stage in 1952 with the news of American use of bacteriological weapons in the Korean War. In January and February, the North Korean army reported that US aircraft had repeatedly dispersed flies, fleas, grasshoppers, and other insects that carried pathogenic bacteria in several locations on the front lines and in rear areas. China confirmed the appearance of infected insects, and Zhou Enlai, then the foreign minister, made a statement in February to support North Korea and denounce the United States.[31] In spite of this, according to PRC official documents, the US Army kept using biological weapons in Korea and extended its attack to China. From February to April, American planes allegedly made more than one thousand sorties and dropped germ-infected pests in various locations in Manchuria and near Qingdao. China made an official protest and presented an open letter to the International Court of Justice.[32] Although American and Western authorities dismissed this allegation, China claimed that neither the Red Cross nor the World Health Organization was free from political bias. Harsh remarks such as "Monstrous American aggressors, whose hands are already steeped in blood" and "Punish the American Butchers Who Are Bombing and Spreading Germs in Northeast China" appeared in Chinese newspapers.[33] To deal with this epidemiological crisis, the central government established the Epidemic Prevention Committee (*fangyi weiyuanhui*), chaired by Zhou Enlai, in March. Following this, provinces and cities in China established similar committees in a quick succession. Shanghai was not a direct target of this alleged attack, but party directives defined the city as part of the "anti-epidemic supervisory region."[34] The city government also created an epidemic prevention committee and established its branches in districts, lanes, counties, and townships, as well as in schools and factories. In addition, the city also

29. *SW,* 270–71.
30. *SWZ,* 44.
31. *Stop U.S. Germ Warfare,* part 1: 5; part 2: 1–4.
32. Ibid., part 1: 8–9, 33–37.
33. Ibid., part 2: 13–32.
34. Lynteris, *Spirit of Selflessness,* 19.

set up the waterway (*shuishang*) epidemic prevention committee to be in charge of disinfection and inspection of docks and ships.[35] These committees and branches circulated information about the perils of biological warfare and instructed how to take precautions and countermeasures. People were urged to immediately notify the authorities in the event that they found any suspected insects or animals. Beginning in the spring, Shanghai organized several citywide campaigns to wipe away dirt and pathogens to protect the city from infection. This was not just ordinary cleaning; this was war against germs, pests, and American imperialists, and the entire Shanghai population was rallied to fight this war. According to *Shanghai weisheng*, in 1952, Shanghai people disposed of a total of 837,000 tons of trash and garbage, filled up 586,000 square meters of depressions, and cleared 400,000 square meters of ditches. They also eradicated 98,000 kilograms of flies, 8,000 kilograms of mosquitoes, and 461,000 mice. At the end of 1952, following directives from the central government, all epidemic prevention committees were renamed to the Patriotic Hygiene Campaign Committee (*aiguo weisheng yundong weiyuanhui*) (PHCC). Until it was transferred to the PHB in 1961, the municipal PHCC was an independent organization with several subordinate departments.[36]

When China first learned about the suspected germ attacks, Western and Chinese scientists visited the sites of the attacks to investigate flora and fauna and endorsed the allegation of the American use of biological weapons. These scientists served as witnesses and expressed anger against American imperialism.[37] The participation of and support from scientists gave credibility to the accusation and legitimated subsequent campaigns. This was an early example of the subjection of science and academia to PRC politics and a harbinger of the persecution of intellectuals in the Anti-Rightist Campaign and during the Cultural Revolution.[38] Even though scientists confirmed the existence of deadly germs, to defend the nation from the threat, instead of employing experts and having them contain and control epidemics, Communists decided to resort to Yan'an-

35. *SWZ*, 218.
36. *SW*, 44–46; *SWZ*, 218.
37. *Stop U.S. Germ Warfare*, part 3: 1–24; part 4.
38. Rogaski, "Nature, Annihilation, and Modernity."

style mass mobilization. It was laypeople who participated in hygiene campaigns and carried out cleaning work. Also, as time progressed, the target of the campaigns shifted from American imperialism to insects and animals that carried pathogens. In this regard, the "Compendium of Agricultural Development" that the central government issued in 1956 is noteworthy. The compendium proclaimed that patriotic hygiene campaigns should be routine (*jingchangxing*) events involving the masses, with productions that were actively promoted and developed. The compendium also featured the eradication of "four pests" (*sihai*) as a goal of the campaign.[39] "Four pests" originally included mice and rats, flies, mosquitoes, and sparrows. In 1960, the government decided to exclude sparrows and to add bedbugs to the list instead. Though small, all these pests are carriers of harmful pathogens and it was emphasized that they should be annihilated by all means: by destroying these pests, people could eliminate sources of infectious diseases and indirectly participate in fighting the war against the United States. However, catching and killing insects and animals and destroying their favorite habitats is not particularly heroic or glorious. Rather, it is a tiresome and physically demanding task. People swept streets and dredged sewage; sealed mouse holes; designed various mouse traps and caught mice; pruned bushes and reclaimed stagnant waters; sprayed insecticides into latrines and removed heaps of waste; and inspected and disinfected hotels, barbershops, and bathhouses.[40] Sometimes work units competed with each other for the highest number of insects and animals killed. The residents' committees and RC health stations played an important role in circulating orders and information and mobilizing local residents.[41] Motivated by patriotism and placed under social pressure, people carried out a variety of cleaning tasks; under the banner of "patriotic hygiene campaign," they were engaged in unpaid manual labor. The campaigns provided an opportunity for the new state to penetrate into the local community and demanded personal dedication through workplace and neighborhood networks.

39. For patriotic hygiene campaigns in Communist Shanghai, see, for example, Shanghai renmin chubanshe bianjibu, ed., *Dali kaizhan yi chusihai wei zhongxin de aiguo weisheng yundong*; SMA B-242-1-535-40; SMA B242-1-805-1; SMA A26-2-243.

40. *SW*, 45–46; *SWZ*, 221–223.

41. *SWZ*, 219; Frolic, ed., *Mao's People*, 228.

Like their Nationalist predecessors, Communist-era hygiene campaigns ran educational programs to spread knowledge on good hygiene and disease prevention. Campaign organizers published brochures, handbills, and posters; dispatched medical and literary workers to factories, schools, and lanes to give talks and perform skits; held slide and film shows; and sent "travel publicity cars" (*xunhui xuanchuanche*) to lanes to give "mini" health exhibitions.[42] In addition to these familiar and tested methods, Communists learned from the Soviet Union the technique of producing propaganda posters. Although posters played only a supplementary role, they were widely used in campaigns and conveyed vivid and lively images and messages.[43]

The patriotic hygiene campaigns emerged out of a mixture of factors. Nationalist precedents, Communist experiences in Yan'an, propaganda techniques imported from the Soviet Union, memories of the Japanese Unit 731, Korean War and Cold War ideologies, and deep anxiety about outbreaks of infectious disease all played a role. Hygiene campaigns had been a prominent feature of Communist strategies to unify and mobilize the masses. However, as time progressed, the very masses that took part in these campaigns increasingly dissolved and economically diversified. Eventually, there no longer existed a unified body to make "joint efforts" to "serve the people." Technological innovations in mass media and communication have changed the way the government communicates with and disseminates instructions among people, and, along with China's medical systems, hygiene campaigns are also changing in the twenty-first century.

Science, Policing, and Mass Mobilization Programs

China's medical system and network in transition were hit by a grave crisis at the beginning of the twenty-first century. Beginning in the autumn of 2002 and continuing through the spring of 2003, SARS (Severe Acute Respiratory Syndrome) struck China. Early cases of this strange

42. SMA B242-1-535-40.
43. Landsberger, "To Spit or Not to Spit."

type of pneumonia caused by an unknown coronavirus were found in Canton and Hong Kong. The development of modern transportation created greater opportunities for the swift dissemination of the virus, and in a short period of time, the disease spread from China throughout East and Southeast Asia as well as to parts of Canada. The case of SARS addresses various issues related to globalization. Obviously SARS was a transnational pandemic, and the virus traveled globally, regardless of national borders. China became a focus of a larger international struggle to contain the disease. Headlines and articles about SARS in China circulated worldwide, and data and information China produced attracted international attention. Conversely, global concerns about SARS profoundly influenced many aspects of social relations and personal experiences in China. Foreign presses reported Chinese customs of selling live animals and raw meat in open markets and raising stock and fowls in small family backyards to sell and to eat, and associated these customs with the disease. The accusation that China's "backward" practices contributed to the outbreak and spread of SARS caused "global embarrassment" and threatened China's status as a modern state.[44]

Research results suggest that SARS was controllable and only moderately infectious, yet the fatality rate among the elderly was higher than 50 percent. Initially Chinese officials denied the prevalence of SARS, despite the fact that China had the largest number of patients and deaths. Concern about political and social stability and the lack of accurate medical knowledge about the disease discouraged Chinese officials from making information public and taking timely action.[45] SARS is believed to have originated in southern China, but many cases also occurred in Beijing. When it became clear that SARS was serious, the Chinese government fired the health minister and the Beijing mayor for covering up SARS cases and for their incompetent handling of the disease. To prevent further spread of the disease and alleviate social anxiety, China's public health administrators took various measures: the new minister of health ordered three major hospitals in Beijing to be cordoned off. Patients as well as medical workers were not allowed to leave the

44. Mason, "Becoming Modern after SARS," 11–13; Mason, "H1N1 Is Not a Chinese Virus," 505–6.

45. Saich, "Is SARS China's Chernobyl," 73–77.

hospitals for a certain period of time. Health officials also ordered those who had had contact with suspected SARS carriers to quarantine themselves at home for twelve days, and suspected cases of SARS were immediately isolated and hospitalized. All SARS patients were required to report to the authorities.

The SARS outbreak affected both social life in Beijing and the sanitary habits of individuals. Schools and dormitories were closed, and public gatherings were cancelled. Because of the fear of being quarantined and hospitalized, students and migrant workers fled the city.[46] The population of Beijing is estimated to have dropped by some 15 to 20 percent.[47] Shops were also closed, and downtown Beijing became desolate. Western media showed schoolchildren and tricycle drivers wearing masks on Beijing streets. Sanitation workers patrolled the city to prohibit spitting in public, and fines for spitting increased tenfold. Volunteers stood on the streets to distribute tissues and spittle bags. Health officials ordered the RCs to monitor local communities, and residents were required to report to their committee when they discovered SARS patients in their neighborhood. Officials also arrested those who spread "unauthorized rumors" through the Internet and on cell phones.[48] Moreover, the Propaganda Department organized a "Struggle against SARS" campaign and rallied citizens to participate in measures to enhance the national spirit.[49] The implementation of SARS-control programs exemplifies a full-scale administrative effort to protect individual and community health as well as the national reputation.

Chinese responses to the SARS outbreak and its repercussions reveal historical continuities in epidemic prevention work as well as state efforts to restructure the public health apparatus. These SARS-control measures are quite understandable when interpreted against the story of health and diseases covered in this study. Health administrators in early twenty-first-century Beijing carried out epidemic-control programs in a manner similar to their counterparts in Republican Shanghai. Beijing administrators provided medical and social services, but they also enforced regulations,

46. Kaufman, "SARS and China's Health-Care Responses," 53.
47. Rawski, "SARS and China's Economy," 111.
48. Saich, "Is SARS China's Chernobyl," 89.
49. Ibid., 86–87.

confinement, quarantines, and even used policing to control SARS. The idea of protecting physical health from contagion using the theories of modern biomedicine granted these administrators the ability and authority to obtrude on people's lives and constrain their activities. We can locate the beginning of an intrusive pattern of state intervention in private bodies and behavior as far back as the Nationalists' handling of cholera injection drives and their promulgation of hygiene emergency laws. Outbreaks of infectious diseases provided both the Nationalists and the Communists with opportunities to expand their authority through disciplinary techniques and to order the people to follow detailed instructions. In their responses to such crises, Nationalists and Communists both championed science, organized campaigns, and sought to co-opt local grassroots organizations, whether the *baojia* system or the residents' committee, as state agents. Fighting against an epidemic was still analogous to defending the nation, and the body was still a site that merged national desires to be strong with individual desires to be healthy.

At the same time, the SARS crisis marked a turning point for China's public health work: from the socialist model of "to serve the people" to professional service to protect the community. As Katherine Mason's study has demonstrated, around and after the time of the SARS crisis, health stations have been gradually replaced by disease-prevention centers operated by white-collar professionals to carry out epidemiological research. The goal of these professionals of the new generation has not been simply to help the masses. Rather they have divided the "people" into categories: those who have been infected and need to be examined, and those who need to be protected and served. What matters most to them is not voluntarism or political correctness, but academic achievement, career advancement, international recognition, and material rewards. By adhering to universal scientific procedures and protocols, they have been striving to participate in and contribute to the global common good, which has excluded those who were "backward" and "dirty." Although the state organized the campaigns against SARS, as the Chinese population has become more mobile and stratified, it has been increasingly difficult to organize government-sponsored mass gatherings and marches. Failure of the state to offer affordable medical services and insurances further contributed to the general lack of coherence and political enthusiasm. The advent of new mass media, such as TV and the

Internet, has made conventional campaign methods less effective and appealing.[50]

These accounts also call attention to the meanings and power of medical science. Scholars have pointed out the subordination of science to politics in China during the Maoist era.[51] Yet such subordination is not unique to that era. As Ming-cheng Lo puts it, modernity and science "can never exist outside of the culturally specific plans of its deliverers and the culturally specific evaluations of its receivers."[52] In both the past and the present, medical science is rarely culturally and politically neutral. Moreover, the authority of medical science itself is not always well established: it is continually changing and developing, and outbreaks of new unknown diseases (such as AIDS and Ebola fever) present ongoing challenges. Nonetheless, health administrators of different regimes, including those of the Shanghai PHB during the Nationalist period, those who worked under the Japanese occupation, and those of Communist China, all assumed that modern medical science could overcome communicable diseases. The lesson from "the gospel of germs" endures, and the conviction that biomedicine can effectively kill germs and viruses and save human lives continues to give power and legitimacy to administrators and doctors with different political goals and visions.

It is also noteworthy that not only doctors of biomedicine but also those who specialized in traditional Chinese medicine were mobilized to treat a large number of SARS patients; sometimes they worked together side by side in the same institution. Doctors of Chinese medicine validated the presence of viruses and championed the efficacy of biomedicine, while observing and diagnosing SARS cases using the framework of the environment, climate, and physical constitutions. They paid special attention to regional diversities of symptoms and different stages of severity, and prescribed and administered herbal drugs accordingly. With state sponsorship, Chinese medicine is re-created and reestablished as a new tradition, and Chinese doctors participated in national efforts to defend people from the SARS threat in the early twenty-first century.[53]

50. Mason, *Infectious Change.*
51. For example, Laurence Schneider, *Biology and Revolution*; Shapiro, *Mao's War against Nature*; Rogaski, "Nature, Annihilation, and Modernity."
52. Lo, *Doctors within Borders,* 197.
53. Hanson, "Conceptual Blind Spots," 228–54.

Such a reliance on Chinese doctors indicates that Chinese medicine has not simply persisted or endured. Rather it points to China's medical integration and pluralism: Western medicine and Chinese medicine could coexist and interact with each other, and Chinese medicine continues to reinvent itself. China's "tradition" is never fixed or secure. It is always appropriated and accommodated to respond to social and political needs.

This study of health and hygiene is intertwined with various themes that have punctuated Shanghai's history and have shaped its society. Situated in Shanghai and focused on local affairs, local actors, and their perspectives and practices, much of my narrative highlights what is distinctive about Shanghai's urban life. This study of health and hygiene suggests the overlaps and interconnections between Western ideas and local customs in the city as well as the common threads that tie commercial promotion and intellectual discourse together in Shanghai. Shanghai people of all walks of life coped with Western institutions, governmental directives, and commercial advertisement in a sensible manner, and they were flexible and pragmatic in their adoption of and accommodation to different values and practices. They embraced what Hanchao Lu has called "a pragmatism of incorporating whatever was appealing and available to make life better (or in some cases to make life possible)"[54] to protect their lives and stay well. The power of hygienic modernity derived from the diverse views and behavior of Shanghai people and the breadth and reach of the cultural capital of the city.

During the last two centuries, Shanghai has served as a model for the economic development of China and has attracted people from all over China and the world. The city continues to be emulated, admired, and feared by people from other places; at times, it is an object of disgust. An examination of the history of health and hygiene in Shanghai has important implications for our understanding of modern Chinese cities. Yet such an examination might raise some methodological questions. How typical or exceptional was Shanghai? There is much about Shanghai that is distinctive, and we need to avoid the risk of singularity. How can Shanghai be compared and contrasted with other Chinese cities in the early twentieth century? Scholarship on other Chinese cities is growing

54. Hanchao Lu, *Beyond the Neon Lights*, 295.

rapidly. For example, *Remaking the Chinese City* was published as a result of the conference "Beyond Shanghai: Imagining the City in Republican China." Articles in this volume discuss nine Chinese cities, and deliberately exclude Shanghai from their investigations.[55] This purposeful exclusion allows these articles to modify the existing Shanghai-centered approach of Chinese urban studies. Such a trend is highly welcomed. Studies of other cities will introduce comparative perspectives and help us understand what is and is not unique to Shanghai and will illuminate the diversity of modern China's urban culture. Such research also facilitates academic conversations among scholars who study different cities and provide fresh insight into urban studies. In studying other cities and comparing them with Shanghai, health, hygiene, and medicine can provide useful reference points. Staying well is everyone's concern, but in their efforts to create salubrious urban environments, different cities have encountered different situations and problems and have employed diverse strategies to overcome particular challenges. How did residents of interior cities (such as Chengdu) and colonial cities (such as Changchun and Taipei) understand Western and Japanese medical ideas and models and apply them to their cities? How did administrators of capital cities (such as Beijing and Nanjing) create public health administrations and enforce their regulations? What medical institutions did they operate? How did merchants of hygiene items in other treaty ports (such as Canton) operate their businesses and advertise their products? What sort of commercial culture developed there? Exploring these questions will help us understand not only the diverse urban experiences of modern China but also the various ways in which people have made sense of their physical health in different contexts.

55. Esherick, ed., *Remaking the Chinese City.*

APPENDIX I

Shanghai and Its Foreign Concessions

To understand Shanghai's unique position in China, the history of the city's foreign concessions cannot be ignored.[1] Shanghai is a port city located at the junction of the Yangzi and Huangpu Rivers. It had been an important commercial town and a center of cotton trade in the Jiangnan area since the late Song period.[2] In the early nineteenth century, as proper maintenance of the Grand Canal became difficult, the Qing decided to switch from canal-based transportation to sea routes; this shift significantly invigorated Shanghai's rise as a commercial center.[3] However, the modern development of Shanghai began with its opening as a treaty port. At the close of the Opium War in 1842, the British and the Qing government of China signed the Treaty of Nanjing. This treaty stipulated British freedom of residence and commercial activity in five treaty ports, including Shanghai. Other foreign countries signed similar treaties, and they, too, were granted privileges of residence and commerce in Shanghai. These treaties also granted foreign extraterritoriality.

The Treaty of Nanjing opened the city to the West, while the Land Regulations (*tudi zhangcheng*), which were signed by the British consul

---

1.   On the foreign concessions in Shanghai, see for example, Xu Gongsu and Qiu Jinzhang, "Shanghai gonggong zujie zhidu"; Hanchao Lu, *Beyond the Neon Lights*, 25–40; Zheng Zu'an, *Bainian Shanghai cheng*, 168–244; Xiong Yuexi, ed., *Shanghai tongshi*, vol. 5, *WanQing shehui*, 17–36.

2.   Linda Johnson, *Shanghai*.

3.   Leonard, *Controlling from Afar*.

and the Shanghai *daotai* (circuit intendant) in 1845, provided the legal basis of the International Settlement. The Land Regulations allowed the British to rent real estate permanently in a designated area. This area, which lay north of the Chinese city and east of the Huangpu River, eventually became the International Settlement. The Land Regulations were revised several times and functioned as a charter for the International Settlement.[4] The Americans also settled to the northeast of the Chinese city, and in 1848 the Shanghai *daotai* verbally agreed to the creation of an American Settlement, which was incorporated into the International Settlement in 1863. Finally, in 1849, after negotiations, the French also acquired control of an area south of the International Settlement that later became the French Concession. As a result of these arrangements, the city of Shanghai was divided into three administrative sectors: the International Settlement, the French Concession, and the Chinese city, which consisted of the old walled city (Nanshi), the Zhabei area (the northeast part of the city proper), and other suburban areas. Altogether the Chinese sections encircled the foreign concessions. Though the foreign concessions were much smaller in area and were completely rural in the 1840s, they developed quickly and eventually became the center of the city's economic activities. Although the foreign sectors continued to expand their areas throughout the nineteenth century, their boundaries were roughly fixed by the early 1910s.[5]

Originally, the Chinese were not allowed to rent properties within the foreign concessions. At first, except for a small number of farmers, most concession residents were Westerners. They constructed Western-style buildings and facilities and enjoyed a Westernized (though isolated) lifestyle within the concessions. At the same time, it was also the Qing's intention to reserve rural areas outside the Chinese city for foreigners and to confine them to these designated areas. From the viewpoint of Qing officials, the presence of the foreign concessions in Shanghai continued

4. Lu Hanchao, "Shanghai tudi zhangcheng yanjiu," 100–145.
5. On the formation of the two foreign concessions, see, for example, Xiong Yuezhi, ed., *Shanghai tongshi*, vol. 5, *WanQing shehui*, 17–36; Xiong Yuezhi, ed., *Shanghai tongshi*, vol. 3, *WanQing zhengzhi*, 19–41.

the old Canton system, which kept the Chinese and Westerners separate.[6]

However, the segregation policy did not last long. The Small Sword Uprising, which broke out in 1853 and lasted seventeen months, marked its end. The Small Sword Society was a secret society that consisted primarily of Cantonese and Fujianese seamen. In September 1853, its members killed the Shanghai *zhixian* (county magistrate) and took over the walled city. They soon occupied other county towns in Shanghai's vicinity. A large number of Chinese refugees, many of whom were wealthy merchants and landlords, fled to the concessions. While some Westerners were concerned about the influx of Chinese into their areas, under the circumstances, it was virtually impossible to stop it. The rapid increase in the Chinese population provided some Westerners an opportunity to make a fortune by subletting residences to wealthy refugees. The Westerners revised the Land Regulations in 1854 and abandoned the segregation policy; doing so officially opened the foreign areas to the Chinese. The suppression of the Small Sword Uprising did nothing to stop the growth of the Chinese population in the concessions. Once again, in the 1850s and 1860s, a large number of Chinese people fleeing from the Taipings entered Shanghai. In fact, over the course of the nineteenth and twentieth centuries, most immigrants to the concessions were Chinese.

Although most residents in the foreign concessions were Chinese, the Chinese authorities did not govern or intervene in the affairs of the concessions; each had its own governing body. The International Settlement was administered by the Shanghai Municipal Council (SMC), first created by the Land Regulations of 1854. The SMC consisted of the representatives of local rate payers, though no Chinese joined until 1928. It was an autonomous body, did not have any formal connection with foreign countries or consulates, and oversaw the International Settlement's administration—including taxation, policing, public work, education, and public health—as well as its legislation. The Settlement also had its own judicial system. In sum, the SMC functioned as a quasi-government

6.   On the Qing's intention, see Lu Hanchao, "Shanghai tudi zhangcheng yanjiu," 17–128.

for the International Settlement until 1943.[7] Similarly, the French Concession was governed by the French Municipal Council (FMC), which, unlike the SMC, was chaired by a French official, the consul-general. While the SMC and the FMC were completely independent of each other, in practice the territories they oversaw were administered in a very similar manner. Despite the fact that most of their residents were Chinese, the two foreign concessions functioned largely as two independent administrative bodies within the Chinese city.

7.   On the SMC, see for example, Linda Johnson, *Shanghai*, 45–98; Xu Gongsu and Qiu Jinzhang, "Shanghai gonggong zujie zhidu," 117–54.

APPENDIX 2

The Lecture Outline for the 1942 Summer Campaign[1]

1. Reasons why you should not dump trash:
   Trash and garbage not only look bad, they will easily breed flies and mosquitoes and attract rats. These insects and animals are vectors of infectious diseases. Dumping trash and feces in the street is immoral behavior. It hurts others and oneself.

2. Since the weather is becoming hot, we should immediately eradicate flies.
   Flies flock together in filthy, smelly places. They carry various pathogenic bacteria, such as typhoid, cholera, and dysentery germs to our food. If we eat food the flies have touched, then we will become infected.

3. We should not eat unsanitary summer refreshments.
   Plum juice, ice cream, soda, water ice, and popsicles are refreshing summer drinks. They can relieve the heat and soothe the spirit. However, if they are made with filthy natural ice, or kept in unclean containers or in facilities that are not fly-proof, they can easily spread diseases.

1. SMA R50-736, 45–48.

4. Reasons why everyone should get cholera-preventive injections:
   Modern medical science has already proved that cholera is caused by the infection of the cholera bacillus. If one receives the cholera-preventive vaccine into one's body before infection sets in, the vaccination can strengthen the [body's] resistance.

5. Several things that individuals can do to prevent cholera:
   Even though cholera is dangerous, modern science is strong, and [so] there are ways to prevent it. Because this disease is transmitted by food, one must be careful in the handling of food and drink, sweep [one's residence] and keep it clean, eliminate flies, receive a cholera-prevention injection, and carry out strict sterilization of patients' discharges. In this way, we can decrease the pathogens and avoid infection.

6. Cleanliness is the foundation of health.
   There is no single way to achieve hygiene (*weisheng zhi dao*), but cleanliness should be understood as the foundation of health. If one's body is unclean and the environment is filthy, this will breed diseases, and they will hurt one's health. Therefore, the clothing one wears, household utensils, and residences all should be clean.

7. Why must one not use a shared towel?
   A shared towel will easily transmit trachoma. If a trachoma patient uses a towel, the pathogen of trachoma stays on the towel. If one does not disinfect the towel (one can boil it [to disinfect it]), one can become infected after using it. Trachoma is a trivial disease, but one can lose one's sight unless properly treated.

8. Benefits of getting sun and fresh air:
   Air and sunlight are free gifts from nature. Fresh air contains a great deal of "vital power." Our breathing is indispensable for circulation. Sunlight can kill germs and strengthen the body. A Western proverb says: "Where sunlight does not reach, germs can always thrive." Isn't this frightening?

9. One should exercise every day.
   The human body is like a machine. A machine will go out of order if it is not used. Human bodies become ill without exercise. Exercise is good for training one's physique and [makes the body] disease resistant. There is a wide range of types of exercise. No doubt, track racing, ball games, boxing, and swimming all provide exercise, but walking, mountain climbing, boating, and pulling carts are also forms of exercise. There is no need to be fashionable.

10. Benefits of getting up early and going to bed early:
    Even though exercise is good for a human body, too much exercise or too much work causes physical and mental fatigue. To recover, sleep is the most important. One's [optimal] daily amount of sleep is related to one's age. In general, ten hours for children and eight hours for adults is appropriate. One should go to bed early at night so that one can get up early the next morning, because the air is fresh in the early morning and it brings health benefits.

11. Significance of school health:
    When one is a child, one's body and mind are in the process of growing. Therefore one cannot develop normally unless one has a proper education [when one is a child]. Without education, one will acquire defects. It is difficult to correct these. Since school is a place where many children come into contact with each other, not only educational facilities but also educational methods should accord with principles of health. Only by doing this can we protect children's health.

12. Why shouldn't we spit?
    Spitting not only spoils cleanliness, spittle also easily transmits infectious diseases. For example, the spittle of a tuberculosis patient contains tuberculosis germs. After the spittle dries, [the germs] will fly with the dust. If one inhales [this dust], one will be infected with tuberculosis.

Glossary

aiguo qiyejia 爱国企业家
aiguo weisheng yundong weiyuanhui 爱国
   卫生运动委员会

baifan 白礬
Bailingji 百龄机
Baiyu 白玉
Bao Guochang 鲍国昌
bao'andui 保安队
baochang weiyuan 包产委员
baojia 保甲
Baojiansi 保健司
baojianzhan 保健站
baowei shengming 保卫生命
biaoyu 标语
binghuan 病患
bingli 病历
bozhi 玻质
bujie 不洁
buwan 补丸
buzhen 补针

changmingpai 长命牌
changpu 菖蒲
changwu weiyuan 常务委员
Chen Diexian 陈蝶仙
Chen Fangzhi 陈方之
Chen Gantang 陈甘棠
Chen Gongbo 陈公博

Chen Yi 陈毅
Chen Zhiqian (C. C. Chen) 陈志潜
chengbao zerenzhi 承包责任制
Chiang Kai-shek (Jiang Jieshi) 蒋介石
choubeihui 筹备会
Choubeiju 筹备局
chuanranbing 传染病
Chun Shengpu zhuzhici 春申浦竹枝词

dadao 大道
Dalu huaxue zhipinchang 大陆化
   学制品厂
dangyi 党义
danwei 单位
daotai 道台
diduan yiyuan 地段医院
Dieshuang 蝶霜
ding 疔
Ding Ganren 丁甘仁
Ding Wenjiang 丁文江
Dōjinkai 同仁会
dongshi 董事
dongshihui 董事会
dongwu 动物
Dongyuan 东院
dou 痘
du 毒
Du Yuesheng 杜月笙
Duanwujie 端午节

fang 坊
Fang Jiyang 方季杨
Fang Yexian 方液仙
fangyi (bōeki) 防疫
Fangyisi 防疫司
Fangyi weiyuanhui / Bōeki iinkai 防疫委员会
fangzhang 坊长
fayang guoyi xueshu 发扬国医学术
fenfang qiwei 芬芳气味
feng 风
Feng Yuxiang 冯玉祥
fenhuigu 粪秽股
fu 妇
fuxing wuminzu er tichang weisheng 复兴吾民族而提倡卫生
fuyong 服用
fu-zhuren weiyuan 副主任委员

geren xingfu 个人幸福
gong nong bing 工农兵
gongchang lianhe baojianzhan 工厂联合保健站
gonggong weisheng 公共卫生
Gongji shantang 公济善堂
gongli 公立
gongtong nuli 共同努力
Gongwuju 工务局
gongyejie 工业界
gongyi 工艺
Gongyongju 公用局
Gongzhong weisheng yundong chengxu 公众卫生运动程序
guai 怪
Guangren yiyuan 广仁医院
Guangyi gongsi 广艺公司
Guangyi zhongyiyuan 广益中医院
Guohuo yundong 国货运动
guojia qiangruo 国家强弱
Guomindang 国民党
guoyi 国医

Heiren 黑人
hou 喉
Hu Hongji 胡鸿基

Hu Yuwei 胡毓威
Hua Tuo 华佗
Hualong yiyuan 华隆医院
Huang Chujiu 黄楚九
Huang Fu 黄郛
Huang Jinrong 黄金荣
Huangpu Qu zhongxin yiyuan 黄埔区中心医院
huaxue gongye 化学工业
huaxue yongpin 化学用品
Huazhong shuidian gongsi 华中水电公司
Hubei 沪北
Hubei gongxunjuanju 沪北工巡捐局
huiqi 秽气
Hujiang shangye shi jingci 沪江商业市景词
Hunan 沪南
Hunan Shenzhou yiyuan 沪南神州医院
huoluan 霍乱
huoluan fangyi shishi guicheng 霍乱防疫实施规程
Huxi weisheng banshichu 沪西卫生办事处

Jiandao (arrow and sword) 箭刀
Jiandao (scissors) 剪刀
Jiangwan 江湾
jiankang 健康
jianshui 碱水
jiating bingchuang 家庭病床
jiating changshi 家庭常识
Jiating gongyeshe 家庭工业社
Jiebai 洁白
jiedao yiyuan 街道医院
Jilian 机联
jin 斤
Jingbaosi 警保司
jingchangxing 经常性
jingsu 精素
jingyan 净盐
jisha 疾痧
jiucha 纠察
jiuzhi yili 救治疫痢
Jizhengshi 技正室
ju 局

jumin weisheng xiaozu 居民卫生小组
jumin weiyuanhui 居民委员会
juwei weishengzhan 居民卫生站

Kang Youwei 康有为
kangjian jiuguo 康健救国
ke 科
Kōain bunkakyoku 興亜院文化局
Kōain kachū renrakubu 興亜院華中
連絡部
Kong Xiangxi (H. H. Kung)
孔祥熙
Kuaijishi 会计室
kulu 苦囵

laji 垃圾
Li Jiuming 李九明
Li Mingyue 李名岳
Li Pingshu 李平书
Li Ting'an (Ting-an Li) 李廷安
Li Xinfu 李新甫
Li Yunshu 李云叔
Li Zufan 李祖范
Li Zuhan 李祖韩
liang 两
Liang Songling 梁嵩龄
lianghao shiyou 良好师友
lianhe fuyou baojianzhan 联合妇幼保
健站
lianhe yiliao jigou 联合医疗机构
lianhe zhensuo 联合诊所
lianhuanhua 连环画
Libai liu 礼拜六
liji 痢疾
Lin Wenqing 林文庆
lingshuizheng 领水证
*linshi fangyi weiyuanhui / rinji bōeki iin
kai* 臨時防疫委員會
Liu Hongsheng 刘鸿生
Liu Ruiheng (J. Heng Liu)
刘瑞恒
Liu Xuzi 刘绪梓
Liu Zhenya 刘振亚
Lixingshe 力行社
Lu Bohong 陆伯鸿

Lu Jiesun 陆介孙
luan 乱
Luoshi zhensuo 雒氏诊所

maixiang 脉象
mei ri shenghuo 每日生活
mingxing shijiu aiyong 明星十九爱用
ming yuanbo 名远播
Mishuchu 秘书处
Mishushi 秘书室
muliao 幕僚

Nagayo Sensai 長与専斎
Nanjing 难经
Nanshi Shanghai yiyuan 南市上海医院
Nanshi weisheng shiwusuo 南市卫生事
务所
Nanyang zhuzaochang 南阳烛皂厂
Nanyuan 南院
nei 内
Neidi 内地
Neijing 内经
Neiwubu 内务部
Neizhengbu 内政部
Ningbo shangren 宁波商人
Niu Huilin 牛惠霖
niuyangyou 牛羊油
Nüzi zhongxi yiliaoyuan 女子中西医疗院
Nüzi zhongxi yixuetang 女子中西医学堂

Pang Jingzhou 庞京周
pianmianxing 片面性
pingmin laogong 平民劳工
Pushan shanzhuang 普善山庄
putong yafen 普通牙粉

qihua 气化
qingdao 清道
qingjie 清洁
Qingjiebu 清洁部
qingjie weisheng yundong 清洁卫生运动
qingqi 清气
qu yiyuan 区医院
quandaodui 劝导队
qudu 去毒

Renji yiguan 仁济医馆
Renji yiyuan 仁济医院
renshu jishi 仁术济世
renti 人体
riyong huaxue gongye 日用化学工业
riyong huaxuepin 日用化学品

Sanxing 三星
Sekizen yōkō 積善洋行
sha 痧
shachong 杀虫
shang 伤
shangdeng weisheng yafen 上等卫生牙粉
Shanghai chengxiang neiwai zong-
    gongchengju 上海城厢内外总工程局
shanghai fangyi weiyuanhui guicheng 上海
    防疫委员会规程
Shanghai gongli yiyuan 上海公立医院
Shanghai jijiu shiyi yiyuan 上海急救时疫
    医院
Shanghai jizhi guohuo gongchang
    lianhehui 上海机制国货工厂联合会
Shanghai rihua fangfang youxiangongsi
    上海日化芳芳有限公司
Shanghai riyong huaxuepinchang 上海日
    用化学品厂
Shanghai Shi gongsuo 上海市公所
Shanghai Shi jiuji fulijie di-yi bingmin
    zhensuo 上海市救济福利界第一病
    民诊所
Shanghai shiyi yiyuan 上海时疫医院
Shanghai xinshenghuo yundong cujinhui
    上海新生活运动促进会
Shanghai yagaochang 上海牙膏厂
Shanghai yushi kabushiki gaisha 上海油
    脂株式会社
Shanghai zhongyi zhuanmen xuexiao 上
    海中医专门学校
Shanghai zizhi gongsuo 上海自治公所
Shanghanlun 伤寒论
Shangwu yinshuguan 商务印书馆
shantang 善堂
shao 少
shehui weisheng zhuangtai 社会卫生状态
Shehuiju 社会局

shen 神
Shen Dunhe 沈敦和
Shenbao zengkan 申报增刊
Shenbao ziyoutan 申报自由谈
sheng weishengchu 省卫生处
shengji 生肌
shetai 舌苔
shi 室
Shi Liangcai 史量才
shijian xinshenghuo er juxing yundong 实践
    新生活而举行运动
shijij yiyuan 市级医院
*shixing xinshenghuo xu cong qingjie
    weisheng zuoqi* 实行新生活须从清洁卫生
    做起
shiye jiuguo 实业救国
shiyi 时疫
shiyi bingfang 时疫病房
shiyi yiyuan 时疫医院
shou 守
shuishang 水上
sida youdian 四大优点、
sihai 四害
sili 私立
Song Zejiu 宋则久
Song Ziwen (T. V. Soong) 宋子文
Songhu jingchating 淞沪警察厅
Songhu shangbu weishengju 淞沪商埠卫
    生局
Songhu weishengju 淞沪卫生局
Sun Chuanfang 孙传芳
Sun Yat-sen 孙逸仙

Taipingyang feizaochang 太平洋
    肥皂厂
tanci 弹词
tansuangai 碳酸钙
tansuanmei 碳酸镁
tebieshi weishengju 特别市卫生局
Tewu jiguan/ Tokumu kikan 特務機關
Tianjin zhiyi gongsi 天津制胰公司
Tianxu Wosheng 天虚我生
tichang guoyao gongneng 提倡国药功能
tigong 体功
Tongjisi 统计司

Tongmenghui 同盟会
Tongren yiyuan 同仁医院
tudi zhangcheng 土地章程
tuiguang gongyi liji bingren 推广公益利济
  病人
tujian 土硷
tuxie 吐泻
tuzao 土皂

wai 外
Wang Qizhang 汪企张
Wang Yiting 王一亭
wei 卫
weisheng / eisei 卫生
weisheng biaoyan 卫生表演
Weisheng jiaoyuhui 卫生教育会
weisheng jichayuan 卫生稽查员
weisheng jieyanling 卫生戒严令
weisheng shebeifei 卫生设备费
weisheng shiwusuo 卫生事务所
weisheng xingzheng xitong dagang 卫生行
  政系统大纲
weisheng xuanshi 卫生宣誓
weisheng yundong 卫生运动
weisheng zhanlanhui 卫生展览会
weisheng zhi dao 卫生之道
Weishengchu 卫生处
weishengge 卫生歌
Weishengju 卫生局
Weishengke 卫生科
Weishengshu 卫生署
Weishengsi 卫生司
Weita cibaoming 维他赐保命
weiyuan 委员
Wu Hongyu 吴虹玉
Wu Juemi 吴觉迷
Wu Liande 伍连德
Wu Tiecheng 吴铁城
Wu Yaodong 吴耀东
Wudi 无敌
Wudipai camian yafen de shida
  gongyong 无敌牌擦面牙粉
  的十大功用
wuguan 五官
wumei lianjia 物美廉价

Wuzhou guben zaochang 五洲固本
  皂厂
Wuzhou yaofang 五洲药房

Xia Yingtang 夏应堂
xiaji weisheng yundong dahui shishi
  dagang 夏季卫生运动大会实施大纲
xian 县
xian weishengyuan 县卫生院
xian yiyaun 县医院
Xiang Songmao 项松茂
xiang weishengyuan 乡卫生院
xiangyi 香胰
xiaoshimin 小市民
Xie Guan 谢观
xifa 西法
xinshenghuo gongyue 新生活公约
Xinyi 信谊
xiyao 西药
xiyi 西医
xiyi feizao 洗衣肥皂
Xiyuan 西院
Xu Huafeng 徐华封
Xu Shou 徐寿
Xu Wancheng 许晚成
Xu Xiaochu 许晓初
xuanchuan duiwu 宣传队伍
Xue Dubi 薛笃弼
Xue Kunming 薛坤明
xuelun 血轮
xunhui xuanchuanche 巡回宣传车

yagao 牙膏
yan 眼
Yan Chunyang 严春阳
Yan Fu 严复
Yan Fuqing 颜福庆
Yang Chongrui (Marion Yang) 杨崇瑞
Yang Ximeng 杨西孟
yangjian 洋硷
Ye Jiting 叶吉廷
Ye Xiangting 叶翔廷
Ye Zhongting 叶钟廷
ying 应
yinshi 饮食

yinxing xiangzao 银星香皂
yiwu zhuren 医务主任
yiyuan 医院
Yizhengsi 医政司
Yonghe shiye gongsi 永和实业公司
you 幼
Youxi shijie 游戏世界
Yu Fengbin 俞凤宾
Yu Qiaqing 虞洽卿
Yu Yunxiu 余云岫
Yuan Jufan 袁矩范
Yuan Lüdeng 袁履登
Yueli chang'e 月里嫦娥
Yuhua huaxue gongye gufen youxian gongsi 裕华化学工业股份有限公司
yun 运

Zang Boyong 臧伯庸
zangqi de xing tezheng 脏器的形特征
zaojia 皂荚
Zhang Bingrui 张炳瑞
Zhang Changfu 张长福
Zhang Jinqing 张晋卿
Zhang Meixuan 张梅轩
Zhang Xueliang 张学良
Zhang Zhujun 张竹君
zhangcheng 章程
zhangnao 樟脑
zhuangxiamei 装匣美
zhen 针
zhen weishengyuan 镇卫生院
zhengqi qingjie 整齐清洁
zhenliaozhan 诊疗站
zhensuo 诊所

zhixian 知县
Zhiyaoye tongyehui 制药业同业会
Zhong Kui 钟馗
Zhongguo huaxue gongyeshe 中国化学工业社
Zhongguo kexue yiquguan 中国科学仪器馆
Zhongguo renmin jiuji fulihui 中国人民救济福利会
Zhongguo zhizaochang 中国制皂厂
Zhonghua boyihui 中华博医会
Zhonghua guohuo weichihui 中华国货维持会
Zhonghua yixue chuanjiaohui 中华医学传教会
Zhongshan 中山
zhongxiyi jiehe 中西医结合
Zhongyang fangyichu 中央防疫处
Zhongyang weisheng shiyansuo 中央卫生实验所
zhongyi 中医
Zhou Enlai 周恩来
zhouchang 粥厂
Zhu Baosan 朱葆三
Zhuayuanshi 专员室
zhuren weiyuan 主任委员
zhushe zhengshu 注射证书
zhushedui 注射队
zhuyi 猪胰
zhuyi zhixu 注意秩序
zhuyou 猪油
zhuzhici 竹枝词
zongwu zhuren 总务主任
Zongwusi 总务司
zu 组

Bibliography

Some Chinese archives and books have both Chinese and English titles. Original English titles are in brackets; my translations are in parentheses.

Shanghai Shi Dang'anguan 上海市档案馆
Shanghai Municipal Archives (SMA)

A26-2-243: Zhonggong Shanghai Shi gaodeng xuexiao weiyuanhui guanyu kaizhan aiguo weisheng yundong de zhishi he xuexi xuanjufa de tongzhi baogao jilu (1953) 中共上海市高等学校委员会关于开展爱国卫生运动的指示和学习选举法的通知报告记录 (Chinese Communist Party, Committee of Higher Educational Institutions in Shanghai, records of instructions on launching a patriotic hygiene campaign and notification of learning and election methods).

A38-2-242: Qinghua gongye xitong Zhongguo huaxue gongye Daming zaozhi deng siying gongchang de jiben qingkuang diaocha baogao (1954) 轻化工业系统中国化学工业大明造纸等私营工厂的基本情况调查报告 (Investigation report concerning the basic circumstances of light chemical industries, including China Chemical Industries, Daming Paper Manufacturer, and other private factories).

A38-2-255: Guanyu gongsi heyingchang renshi anpai wenti (1954) 关于公私合营厂人事安排问题 (Regarding personnel arrangement issues in public-private joint operation factories).

B241-1-377: Shanghai Renji yiyuan jieguan qian diaocha dengji de yiyuan de gaikuang, gongzuo baogao, ji zuzhi zhangcheng (1950–51) 上海仁济医院接管前调查登记的医院的概况，工作报告及组织章程 (Survey, work report, and organizational regulations of Shanghai Renji Hospital, based on the investigation and registration carried out before its acquisition).

B241-1-502-30: Zhongguo Hongshizihui Shanghai Shi fenhui 中国红十字会上海市分会 (The Chinese Red Cross Society Shanghai Branch Office).

B242-1-131-35: Shanghai Renji yiyuan chuangli qingkuang (1949) 上海仁济医院创立情况 (Circumstances surrounding the founding of Shanghai Renji Hospital).

B242-1-146: Shanghai Renji yiyuan gaikuang (1949) 上海仁济医院概况 (An overview of Shanghai Renji Hospital).

B242-1-351-107: Shanghai Renji yiyuan tianbao Shanghai Shi jieshou waiguo jintie ji waizi jingying zhi wenhua jiaoyu jiuji jiguan ji zongjiao tuanti dengji zongbiao (1951) 上海仁济医院填报上海市接受外国津贴及外资经营之文化教育救济机关及宗教团体登记总表 (Comprehensive registration charts of cultural, educational, and social welfare organizations and religious institutions in Shanghai subsidised and/or managed by foreigners, a report filled by Shanghai Renji Hospital).

B242-1-476-1: Shanghai Shi renmin zhengfu weishengju guanyu wei Gaungyi zhongyiyuan, Gongji shantang deng hebing zuzhi baoqing heshi de han (1953) 上海市人民政府卫生局关于为广益中医院，公济善堂等合并组织报请核示的函 (Shanghai Municipality People's Government Public Health Bureau, a letter of request for investigation and guidance on the amalgamation of Guangyi Chinese Hospital, Gongji Benevolent Hall, and other institutions).

B242-1-476-3: Shanghai Shi Yimiao Qu renmin zhengfu guanyu Guangyi zhongyiyuan hebing zuzhi tianshe bingchuang gaiwei Shanghai Shi jiuji fulijie di-yi bingmin zhensuo buban shenqing shouxu de han (1953) 上海市邑庙区人民政府关于广益中医院合并组织添设病床改为上海市救济福利界第一病民诊所补办申请手续的函 (Shanghai Municipality Yimiao District People's Government, a letter on completing the application procedures for Guangyi Chinese Hospital; concerning adding more beds and its incorporation [with other institutions] and reorganization into the Shanghai Social Welfare Society Number One Clinic for the Sick).

B242-1-535-40: Shanghai Shi aiguo weisheng yundong weiyuanhui guanyu Shanghai Shi aiguo weisheng yundong 1953 nian di-er jidu gongzuo zongjie 上海市爱国卫生运动委员会关于上海市爱国卫生运动 1953 年第二季度工作总结 (The Shanghai Municipality Patriotic Hygiene Campaign Committee, a summary of the 1953 Shanghai second patriotic hygiene campaign work).

B242-1-805-1: Shanghai Shi weishengju guanyu Shanghai Shi aiguo weisheng yundong sannianlai gongzuo baogao (1955) 上海市卫生局关于上海市爱国卫生运动三年来工作报告 (Shanghai Municipality Public Health Bureau regarding Shanghai patriotic hygiene campaign work report for the past three years).

B242-1-899: Shanghai Shi weishengju guanyu jieguan Guangyi zhongyiyuan Hubei menzhensuo han (1956) 上海市卫生局关于接管广益中医院沪北门诊所函 (Shanghai Public Health Bureau, a letter concerning the acquisition of Guangyi Chinese Hospital Hubei Clinic).

B242-1-899-1: Shanghai Shi minzhengju guanyu Guangyi zhongyiyuan Hubei menzhensuo de chuli yijian qingxun yujian fuhan (1956) 上海市民政局关于广益中医院沪北门诊所的处理意见请讯预见复函 (Shanghai Municipality Civil Affairs Bureau: A reply letter on the opinions regarding how to manage Guangyi Chinese Hospital Hubei Clinic and asking expectations).

B3-1-12-1: Shanghai Shi weishegju guanyu ni jiebanqian Guangyi zhongyiyuan Hubei menzhenbu de qingshi he Shanghai Shi renwei de pifu 上海市卫生局关于拟接办前广益中医院沪北门诊部的请示和上海市人委的批复 (Shanghai Public Health Bureau's inquiry regarding instructions on Guangyi Chinese Hospital Hubei Clinic before its take-over; reply [to this inquiry] by Shanghai Municipality People's Committee).

Q113-4-1: Shanghai Guangyi zhongyiyuan guanyu chengqing li'an wenti de han he Shanghai Shi shehuiju, Shanghai Shi dangbu de pifu, dengji xuke zhengshu ji gai yuan zhangcheng qingkuang diaochabiao (1929–1946) 上海广益中医院关于呈请立案问题的函和上海市社会局，上海市党部的批复，登记许可证书及该院章程情况调查表 (Shanghai Guangyi Chinese Hospital's letter to request approval of filing a case; official replies from the Shanghai Social Affairs Bureau and the Party, permit for registration, and charters and investigation charts of the stated hospital's regulations and circumstances).

Q113-4-4: Shanghai Guangyi zhongyiyuan guanyu Shanghai Shi shehuiju, Shanghai Shi weishengju de ge zhong xunling, tongzhihan, 1931–43 上海广益中医院关于上海市社会局，上海市卫生局的各种训令，通知函，1931–43 (Various instructions and notification letters from Shanghai Social Affairs Bureau and Public Health Bureau on Shanghai Guangyi Chinese Hospital).

Q6-9-190: Shanghai Shi shehuiju shiyi yiyuan juan (1947) 上海市社会局时疫医院卷 (Shanghai social affairs bureau, the file for epidemic hospitals).

Q6-9-190-12: Shanghai shiyi yiyuan faqi zuzhi liyoushu ji shiye jihuashu (liyoushu) (1947) 上海时疫医院发起组织理由书及事业计划书 (理由书) (Chinese Infectious Hospital, the statement of rationale for launching the organization and the business plan) (the statement of rationale).

Q6-9-190-13: Shanghai shiyi yiyuan faqi zuzhi liyoushu ji shiye jihuashu (jihuashu) (1947) 上海时疫医院发起组织理由书及事业计划书 (计划书) (Chinese Infectious Hospital, the statement of rationale for launching the organization and the business plan) (the business plan).

Q6-9-192: Shanghai shehuiju guanyu Hunan Guangyi zhongyiyuan zhuce dengji deng wenjian (1945) 上海社会局关于沪南广益中医院注册登记等文件 (Shanghai Social Affairs Bureau, Hunan Guangyi Chinese Hospital's certification and registration, and other documents).

R1-12-105: Jieshou shizhengfu weishengke ji jingchaju weishengke yijiao qingce 接收市政府卫生科及警察局卫生科移交清册 (Taking over the public health office of the municipal government and public health office of the police, inventory of transfer).

R1-12-11: Riwei Shanghai tebieshi zhengfu weisheng xingzheng zhuangtai ji shishi gongzuo baogaobiao (1943) 日伪上海特别市政府卫生行政状态暨实施工作报告表 (The condition of public health administration of the Japanese Puppet Government of the Shanghai Special Municipality and business report charts).

R1-12-133: Riwei Shanghai tebieshi zhengfu fangyi huiyi min sanshi nian si yue 日伪上海特别市政府防疫会议民 30 年 4 月 (The Japanese Puppet Government of Shanghai Special Municipality, epidemic control meeting, April 1941).

R1-12-15: Choubei chengli weishengju 筹备成立卫生局 (Preparations for the founding of the public health bureau).

R1-12-341: Nanshi zhuangzhi fangyi zilaishui (1942) 南市装置防疫自来水 (Installing tap water facilities in Nanshi for epidemic prevention).

R1-12-343: Fangyi zhushe (1941) 防疫注射 (Anti-epidemic injections).

R1-12-387: Xialing juxing di-yi jie weisheng yundong dahui 夏令举行第一届卫生运动大会 (Holding the first summer hygiene campaign mass meeting).

R1-12-388: Riwei tebieshi zhengfu xialing di-er jie weisheng yundong dahui juan 日伪特别市政府夏令第二届卫生运动大会卷 (The file for the Japanese Puppet Government Special Municipality second summer hygiene campaign mass meeting).

R1-12-389: Riwei Shanghai tebieshi zhengfu xialing weisheng yundong di-san jie dahui 日伪上海特别市政府夏令卫生运动第三届大会 (The Japanese Puppet Government of Shanghai Special Municipality, third summer hygiene campaign mass meeting).

R1-12-406: Riwei Shanghai tebieshi zhengfu dongling di-yi jie weisheng yundong dahui juan 日伪上海特别市政府冬令第一届卫生运动大会卷 (The file for the Japanese Puppet Government of Shanghai Special Municipality first winter hygiene campaign mass meeting).

R50-1142: Choubei weishengju shiyi juan (1941) 筹备卫生局事宜卷 (The file of relevant matters on preparing the public health bureau).

R50-1151: Chengli weishengju juan (1941) 成立卫生局卷 (The file for the founding of the public health bureau).

R50-1183: Weisheng xingzheng shishi gongzuo baogaobiao (1941–43) 卫生行政实施工作报告表 (The business report forms of public health administration implementation).

R50-1203: Shanghai tebieshi weishengju zongwulei ershijiu Nanshi linshi fangyi weiyuanhui huiyilu (1942) 上海特别市卫生局总务类29 南市临时防疫委员会会议录 (Shanghai Special Municipality Public Health Bureau General Affairs Section 29, Nanshi provisional epidemic control committee meeting minutes).

R50-1254: Jingchaju weishengke yijiao yuanyi qingce, qiju (1941) 警察局卫生科移交员役清册, 器具 (The public health office of the police transfers inventory of staff and servants and utensils).

R50-1384: Shanghai tebieshi weishengju gongzuo yuebao 1944–45 nian (yi) 上海特别市卫生局工作月报 1944–45 年 (一) (Shanghai Special Municipality Public Health Department monthly business report, number one).

R50-289: Korera bōeki jisshi kitei コレラ防疫实施规定 (Regulations on cholera prevention measures).

R50-299: Bōeki kaigi / Fangyi huiyi (1941–43) 防疫会议 (Epidemic prevention meetings).

R50-304: Nanshi Huininglu faxian huoluan jinxing pumie gongzuo'an (1942) 南市徽宁路发现霍乱进行扑灭工作案 (Plan for implementing works to eradicate cholera found in Nanshi Huininglu).

R50-305: Baoshan Qu faxian huoluanyi 宝山区发现霍乱疫 (Cholera cases found in Baoshan District).

R50-731: Weisheng yundong dahui (1942) 卫生运动大会 (Hygiene campaign mass meeting).

R50-732: Guanyu di-yi jie dongji weiyun (1942–43) 关于第一届冬季卫运 (Regarding the first winter hygiene campaign).

R50-735: Shanghai tebieshi weishengju weishenglei youguan juban di-er jie xialing weisheng yundong wenti de laihan wenshu (1942) 上海特别市卫生局卫生类有关举办第二届夏令卫生运动问题的来函文书 (The Shanghai Special Municipality Public Health Bureau, correspondences on holding the second summer hygiene campaign).

R50-736: Di-san jie xiaji weisheng yundong dahui fu gaisuanshu 第三届夏季卫生运动大会付概算书 (A rough estimate of the cost of the third hygiene campaign).

R50-738: Ge ji xiaoxuexiao weisheng jiangyan chengjibiao 各级小学校卫生讲演成绩表 (Grade cards of hygiene lectures from elementary schools at all levels).

R50-872: Gonggong weisheng xunlianban quanjuan (1942) 公共卫生训练班全卷 (Comprehensive files for public health training classes).

S59-1-39-146: Shanghai Zhongguo huaxue gongyeshe pifa jiemubiao (1937) 上海中国化学工业社批发价目表 (Shanghai China Chemical Industries wholesale price tables).

S86-1-10: Shanghai Shi riyong huaxuepin gongye gaikuang jianshi (1948) 上海市日用化学品工业概况简史 (An overview and brief history of daily use chemical product industries in Shanghai).

U1-16-2192: Jinzhi suidi tutan zhi guize 1941–43 禁止随地吐痰之规则 [Spitting].

U1-16-289: Shanghai Shi weishengju zuzhi xitongbiao, zhizhang fengong, zhiyuan deng cailiao (1927–37) 上海市卫生局组织系统表，职掌分工，职员等材料 [Organization of the Department Activities of the Various Branches and Staff Record].

U1-16-290: Shanghai Shi weishengju yu gongbuju weishengchu zhi guanxi de fuzhi yu jianbao cailiao (1926–35) 上海市卫生局与工部局卫生处之关系的复制与剪报材料 (Copies and newspaper clippings on the relationships between the Shanghai Municipality Public Health Bureau and Shanghai Municipal Council Public Health Department).

U1-16-291: Shanghai Shi weishengju 1926–35 nian gongzuo dongtai jianbao 上海市卫生局1926–1935 年 工作动态剪报 [Activities—Miscellaneous News Cutting].

U1-16-292: Shanghai Shi weishengju juzhang cheng shizhang guanyu shizheng weisheng gaige 上海市卫生局局长呈市长关于市政卫生改革 [Municipality of Greater Shanghai Activities Reform of Municipal Sanitation Hu Hung-chi's Petition to Mayor].

U1-16-293: Shanghai Shi gongzuo dongtai he Shanghai Shi weisheng jihua ji yijianshu 上海市工作动态和上海市卫生计划及意见书 [Plans and Ideas for the Health of Greater Shanghai by Hu Hung-chi].

U1-16-298: Da Shanghai shizhengfu gongzuo dongtai guanyu Shanghai Shi weishengju 1934 nian tuixing di-shisan jie weisheng yundong de laiwangjian ji cailiao 大上海市政府工作动态关于上海市卫生局 1934 年推行第 13 届卫生运动的来往件及材料 (1934) [13th Health Campaign—1934].

U1-16-299: Da Shanghai shizhengfu gongzuo dongtai 1935 nian di-shisi ci weisheng yundong 大上海市政府工作动态 1935 年第 14 次卫生运动 [14th Health Campaign—1935].

U1-16-300: Da Shanghai shizhengfu gongzuo dongtai 1936 nian di-shiwu qi weisheng yundong 大上海市政府工作动态 1936 年第 15 期卫生运动 [15th Health Campaign—1936].

U1-16-301: Di-shiliu qi weisheng yundong 第 16 期卫生运动 [16th Health Campaign—1937].

U1-16-318: Huazu liangjie guanyu weisheng gongzuo de laiwangjian (1929–33) 华租两界关于卫生工作的来往件 [Disagreement—Miscellaneous].

U1-16-319: Huazu liangjie guanyu weisheng gongzuo baogao de jian laiwang xinjian ji youguan cailiao (1925–34) 华租两界关于卫生工作报告的件来往信件及有关材料 (Correspondences between Chinese Shanghai and the International Settlement regarding public health work reports and other documents).

U1-16-4651: Weishengchu nianbao 卫生处年报 [Shanghai Municipal Council Public Health Department Annual Report].

U1-16-519: Guanyu 1930 nian yiyuan ji yiwu gongzuo weiyuanhui deng gongzuo baogao wenjian 关于 1930 年医院及医务工作委员会等工作报告文件 [Hospital and Nursing Service Commission, 1930].

U1-16-520: Yiwu weiyuanhui 医务委员会 [Hospital Commission Report].

U1-16-542: Shanghai gonggong zujie gongbuju weishengchu youguan yiyuan quanshi diaocha cailiao, sheli funü ertong yiyuan ji yufang chuanranbing yu chuanranbingren guanli xize deng wenjian 上海公共租界工部局卫生处有关医院全市调查材料，设立妇女儿童医院及预防传染病与传染病人管理细则等文件 (Shanghai International Settlement Municipal Council Public Health Department, regarding investigation materials on hospitals in the entire city, establishing women's and children's hospitals, detailed regulations on infectious disease prevention and infectious disease patient management, and other documents).

U1-16-548: Benshi yiyuan diaochabiao 本市医院调查表 (Investigation forms of hospitals in the city).

U1-16-549: Youguan qita yiyuan yewu qingkuang de baogao 有关其他医院业务情况的报告 (Reports on business conditions of other hospitals).

U1-16-737: Shanghai shiyi yiyuan jianshi nianbao deng shiyi, 1935–43 上海时疫医院简史年报等事宜 (Chinese Infectious Disease Hospital's brief history, annual reports, and other relevant materials).

U1-16-738: Shanghai shiyi yiyuan yiwu baogao ji jingfei buzhu deng cailiao (1920–43) 上海时疫医院医务报告及经费补助等材料 (Chinese Infectious Disease Hospital business report and materials on outlay, subsidies, and other issues).

U1-16-749: Shanghai gonggong zujie weishengchu guanyu Shanghai Hongshizihui Shanghai zhiyaoye tongyehui deng danwei zhuban Shanghai jiuji shiyi yiyuan de wenjian (1940–42) 上海公共租界卫生处关于上海红十字会，上海制药业同业会等单位主办上海救济时疫医院的文件 (Shanghai International Settlement Public Health Department, documents on Shanghai Emergency Hospital sponsored by Shanghai Red Cross Society, Shanghai Drug Manufacturers' Association, and other units).

U1-16-822: Shanghai gonggong zujie weishengchu guanyu Renji yiyuan de jianzhang, jianshi deng wenjian 上海公共租界卫生处关于仁济医院的简章，简史等文件 (Shanghai International Settlement Public Health Department, documents on Renji Hospital's brief rules, brief history, and other matters).

U1-16-823: Shanghai gonggong zujie weishengchu guanyu Renji yiyuan linian buzhujin shixiang ji Riben Tongrenhui jieban jiankuang de wenjian 上海公共租界卫生处关于仁济医院历年补助金事项及日本同仁会接办简况的文件 (Shanghai International Settlement Public Health Department, documents on Renji Hospital's subsidies from past years as well as a short explanation of its acquisition by Dōjinkai of Japan).

U1-4-212: Tongren yiyuan youguan shenling buzhujin deng shi Shanghai gonggong zujie zongban deng laiwanghan (1939–42) 同仁医院有关申领补助金等事上海公共租界总办等来往函 (Grant applications and correspondences from Tongren Hospital with the general manager of the Shanghai International Settlement).

U1-4-213: Tongren yiyuan youguan shenling buzhujin deng shi Shanghai gonggong zujie zongban deng laiwanghan (1943) 同仁医院有关申领补助金等事上海公共租界总办等来往函 (Grant applications and correspondences from Tongren Hospital with the general manager of the Shanghai International Settlement).

U1-4-216: Renji yiyuan youguan shenling buzhujin yu Shanghai gonggong zujie gongbuju zongban laiwanghan (1933–41) 仁济医院有关申领补助金与上海公共租界工部局总办
来往函 (Grant applications and correspondences from Renji Hospital with the general manager of the Shanghai Municipal Council).

U1-4-220: Commission of Public Health, Chinese Infectious Disease Hospital.

U1-4-259: Shanghai jijiu shiyi yiyuan 上海急救时疫医院 (Shanghai Emergency
Hospital).

Y9-1-37: Shanghai Shi chengli shizhounian jinian gongye zhanlanhui tekan. 上海市成立
十週年紀念工業展覽會特刊 (The special issue about the industrial exhibition to commemorate the tenth anniversary of the opening of the Shanghai Municipality).

Y9-1-78: Xiandai shiyejia 現代實業家 (Contemporary businessmen).

Y9-1-101-38: Gongshang shiliao di-er ji 工商史料第二集 (1935) (Historical records of industry and commerce, vol. 2).

Y9-1-101-114: Gongshang shiliao di-yi ji 工商史料 第一集 (1935) (Historical records of industry and commerce, vol. 1).

Gaimushō kiroku 外務省記録 (GK) (Records of the Ministry of Foreign Affairs)

H-4-1-0-1-18:
H-men: Tōhō bunka jigyō
H 門　東方文化事業
(Division H: Activities on eastern culture)
4-rui: Hojo (byōin, gakkai, mindan, gakkō)
4 類　補助（病院、学会、民団、学校）
(Section 4 Subsidies—hospitals, academic associations, civil organizations, and schools)
1-kkō Byōin
1 項　病院
(Class 1: Hospitals)
0-moku
0 目
(Order 0)
18: Byōin kankei zakken/Shanghai mindan ritsu shinryōjo kankei
18. 病院関係雑件　上海民立診療所関係
(No. 18: Miscellaneous documents related to hospitals/concerning the clinic sponsored
by the Shanghai Residents Association).

I-men: Bunka, shūkyō, eisei, rōdō oyobi shakai mondai
I 門　文化、宗教、衛生、労働及社会問題
(Division I: Culture, religion, public health, labor, and social problems)
3-rui: Eisei
3 類　衛生
(Section 3: Public health)
2-kō: densenbyō, ken'eki, bōeki
2 項　伝染病、検疫、防疫

(Classs 2: Infectious Diseases, quarantine, and epidemic prevention)
0 目 (Order 0)
7: Densenbyō hōkoku zassan Chūgoku no bu dai 2 kan
7: 伝染病報告雑編纂、中国の部（満蒙を除く）第 2 巻
(7: Miscellaneous Reports of Epidemic Diseases in China—Excluding Manchuria and Mongol) Volume 2.
8: Volume 3
11: Volume 6
12: Volume 7
13: Volume 8

Anderson, Warwick. *Colonial Pathologies: American Tropical Medicine, Race, and Hygiene in the Philippines.* Durham, NC: Duke University Press, 2006.

Andrews, Bridie J. "In Republican China, Public Health by Whom, for Whom?" In *Science, Public Health, and the State in Modern Asia,* edited by Liping Bu, Darwin H. Stapleton, and Ka-Che Yip, 177–194. New York: Routledge, 2012.

———. *The Making of Modern Chinese Medicine, 1850–1960.* Vancouver: University of British Columbia Press, 2014.

———. "Tuberculosis and the Assimilation of Germ Theory in China, 1895–1937." *Journal of the History of Medicine* 52 (1997): 114–57.

Andrews, Bridie, and Mary Brown Bullock, eds. *Medical Transitions in Twentieth-Century China.* Bloomington: Indiana University Press, 2014.

Appadurai, Arjun, ed. *The Social Life of Things: Commodities in Cultural Perspective.* Cambridge, UK: Cambridge University Press, 1986.

Arnold, David. *Colonizing the Body: State, Medicine, and Epidemic Disease in Nineteenth-Century India.* Berkeley: University of California Press, 1993.

———, ed. *Imperial Medicine and Indigenous Societies.* Manchester, UK: Manchester University Press, 1988.

Bao Xiang'ao 鮑相璈, and Mei Qizhao 梅啓昭. *Meishi yanfang xinbian* 梅氏驗方新編 (A new compilation of Mr. Mei's recipes). Edited and annotated by Tianxuwosheng 天虛我生. Shanghai: Jiating gongyeshe, 1937.

Barlow, Tani E., ed. *Formations of Colonial Modernity in East Asia.* Durham, NC: Duke University Press, 1997.

———. "Introduction: On 'Colonial Modernity.' " In *Formations of Colonial Modernity in East Asia,* edited by Tani E. Barlow, 1–20. Durham, NC: Duke University Press, 1997.

———. "Wanting Some: Commodity Desire and the Eugenic Modern Girl." In *Women in China: The Republican Period in Historical Perspective,* edited by Mechthild Leutner and Nicola Spakowski, 312–50. Münster: LIT Verlag, 2005.

Barret, David P., and Larry N. Shyu, eds. *Chinese Collaboration with Japan, 1932–1945: The Limits of Accommodation.* Stanford, CA: Stanford University Press, 2001.

Bashford, Alison. *Imperial Hygiene: A Critical History of Colonialism, Nationalism and Public Health.* New York: Palgrave Macmillan, 2004.

Bayly, C. A. "The Origins of Swadeshi (Home Industry): Cloth and Indian Society, 1700–1930." In *The Social Life of Things: Commodities in Cultural Perspective,* edited by Arjun Appadurai, 285–321. Cambridge, UK: Cambridge University Press, 1988.

Benedict, Carol. *Bubonic Plague in Nineteenth-Century China.* Stanford, CA: Stanford University Press, 1996.

Bennett, Adrian Arthur. *John Fryer: The Introduction of Western Science and Technology into Nineteenth-Century China.* Cambridge, MA: East Asian Research Center, Harvard University, 1967.

Benson, Carlton. "The Manipulation of Tanci in Radio Shanghai during the 1930s." *Republican China* 20, no. 2 (1995): 117–46.

Bèrgere, Marie-Claire. "Civil Society and Urban Change in Republican China." In *Reappraising Republican China,* edited by Frederic Wakeman and Richard Louis Edmonds, 55–74. Oxford: Oxford University Press, 2000.

———. *The Golden Age of the Chinese Bourgeoisie, 1911–1937.* Translated by Janet Lloyd. Cambridge, UK: Cambridge University Press, 1986.

Bickers, Robert, and Christian Henriot. "Introduction." In *New Frontiers: Imperialism's New Communities in East Asia, 1842–1953.* Edited by Robert Bickers and Christian Henriot, 1–11. Manchester, UK: Manchester University Press, 2000.

———, eds. *New Frontiers: Imperialism's New Communities in East Asia, 1842–1953.* Manchester, UK: Manchester University Press, 2000.

Bodenhorn, Terry, ed. *Defining Modernity: Guomindang Rhetorics of a New China, 1920–1970.* Ann Arbor: Center for Chinese Studies, University of Michigan, 2002.

Bōeki hō 30 防疫報 (Report on epidemic prevention) (July 8, 1942). Filed in GK I-3-2-0-13, vol. 8.

Bowers, John Z. "American Private Aid at Its Peak: Peking Union Medical College." In *Medicine and Society in China,* edited by John Z. Bowers and Elizabeth Purcell, 82–98. New York: Josiah Macy Jr. Foundation, 1974.

Bowers, John Z., and Elizabeth Purcell, eds. *Medicine and Society in China.* New York: Josiah Macy Jr. Foundation, 1974.

Bracken, Gregory. *The Shanghai Alleyway House.* New York: Routledge, 2013.

Bretelle-Establet, Florence. "French Medicine in Nineteenth and Twentieth Century China: Rejection or Compliance in Far South Treaty Ports, Concessions and Leased Territories." In *Twentieth Century Colonialism and China: Localities, the Everyday and the World,* edited by Bryna Goodman and David S. G. Goodman, 134–50. New York: Routledge, 2012.

Britton, Roswell S. *The Chinese Periodical Press 1800–1912.* Shanghai: Kelly & Walsh, 1933.

Brook, Timothy. *Collaboration: Japanese Agents and Local Elites in Wartime China.* Cambridge, MA: Harvard University Press, 2005.

———. *The Confusions of Pleasure: Commerce and Culture in Ming China.* Berkeley: University of California Press, 1999.

Bu, Liping. "Beijing First Health Station: Innovative Public Health Education and Influence on China's Health Profession." In *Science, Public Health, and the State in Modern Asia,* edited by Liping Bu, Darwin H. Stapleton, and Ka-Che Yip, 129–43. New York: Routledge, 2012.

————. "Public Health and Modernisation: The First Campaigns in China, 1915–1916." *Social History of Medicine* 22, no. 2 (2009): 305–19.

Bu, Liping, Darwin H. Stapleton, and Ka-Che Yip, eds. *Science, Public Health, and the State in Modern Asia.* New York: Routledge, 2012.

Bullock, Mary Brown. *An American Transplant: The Rockefeller Foundation of the Peking Union Medical College.* Berkeley: University of California Press, 1980.

Burke, Timothy. *Lifebuoy Men, Lux Women: Commodification, Consumption and Cleanliness in Modern Zimbabwe.* Durham, NC: Duke University Press, 1996.

Bush, Richard C. *The Politics of Cotton Textiles in Kuomintang China, 1927–1937.* New York: Garland, 1982.

Bushman, L. Richard, and Claudia L. Bushman. "The Early History of Cleanliness in America." *Journal of American History* 74, no. 4 (1998): 1213–38.

Campbell, Cameron. "Mortality Change and the Epidemiological Transition in Beijing, 1644–1990." In *Asian Population History,* edited by Liu Ts'ui-jung, James Lee, David Sven Reher, Osamu Saito, and Wang Feng, 221–47. Oxford: Oxford University Press, 2001.

————. "Public Health Efforts in China before 1949 and Their Effects on Mortality: The Case of Beijing." *Social Science History* 21, no. 2 (1997): 179–218.

Chan, Gilbert F., ed. *China at the Crossroads: Nationalists and Communists, 1927–1949.* Boulder, CO: Westview Press, 1980.

Changwu weiyuanhui 常務委員會 (Standing Committee). "Shanghai Shi di-shisan jie weisheng yundong baogaoshu" 上海市第十三屆衛生運動報告書 (Shanghai Municipality thirteenth hygiene campaign report). *Weisheng Yuekan* 衛生月刊 4, no. 10 (1934): 405–14.

Chao, Yüan-ling. *Medicine and Society in Late Imperial China: A Study of Physicians in Suzhou, 1600–1850.* New York: Peter Lang, 2009.

Chen, Bin, Terry L. Cooper, and Rong Sun. "Spontaneous or Constructed? Neighborhood Governance Reforms in Los Angeles and Shanghai." *Public Administration Review,* December (2009): S108–S114.

Chen Diexian. *The Money Demon: An Autobiographical Romance.* Translated by Patrick Hanan. Originally published in Chinese in 1913. Honolulu: University of Hawai'i Press, 1999.

Chen Diexian 陳蝶仙, ed. *Jiating changshi huibian* 家庭常識彙編 (A collection of household common knowledge). Shanghai: Wenming shuju, 1940.

Chen Fangzhi 陳方之. "Shanghai Shi de gonggong weisheng wenti" 上海市的公共衛生問題 (Public health problems in Shanghai). *Xinyi yu shehui huikan* 新醫與社會彙刊 1 (1928): 106–24.

Chen Gao 沈誥. "Shanghai Shi di-shiwu jie weisheng yundong choubei jingguo" 上海市第十五屆衛生運動籌備經過 (Shanghai Municipality thirteenth hygiene campaign preparation process). *Weisheng Yuekan* 6, no. 7 (1936): 357–59.

Chen Haifeng 陈海峰, ed. *Zhongguo weisheng baojianshi* 中国卫生保健史 (A history of public health and hygiene in China). Shanghai: Shanghai kexue jishu chubanshe, 1992.

Chen Hanzhang 陳翰章. "Xianzai Zhongguo xuexiaozhong weishengshang liang da wumiu" 現在中國學校中衛生上兩大誤謬 (Two great mistakes in today's school health).
Shehui yibao 社會醫報 125 (1930): 97–100.

Chen, Kaiyi. *Seeds from the West: St. John's Medical School, Shanghai, 1880–1952*. Chicago: Imprint Publications, 2001.

Chen, Nancy. "Health, Wealth, and the Good Life." In *China Urban: Ethnographies of
Contemporary Culture*, edited by Nancy Chen, 165–82. Durham, NC: Duke University Press, 2001.

Chen Pei 陈佩, and Fan Guanrong 范关荣, eds. *Renshu jishi: Shanghai di-yijia xiyi yiyuan
de bainian gushi* 仁术济世: 上海第一家西医医院的百年故事 (Arts of benevolence save society: A hundred years of stories from Shanghai's first Western hospital). Shanghai:
Fudan daxue chubanshe, 2010.

Chen Xinwen 陈歆文. *Zhongguo jindai huaxue gongyeshi* 中国近代化学工业史 (History of
modern chemical industry in China). Beijing: Huaxue gongye she, 2006.

Cheng Gang. "The Neighborhood Committee—Residents' Own Organization." *Beijing Review*, April 9–15 (1990): 30–32.

China Contribution Committee, Special Committee on Survey and Occupation. *The
Christian Occupation of China, A General Survey of the Numerical Strength and Geo-
graphical Distribution of the Christian Forces in China, Made by the Special Committee
on Survey and Occupation China Continuation Committee, 1918–1921*. Shanghai: China
Continuation Committee, 1922.

China Weekly Review 1927. Shanghai.

China Year Book 1933. Tianjin and Shanghai: Tianjin Press and the North China Daily
Press, 1933.

Chinese Medical Association, ed. *Chinese Medical Directory* 1932, 1934, 1937, 1939, 1940,
1941. Shanghai: Chinese Medical Association.

Chinese Posters Foundation, http://chineseposters.net/themes/shanghai.php.

"Cholera in 1932." *Chinese Medical Journal* 46 (1932): 1207–9.

"Chūshi ni okeru korera ryūko jyōkyō ni kansuru ken" 中支におけるコレラ流行に関す
る件 (On the prevalence of cholera in Central China). Filed in GK I-3-2-0-12, vol. 7.

Claypool, Lisa. "Zhang Jian and China's First Museum." *Journal of Asian Studies* 64,
no. 3 (2005): 567–604.

Coble, Parks M. *Chinese Capitalists in Japan's New Order: The Occupied Lower Yangzi,
1937–1945*. Berkeley: University of California Press, 2003.

———. *The Shanghai Capitalists and the Nationalist Government, 1927–1937*. Cambridge, MA: Council on East Asian Studies, Harvard University, 1980.

Cochran, Sherman. *Big Business in China: Sino-Foreign Rivalry in the Cigarette Industry, 1890–1930*. Cambridge, MA: Harvard University Press, 1980.

———. *Chinese Medicine Men: Consumer Culture in China and Southeast Asia*. Cambridge, MA: Harvard University Press, 2006.

———. *Encountering Chinese Networks: Western, Japanese, and Chinese Corporations in
China, 1880–1937*. Berkeley: University of California Press, 2000.

———, ed. *Inventing Nanjing Road: Commercial Culture in Shanghai, 1900–1945*.
Ithaca, NY: East Asia Program, Cornell University, 1999.

———. "Marketing Medicine and Advertising Dreams in China, 1900–1950." In *Becoming Chinese: Passages to Modernity and Beyond*, edited by Wen-hsin Yeh, 62–97. Berkeley: University of California Press, 2000.

Cochran, Sherman, and Andrew Hsieh. *The Lius of Shanghai*. Cambridge, MA: Harvard University Press, 2013.

Cohen, Paul. "The Post-Mao Reforms in Historical Perspectives." *Journal of Asian Studies* 47, no. 3 (1988): 519–40.

Cohen, William, and Ryan Johnson, eds. *Filth: Dirt, Disgust, and Modern Life*. Minneapolis: University of Minnesota Press, 2005.

Croizier, Ralph. *Traditional Medicine in Modern China: Science, Nationalism, and the Tensions of Cultural Change*. Cambridge, MA: Harvard University Press, 1968.

Culp, Robert. *Articulating Citizenship: Civic Education and Student Politics in Southeastern China, 1912–1940*. Cambridge, MA: Harvard University Asia Center, 2007.

Cunningham, Andrew, and Bridie Andrews. "Introduction." In *Western Medicine as Contested Knowledge*, edited by Andrew Cunningham and Bridie Andrews, 1–23. Manchester, UK: Manchester University Press, 1997.

———, eds. *Western Medicine as Contested Knowledge*. Manchester, UK: Manchester University Press, 1997.

"Dahui biaoyu ji jieyanling" 大會標語及戒嚴令 (Hygiene campaign slogans and emergency law). *Weisheng yuekan* 4, no. 7 (1934): 294.

"Dahui jishi: jiesuan baogaoshu" 大會紀實：決算報告書 (Campaign records: statement of accounts). *Weisheng yuekan*, no. 5 (1928): 66–67.

Daitōashō 大東亞省 (The Ministry of Great East Asia). "Kōso, Sekkō, Anki sanshō no suidō jigyō narabini denki jigyō" 江蘇、浙江、安徽三省の水道事業並びに電気事業 (A general situation on the waterworks and electric businesses in Jiangsu, Zhejiang, and Anhui provinces). *Chōsa geppō* 調査月報 2, no. 3 (1941): 135–62.

"Damages to Medical Institutes in Shanghai." *Chinese Medical Journal* 46 (1932): 332–33.

de Certeau, Michel. *The Practice of Everyday Life*. Translated by Steven Rendall. Berkeley: University of California Press, 1984.

Dikötter, Frank. *The Age of Openness: China before Mao*. Berkeley: University of California Press, 2008.

———. "A Cultural History of the Syringe in Modern China." *Twentieth-Century China* 28, no. 1 (2002): 37–56.

———. *Exotic Commodities: Modern Objects and Everyday Life in China*. New York: Columbia University Press, 2006.

———. *Sex, Culture, and Modernity in China: Medical Science and the Construction of Sexual Identities in the Early Republican Period*. Honolulu: University of Hawai'i Press, 1995.

Dirlik, Arif. "Reversals, Ironies and Hegemonies: Notes on the Contemporary Historiography of Modern China." *Modern China* 22, no. 3 (1996): 243–84.

"Di-shier jie weisheng yundong baogao" 第十二屆衛生運動報告 (The twelfth hygiene campaign report). *Weisheng yuekan* 4, no. 2 (1934): 87–90.

Eastman, Lloyd. "Fascism in Kuomintang China: The Blue Shirts." *China Quarterly* 80 (1979): 1–31.

Elman, Benjamin. *On Their Own Terms: Science in China, 1550–1900*. Cambridge, MA: Harvard University Press, 2005.

Elvin, Mark. "The Administration of Shanghai, 1905–1914." In *The Chinese City between Two Worlds*, edited by Mark Elvin and William Skinner, 239–62. Stanford, CA: Stanford University Press, 1974.

———. "The Gentry Democracy in Chinese Shanghai, 1905–1914." In *Modern China's Search for A Political Form*, edited by Jack Gray, 41–65. Oxford: Oxford University Press, 1969.

Elvin, Mark, and G. William Skinner. *The Chinese City between Two Worlds*. Stanford, CA: Stanford University Press, 1974.

Esherick, Joseph W. "Modernity and Nation in the Chinese City." In *Remaking the Chinese City: Modernity and National Identity, 1900–1950*, edited by Joseph Esherick, 1–16. Honolulu: University of Hawai'i Press, 2000.

———, ed. *Remaking the Chinese City: Modernity and National Identity, 1900–1950*. Honolulu: University of Hawai'i Press, 2000.

Esherick, Joseph W., and Jeffrey N. Wasserstrom. "Acting Out Democracy: Political Theater in Modern China." In *Popular Protest and Political Culture in Modern China*, edited by Jeffrey N. Wasserstrom and Elizabeth J. Perry, 32–70. Boulder, CO: Westview Press, 1994.

Fagui 法規 (Statutes). *Weisheng gongbao* 衛生公報 (Public health gazette) 1, no. 1 (1929): 1–5.

Fagui 法規 (Statutes). *Weisheng gongbao* 衛生公報 (Public health gazette) 2, no. 1 (1930): 133–46.

Fang Zhixiong 方之雄. "Zhongguo riyong huaxuepin gongye de dianjiren Fang Yexian" 中国日用化学品工业的奠基人方液仙 (Fang Yexin, the founder of China's eveyday use chemical industry). In *Chuangye Shanghaitan*, edited by Shanghai shi Ningbo jingji jianshe cujinhui xiehui, Shanghai Shi Ningbo tongxiang lianyihui, and *Ningboren zai Shanghai* xilie congshu bianweihui, 359–68. Shanghai: Shanghai shi Ningbo jingji jianshe cujinhui xiehui, 2003.

Farquhar, Judith. "Market Magic: Getting Rich and Getting Personal in Medicine after Mao." *American Ethnologist* 23, no. 2 (1996): 239–57.

Ferlanti, Federica. "The New Life Movement in Jiangxi Province, 1934–1938." *Modern Asian Studies* 44, no. 5 (2010): 961–1000.

Fewsmith, Joseph. *Party, State, and Local Elite in Republican China: Merchant Organizations and Politics in Shanghai, 1890–1930*. Honolulu: University of Hawai'i Press, 1985.

Field, Andrew David. *Shanghai's Dancing World: Cabaret Culture and Urban Politics, 1919–1954*. Hong Kong: Chinese University Press, 2010.

"Foreign Settlement of Shanghai, Census 1930." Filed in SMA U1-16-519.

Foucault, Michel. *Power. The Essential Works of Foucault, 1954–1984*, vol. 3, edited by James D. Faubion. New York: New Press, 2000.

Frolic, B. Michael, ed. *Mao's People: Sixteen Portraits of Life in Revolutionary China*. Cambridge, MA: Harvard University Press, 1980.

Fu Hui 傅惠, and Deng Zongyu 邓宗禹. "Yixuejie de yingmeipai yu deripai zhi zheng" 医学界的英美派与德日派之争 (Conflicts within the medical circle between the Anglo-American group and the German-Japanese group). In *Wenshi ziliao xuanji*, no. 119, edited by Quanguo zhengxie wenshi ziliao weiyuanhui, 64–74. Beijing: Zhongguo wenshi chubanshe, 1989.

Fu, Poshek. *Passivity, Resistance, and Collaboration: Intellectual Choice in Occupied Shanghai, 1937–1945*. Stanford, CA: Stanford University Press, 1993.

Fukushi Yuki 福士由紀. "Nicchu sensōki Shanghai ni okeru kōshū eisei to shakai kanri: korera yobō undo o chūshin to shite" 日中戦争期上海における公衆衛生と社会管理：コレラ予防運動を中心として (Public health and social control in Shanghai during the Sino-Japanese War: A case study of the cholera prevention campaign). *Gendai Chūgoku* 現代中国 77 (2003): 53–66.

Furth, Charlotte. "Introduction: Hygienic Modernity in Chinese East Asia." In *Health and Hygiene in Chinese East Asia*, edited by Angela Ki Che Leung and Charlotte Furth, 1–21. Durham, NC: Duke University Press, 2010.

Furth, Charlotte. *Ting Wen-chiang: Science and China's New Culture*. Cambridge, MA: Harvard University Press, 1970.

Gaimushō kiroku 外務省記録 (Records of the Ministry of Foreign Affairs).

Gamewell, Mary Ninde. *The Gateway to China: Pictures of Shanghai*. New York: Revell, 1916.

Garrett, Shirley. "The Chamber of Commerce and the YMCA." In *The Chinese City between Two Worlds,* edited by Mark Elvin and William G. Skinner, 211–61. Stanford, CA: Stanford University Press, 1974.

———. *Social Reformers in Urban China: The Chinese YMCA, 1895–1926*. Cambridge, MA: Harvard University Press, 1970.

Ge Zhuang 葛壮. *Zongjiao he jindai Shanghai shehui de bianqian* 宗教和近代上海社会的变迁 (Religions and the transformation of modern Shanghai society). Shanghai: Shanghai shudian chubanshe, 1998.

Gerth, Karl. *China Made: Consumer Culture and the Creation of the Nation*. Cambridge, MA: Harvard University Asia Center, 2003.

Gezhi huibian 格致彙編 (*The Chinese Scientific Magazine*).

Glosser, Susan L. *Chinese Visions of Family and State, 1915–1953*. Berkeley: University of California Press, 2003.

Gluck, Carol. *Japan's Modern Myths: Ideology in the Late Meiji Period*. Princeton: Princeton University Press, 1985.

"Gongyi cishan tuanti dengjibiao, 1930" 公益慈善團體登記表 (Registration chart of public welfare and charitable organizations). Filed in SMA Q113-4-1.

Gongzuo baogao 工作報告 (Business report). Filed in SMA R50-1384.

Goodman, Bryna. "Improvisations on a Semicolonial Theme, or, How to Read Multi-ethnic Participation in the 1893 Shanghai Jubilee." *Journal of Asian Studies* 59, no. 4 (2000): 889–926.

———. *Native Place, City, and Nation: Regional Networks and Identities in Shanghai, 1853–1937*. Berkeley: University of California Press, 1995.

Goodman, Bryna, and David S. G. Goodman. "Colonialism and China." In *Twentieth-Century Colonialism and China: Localities, the Everyday and the World*, edited by Bryna Goodman and David S. G. Goodman, 1–22. New York: Routledge, 2012.

———, eds. *Twentieth-Century Colonialism and China: Localities, the Everyday and the World*. New York: Routledge, 2012.

Grant, John B., and T. M. P'eng. "Survey of Urban Public Health Practice in China." *Chinese Medical Journal* 48 (1934): 1074–79.

Gray, Jack, ed. *Modern China's Search for a Political Form*. Oxford: Oxford University Press, 1969.

Greene, J. Megan. "GMD Rhetoric of Science and Modernity (1927–70): A Neo-traditional Scientism?" In *Defining Modernity: Guomindang Rhetoric of a New China, 1920–1970*, edited by Terry Bodenhorn, 223–61. Ann Arbor, MI: Center for Chinese Studies, 2002.

Gu Bingquan 顾炳权, ed. *Shanghai yangchang zhuzhici* 上海洋场竹枝词 (Local popular verse from Shanghai). Shanghai: Shanghai shudian chubanshe, 1996.

Guo Dewen 郭德文. "Mingyi de yaolan: Sheng Yuehan daxue yixueyuan" 名医的摇篮：圣约翰医学院. (Cradle of great doctors: Shanghai St. John's medical school). In *Shanghai Sheng Yuehan daxue*, edited by Xu Yihua, 335–40. Shanghai: Shanghai renmin chubanshe, 2007.

Guo Hongxiao 果鸿孝. "Song Zejiu 宋则久." In *Zhongguo jindai qiye de kaituozhe*, vol. 1, edited by Kong Lingren and Li Dezheng, 426–35. Jinan: Shandong renmin chubanshe, 1991.

Guohuo shiye chubanshe bianjibu 國貨事業出版社編輯部 (National product business publisher editorial department), ed. *Zhongguo guohuo gongchang shilüe* 中國國貨工廠史略 (A brief history of China's national product manufacturing business). Shanghai: Guohuo shiye chubanshe bianjibu, 1935.

Guomin zhengfu 國民政府 (The National Government). "Xiaji weisheng yundong dahui shishi dagang" 夏季衛生運動大會實施大綱 (An outline for summer hygiene campaign implementation meetings). Academia Historica, file 001-012161-007.

Guomin zhengfu zhujichu tongjiju 國民政府主計處統計局 (The Statistic Bureau of the Department of Accounting, the National Government), ed. *Zhonghua minguo tongji tiyao* 中華民國統計提要 (A summary of statistics of the Republic of China). n.p., 1935.

Hanan, Patrick. "Introduction." In *The Money Demon: An Autobiographical Romance* by Chen Diexian, 1–10. Honolulu: University of Hawai'i Press, 1999.

Hanson, Marta E. "Conceptual Blind Spots, Medical Blindfolds: The Case of SARS and Traditional Chinese Medicine." In *Health and Hygiene in Chinese East Asia: Politics and Publics in the Long Twentieth Century*, edited by Angela Ki Che Leung and Charlotte Furth, 228–54. Durham, NC: Duke University Press, 2010.

Harrison, Henrietta. *The Making of the Republican Citizen: Political Ceremonies and Symbols in China 1911–1929*. Oxford: Oxford University Press, 2002.

Harrison, Mark. *Public Health and Preventive Medicine in British India, 1859–1914*. Cambridge, UK: Cambridge University Press, 1994.

Hauser, Ernest O. *Shanghai: City for Sale*. New York: Harcourt, Brace and Company, 1940.

Hayford, Charles W. *To the People: James Yen and Village China.* New York: Columbia University Press, 1990.

He Kuang 何况. *Huochai dawang Liu Hongsheng* 火柴大王刘鸿生 (Liu Hongsheng, the majordomo of the match industry). Beijing: Jeifang chubanshe, 1995.

He, Qiliang. "Spectacular Death: Sheng Xuanhuai's Funeral Procession in 1917." *Twentieth-Century China* 41, no. 2 (2016): 136–58.

He Shixi 何时希. *Jindai yilin yishi* 近代医林轶事 (Anecdotes about medical doctors in modern era). Shanghai: Shanghai zhongyiyao daxue chubanshe, 1995.

———. "Menghe Dingshi sandai mingyi" 孟河丁氏三代名医 (The Ding family from Menghe: Three generations of eminent physicians). In *Haishang yilin,* edited by Zhongguo renmin zhengzhi xieshang huiyi Shanghai Shi weiyuanhui wenshi ziliao gongzuo weiyuanhui. Shanghai: Shanghai renmin chunbanshe, 1991.

"Health Commissioner in Shanghai." *Chinese Medical Journal* 46 (1932): 1220.

Henriot, Christian. "The Colonial Space of Death: Shanghai Cemeteries, 1844–1949." In *Twentieth-Century Colonialism and China: Localities, the Everyday and the World,* edited by Bryna Goodman and David S. G. Goodman, 108–33. New York: Routledge, 2012.

———. "'Invisible Deaths, Silent Deaths': 'Bodies without Masters' in Republican Shanghai." *Journal of Social History* 43, no. 2 (2009): 407–37.

———. *Prostitution and Sexuality in Shanghai: A Social History, 1849–1949.* Cambridge, UK: Cambridge University Press, 2001.

———. *Shanghai, 1927–1937: Municipal Power, Locality, and Modernization.* Translated by Noel Castelino. Berkeley: University of California Press, 1993.

Henriot, Christian, and Wen-shin Yeh, eds. *In the Shadow of the Rising Sun: Shanghai under Japanese Occupation.* Cambridge, UK: Cambridge University Press, 2004.

Hershatter, Gail. *Dangerous Pleasures: Prostitution and Modernity in Twentieth-Century Shanghai.* Berkeley: University of California Press, 1997.

Hevia, James. *English Lessons: The Pedagogy of Imperialism in Nineteenth-Century China.* Durham, NC: Duke University Press, 2003.

Hinrichs, TJ, and Linda L. Barnes, eds. *Chinese Medicine and Healing: An Illustrated History.* Cambridge, MA: Belknap Press of Harvard University Press, 2013.

Ho, Ping-ti. *Studies on the Population of China, 1368–1953.* Cambridge, MA: Harvard University Press, 1959.

Hu Hongji 胡鸿基 (Hou-ki Hu). *Gonggong weisheng gailun* 公共衛生概論 (Introduction to public health). Shanghai: Shangwu yinshuguan, 1929.

———. "Shanghai Shi wunianlai zhi weisheng xingzheng huigu" 上海市五年來之衛生行政回顧 (Reminiscing about Shanghai's public health administration for the last five years). In *Hu juzhang Hongji boshi jiniance,* edited by Hu juzhang Hong Xing Ji zhuidaohui, 4–18. Shanghai, n.p., 1932.

Hu, Hou-ki (Hu Hongji). "The New Department of Health, Port of Shanghai and Woosong." *Chinese Medical Journal* 41 (1927): 429–38.

———. "Plans and Ideas for the Health of Greater Shanghai." Filed in SMA U1-16-293.

Hu juzhang Hong Xing Ji zhuidaohui 胡局長鴻興基追悼會 (The association to commemorate the late director Hu Hongji), ed. *Hu juzhang Hongji boshi jiniance* 胡局長鴻基博士紀念冊 (A volume to commemorate Dr. Hu Hongji). Shanghai, n.p., 1932.

Huang Hanmin 黄汉民, and Lu Xinglong 陆兴龙. *Jindai Shanghai gongye qiye fazhanshilun* 近代上海工业企业发展史论 (Study on the history of the development of industry in modern Shanghai). Shanghai: Shanghai caijing daxue chubanshe, 2000.

Huang, Philip. "Public Sphere/Civil Society in China? A Third Realm between State and Society." *Modern China* 19, no. 2 (1993): 216–40.

Huang Shuze, and Lin Shixiao, eds. *Contemporary China: Health Career*. Beijing: Dangdai Zhongguo chubanshe, 2009.

Huang Zhiwei 黄志伟, and Huang Ying 黄莹, eds. *Wei shiji daiyan: Zhongguo jindai guanggao* 为世纪代言：中国近代广告. (Speaking for the times: Modern advertising in China). Shanghai: Shanghai xuelin chuban jituan, 2004.

Hui Xicheng 惠西成, and Shi Zi 石子. *Zhongguo minsu daguan xia* 中国民俗大观下 (A panorama of Chinese folk customs, vol. 2). Guangzhou: Guangdong lüyou chubanshe, 1988.

"Huxiang wenda" 互相問答 (Questions and answers). *Gezhi huibian* 1, no. 10 (1876): 10–11.

"Huxiang wenda" 互相問答 (Questions and answers). *Gezhi huibian* 3, no. 12 (1880): 15–16.

"Hygiene and Public Health: The Cholera Epidemic." *Chinese Medical Journal* 46 (1932): 932.

Jen, P. Y. (Ren Peiyuna). "A Survey of the Water Supply Companies in China." *Quarterly Review of Social Science* 7, no. 2 (1936): 267–86.

Jijiu shiyi yiyuan shiwuchu 急救時疫醫院事務處 (Shanghai Emergency Hospital Administration), ed. *Shanghai jijiu shiyi yiyuan gongzuo baogao fu zhengxinlu* 上海急救時疫醫院工作報告付徵信錄 (Shanghai Emergency Hospital business report and financial statement). n.p., 1940.

Jin Baoshan 金宝善. "Weisheng yu jiuguo" 衛生與救國 (Health and national salvation). *Weisheng yuekan* 4, no. 4 (1934): 65–68.

Johnson, David, Andrew J. Nathan, and Evelyn S. Rawski, eds. *Popular Culture in Late Imperial China*. Berkeley: University of California Press, 1974.

Johnson, Linda Cooke. *Shanghai: From Market Town to Treaty Port, 1074–1858*. Stanford, CA: Stanford University Press, 1995.

Jordan, J. H. "Shanghai Municipal Council—Public Health Department." *Chinese Medical Journal* 49 (1935): 993–97.

Kaufman, Joan. "SARS and China's Health-Care Responses: Better to Be Both Red and Expert!" In *SARS in China: Prelude to Pandemic?* edited by Arthur Kleinman and James L. Watson, 53–68. Stanford, CA: Stanford University Press, 2006.

Keren 可人. "Woguo gonggong weisheng shiye xianqu Yan Fuqing" 我国公共卫生事业先驱颜福庆 (Yan Fuqing: A pioneer of public health activities in our country). In *Shanghai renwu shiliao*, edited by Zhongguo renmin zhengzhi xieshang huiyi Shanghai Shi weiyuanhui wenshi ziliao gongzuo weiyuanhui. Shanghai: Shanghai zhengxie wenshi ziliao bianjibu, 1992.

Kim, C. S. "A Brief Survey of Public Health Activities in Shanghai." *Chinese Medical Journal* 42 (1928): 162–80.

"Kimitsu 1109: Gokuhi Chūshi korera ryūkō jōhō" 機密 1109: 極秘中支コレラ流行情報 (Confidential report, no. 1109: General information about the cholera outbreak in Central China). Filed in GK I-3-2-0-8, vol. 3.

Kleinman, Arthur, and James L. Watson, eds. *SARS in China: Prelude to Pandemic?* Stanford, CA: Stanford University Press, 2006.

Kleinman, Arthur, Yunxiang Yan, Jing Jun, Sing Lee, Everett Zhang, Pan Tianshu, Wu Fei, and Guo Jinhua. *Deep China: The Moral Life of the Person: What Anthropology and Psychiatry Tell Us about China Today.* Berkeley: University of California Press, 2011.

Kohama Masako 小浜正子. *Kindai Shanghai no kōkyōsei to kokka* 近代上海の公共性と国家 (The "public" and the state in modern Shanghai). Tokyo: Kenbun Shuppan, 2000.

———. "Minkokuki Shanghai no minkan jizen jigyō to kokka kenryoku" 民国期上海の民間慈善事業と国家権力 (Social welfare and state authority in Republican Shanghai). Tōyō *gakuhō* 東洋学報76, nos. 1 and 2 (1994): 1–36.

———. "Minkokuki Shanghai no toshi shakai to jizen jigyō" 民国期上海の都市社会と慈善事業 (Urban society and social welfare in Republican Shanghai). *Shigaku zasshi* 史学雑誌 103, no. 10 (1994): 57–89.

Kojima Shinji 小島晋治, ed. *Taishō Chūgoku kenbunroku shūsei* 大正中国見聞録集成 (Collected reports on travel in China during the Taishō Period). Tokyo: Yumani shobō, 1997.

Kong Lingren 孔令仁, and Li Dezheng 李德征, eds. *Zhongguo jindai qiye de kaituozhe* 中国近代企业的开拓者 (Pioneers of China's modern enterprises). Jinan: Shandong renmin chubanshe, 1991.

Kopytoff, Igor. "The Cultural Biography of Things: Commoditization as Processes." In *The Social Life of Things: Commodities in Cultural Perspective*, edited by Arjun Appadurai, 64–91. Cambridge, UK: Cambridge University Press, 1988.

"Korera bōeki jisshi kitei" コレラ防疫実施規定 (Cholera control enforcement regulations). Filed in SMA R50-289.

Kubo, Toru. "The Kōa-in." In *China at War: Regions of China, 1937–1945*, edited by Stephen R. MacKinnon, Diana Lary, and Ezra F. Vogel, 44–64. Stanford, CA: Stanford University Press, 2007.

Kupinse, William. "The Indian Subject of Colonial Hygiene." In *Filth: Dirt, Disgust, and Modern Life*, edited by William Cohen and Ryan Johnson, 250–76. Minneapolis: University of Minnesota Press, 2005.

Kwok, D. W. Y. *Scientism in Chinese Thought, 1900–1950.* New Haven: Yale University Press, 1965.

Lam, Tong. *A Passion for Facts: Social Surveys and the Construction of the Chinese Nation State, 1900–1949.* Berkeley: University of California Press, 2011.

Lamberton, Mary. *St. John's University: Shanghai 1879–1951.* New York: United Board for Christian Colleges in China, 1955.

Lamson, H. D. "The Problem of Housing for Workers in China." *Chinese Economic Journal* 11, no. 2 (1932): 139–62.

Landsberger, Stefan R. "To Spit or Not to Spit: Health and Hygiene Communication through Propaganda Posters in the PRC—A Historical Overview." http://www.academia.edu/5336077/To_spit_or_not_to_spit_Health_and_Hygiene

_Communication_through_Propaganda_Posters_in_the_PRC_A_Historical
_Overview.

Lean, Eugenia. *Public Passions: The Trial of Shi Jianqiao and the Rise of Popular Sympathy in Republican China.* Berkeley: University of California Press, 2007.

Lee, Leo Ou-fan. "The Cultural Construction in Urban Shanghai: Some Preliminary Explorations." In *Becoming Chinese: Passages to Modernity and Beyond,* edited by Wenhsin Yeh, 31–61. Berkeley: University of California Press, 2000.

———. *Shanghai Modern: Flowering of a New Urban Culture in China, 1930–1945.* Cambridge, MA: Harvard University Press, 1999.

Lee, Leo Ou-fan, and Andrew J. Nathan. "The Beginning of Mass Culture: Journalism and Fiction in the Late Ch'ing and Beyond." In *Popular Culture in Late Imperial China,* edited by David Johnson, Andrew J. Nathan, and Evelyn S. Rawski, 360–95. Berkeley: University of California Press, 1985.

Lei Hsiang-lin (Lei Xianglin) 雷祥麟 (Sean Hsiang-lin Lei). "Weisheng weihe bu shi baowei shengming?—Minguo shiqi linglei de weisheng, ziwo he jibing 衛生為何不是保衛生命?–民國時期另類的衛生，自我和疾病."(Why *weisheng* is not about "defending one's life"—Alternative concepts of *weisheng,* self, and disease in the Republican era). In *Diguo yu xiandai yixue,* edited by Li Shang-jen, 415–54. Taipei: Lianjing chuban shiye gufen youxian gongsi, 2008.

Lei Qili 雷启立, ed. *Ding Wenjiang yinxiang* 丁文江印象 (The impression of Ding Wenjiang). Shanghai: Xuelin chubanshe, 1997.

Lei, Sean Hsiang-lin (Lei Xianglin). "Habituating the Four Virtues: Ethics, Family, and the Body in the Anti-Tuberculosis Campaigns and the New Life Movement." *Bulletin of the Institute of Modern History, Academia Sinica* 74 (2011): 133–77.

———. "Habituating Individuality: Framing Tuberculosis and Its Material Solutions in Republican China." *Bulletin of the History of Medicine* 84 (2010): 248–79.

———. *Neither Donkey nor Horse: Medicine in the Struggle over China's Modernity.* Chicago: University of Chicago Press, 2014.

———. "Sovereignty and Microscope: Constituting Notifiable Infectious Disease and Containing the Manchurian Plague (1910–11)." In *Health and Hygiene in Chinese East Asia,* edited by Angela Leung and Charlotte Furth, 73–106. Durham, NC: Duke University Press, 2010.

———. "When Chinese Medicine Encountered the State: 1910–1949." PhD diss., University of Chicago, 1999.

Leonard, Jane Kate. *Controlling from Afar: The Daoguang Emperor's Management of the Grand Canal Crisis, 1824–1826.* Ann Arbor: Center for Chinese Studies, University of Michigan, 1996.

"Lester Chinese Hospital." Filed in SMA U1-16-822.

The Lester Chinese Hospital Annual Report and Statement Accounts. Various years. Filed in SMA U1-4-216.

Leung, Angela Ki Che. *Leprosy in China: A History.* New York: Columbia University Press, 2009.

———. "Organized Medicine in Ming-Qing China: State and Private Medical Institutions in the Lower Yangzi Region." *Late Imperial China* 8, no. 1 (1987): 134–66.

Leung, Angela Ki Che, and Charlotte Furth, eds. *Health and Hygiene in Chinese East Asia*. Durham, NC: Duke University Press, 2010.

Leutner, Mechthild, and Nicola Spakowski, eds. *Women in China: The Republican Period in Historical Perspective*. Münster: LIT Verlag, 2005.

Lewis, Milton J., and Kerrie L. MacPherson. "Introduction." In *Public Health in Asia and the Pacific: Historical and Comparative Perspectives*, edited by Milton J. Lewis and Kerrie L. MacPherson, 1–9. New York: Routledge, 2008.

———, eds. *Public Health in Asia and the Pacific: Historical and Comparative Perspectives*. New York: Routledge, 2008.

Li Changli 李长莉. *WanQing Shanghai shehui de bianqian: Shenghuo yu lunli de jindaihua* 晚清上海社会的变迁: 生活与伦理的近代化 (Transformation of late-Qing Shanghai society: modernization of the life and ethics). Tianjin: Tianjin chubanshe, 2002.

Li Jingwei 李经纬. *Zhongwai yixue jiaoliushi* 中外医学交流史 (A history of Chinese-foreign medical exchanges). Changsha: Hunan jiaoyu chubanshe, 1998.

Li Pingshu 李平书. *Li Pingshu qishi zixu* 李平书七十自叙 (Autobiography of Li Pingshu: Seventy years). Shanghai, 1924; reprint, Shanghai: Shanghai guji shubanshe, 1989.

Li, Shang-jen (Li Shangren) 李尚仁. "Healing Body, Saving Soul: Medical Missions to Nineteenth-Century China." In *Conference Handbook: Conference on Religion and Healing and the Second Meeting of the Asian Society for History of Medicine*, edited by The Institute of History and Philosophy, Academia Sinica (Taipei, 2004). http://www.ihp.sinica.edu.tw/~medicine/ashm/lectures/paper/paper9.pdf.

———, ed. *Diguo yu xiandai yixue* 帝國與現代醫學 (Empire and modern medicine). Taibei: Lianjing chuban shiye gufen youxian gongsi, 2008.

Li Ting'an 李廷安 (Ting-an Li). "Guomin huiyi yinggai zhuyi weisheng shiye" 國民會議應該注意衛生事業 (The national assembly should pay attention to hygiene). *Yixue zhoukanji* 醫學週刊集 5 (1932): 43–44.

———. "Shanghai Shi weishengju gongzuo zhi gaikuang 上海市衛生局工作之概況" (A general survey of Shanghai Municipal Public Health Bureau's work). *Zhonghua yixue zazhi* 中華醫學雜誌 20, no. 1 (1934): 107–15.

———. "Shanghai Shi zhi gonggong weisheng xingzheng" 上海市之公共衛生行政 (Public health administration in Shanghai). *Weisheng yuekan* 4, no. 1 (1934): 20–24; and *Yishi huikan* 醫事彙刊 19 (1934): 133–39.

———. "Shenme shi 'gonggong weisheng?'" 什麼是公共衛生? (What is "public health"?) *Yixue zhoukanji* 醫學週刊集 1 (1928): 49–52.

———. "Weishengju ji ge qu weisheng shiwusuo zhi zuzhi ji gongzuo" 衛生局及各區衛生事務所之組織及工作 (Organization and works of the Public Health Bureau and District Health Stations). *Weisheng yuekan* 6, no. 10 (1936): 459–63.

———. "Woguo zhongyao dushi weisheng xingzheng jingfei zhi xiankuang" 我國重要都市衛生行政經費之現況 (The state of public health administrative expenditure of important cities in our country). *Weisheng yuekan* 4, no. 11 (1934): 436–42.

Li, Ting-an (Li Ting'an). "Activities of the Bureau of Public Health, City Government of Greater Shanghai." *Chinese Medical Journal* 49 (1935): 990–92.

———. "A Report on the Bureau of Public Health, City Government of Greater Shanghai." Filed in SMA U1-16-319.

Li Zongfa 李宗法. *Feizao* 肥皂 (Soap). Shanghai: Shangwu yinshuguan, 1933.

Li Zufan 李祖范. "Yagao shengchan jianshi" 牙膏生产简史 (A brief history of toothpaste production). In *Gongye shangye*, vol. 6 of *Shanghai wenshi ziliao cungao huibian*, edited by Shanghai Shi zhengxie wenshi ziliao weiyuanhui, 92–104. Originally published in 1959. Shanghai: Shanghai guji chubanshe, 2001.

———. "Zhongguo huaxue gongyeshe jianshi" 中国化学工业社简史 (A brief history of China Chemical Industries). In *Ershi shiji Shanghai wenshi ziliao wenku*, vol. 3, edited by Wu Hanmin, 215–26. Shanghai: Shanghai shudian chubanshe, 1999.

Liangyou 良友 [The Young Companion].

Lin Rukang 林汝康. "Zhongguo huaxue gongyeshe yu Fang Yexian" 中国化学工业社与方液仙 (China Chemical Industries and Fang Yexian). In *Gongye shangye*, vol. 7 of *Shanghai wenshi ziliao cungao huibian*, edited by Shanghai Shi zhengxie wenshi ziliao weiyuanhui, 285–97. Shanghai: Shanghai guji chubanshe, 2001.

Link, Perry Jr. *Mandarin Ducks and Butterflies: Popular Fiction in Early Twentieth-Century Chinese Cities*. Berkeley: University of California Press, 1981.

Lipkin, Zwia. *Useless to the State: "Social Problems" and Social Engineering in Nationalist Nanjing, 1927–1937*. Cambridge, MA: Harvard University Asia Center, 2006.

Liqi Guangzuo 李其光作. "Gonggong weisheng: shenme jiaozuo weisheng yundong" 公共衛生: 甚麼叫做衛生運動 (Public health: What is the hygiene campaign?). *Weisheng zazhi* 衛生雜誌 19 (1934): 12–13.

Liu, Hou, Irene Ssu-chin 劉似錦 (Liu Sijin), ed. *Dr. J. Heng Liu and Health Development in China* 劉瑞恆博士與中國醫藥及衛生事業. Taipei: Taiwan shanwu yinshuguan, 1989.

Liu, J. Heng (Liu Ruiheng). "The Chinese Medical Association First General Conference Address." In *Dr. J. Heng Liu and Health Development in China*, edited by Irene Ssu-chin Liu Hou, 303–6. Taipei: Taiwan shanwu yinshuguan, 1989.

———. "The Ministry of Health." In *Dr. J. Heng Liu and Health Development in China*, edited by Irene Ssu-chin Liu Hou, 287–98. Taipei: Taiwan shanwu yinshuguan, 1989.

Liu, Michael Shiyung. *Prescribing Colonization: The Role of Medical Practices and Policies in Japan-Ruled Taiwan, 1895–1945*. Ann Arbor, MI: Association for Asian Studies, 2009.

Liu Ruiheng 劉瑞恆 (J. Heng Liu). *Xinshenghuo yu jiankang* 新生活與健康 (New Life and health). Nanjing: Zhonghua shuju, 1935.

Liu Shanling 刘善龄. *Xiyang feng: xiyang faming zai Zhongguo* 西洋风: 西洋发明在中国 (Western-style: Western inventions in China). Shanghai: Shanghai guji chubanshe, 1999.

Liu, Ts'ui-jung, James Lee, David Sven Reher, Osamu Saito, and Wang Feng, eds. *Asian Population History*. Oxford: Oxford University Press, 2001.

Lo, Ming-cheng M. *Doctors within Borders: Profession, Ethnicity and Modernity in Colonial Taiwan*. Berkeley: University of California Press, 2002.

Lou, K. Z. 陸幹臣 (Lu Ganchen). *Weisheng yundong shishi jihua* 衛生運動實施計畫 [Policy and Program for Health Campaign]. Shanghai: Association Press of China, 1928.

Lu, Hanchao. "Becoming Urban: Mendicancy and Vagrants in Modern Shanghai." *Journal of Social History* 33, no. 1 (1999): 7–36.

———. *Beyond the Neon Lights: Everyday Shanghai in the Early Twentieth Century.* Berkeley: University of California Press, 1999.

———. "Creating Urban Outcasts: Shantytown in Shanghai, 1920–1950." *Journal of Urban History* 21, no. 5 (1995): 563–96.

Lu Hanchao 卢汉超. "Shanghai tudi zhangcheng yanjiu" 上海土地章程研究 (Study on the land regulations of Shanghai). In *Shanghaishi yanjiu*, edited by Qiao Shuming, 100–145. Shanghai: Xuelin chubanshe, 1984.

Lu Ming 陆明. "Shanghai jindai xiyi yiyuan gaishu" 上海近代西医医院概述 (A brief history of Western hospitals in modern Shanghai). *Zhonghua yishi zazhi* 中华医史杂志 26, no. 1 (1996): 19–26.

Lu Yipei 鲁義培. "Jiankang yu jiuguo" 健康與救國 (Health and national salvation). *Kangjian zazhi* 康健雜誌 1, no. 7 (1933): 1–3.

Lu Zhilian 陆志濂. "Fang Yexian" 方液仙. In *Zhongguo jindai qiye de kaituozhe*, vol. 1, edited by Kong Lingren and Li Dezheng, 27–37. Jinan: Shandong renmin chubanshe, 1991.

Lucas, AnElissa. *Chinese Medical Modernization: Comparative Policy Continuities, 1930s–1980s.* New York: Praeger, 1982.

Lupton, Deborah. *The Imperative of Health: Public Health and the Regulated Body.* London: Sage Publications, 1995.

Lynteris, Christos. *The Spirit of Selflessness in Maoist China: Socialist Medicine and the New Man.* Basingstoke: Palgrave Macmillan, 2013.

Ma Changlin 马长林. *Shanghai de zujie* 上海的租界 (The foreign settlements of Shanghai). Tianjin: Tianjin jiaoyu chubanshe, 2009.

MacLeod, Roy, and Milton Lewis, eds. *Disease, Medicine, and Empire: Perspectives on Western Medicine and the Experience of European Expansion.* New York: Routledge, 1988.

MacPherson, Kerrie. *A Wilderness of Marshes: The Origins of Public Health in Shanghai, 1843–1893.* Oxford: Oxford University Press, 1987.

Martin, Brian. *The Shanghai Green Gang: Politics and Organized Crime, 1919–1937.* Berkeley: University of California Press, 1996.

Mason, Katherine. "Becoming Modern after SARS: Battling the H1N1 Pandemic and the Politics of Backwardness in China's Pearl River Delta." *Behemoth: A Journal on Civilisation* 3, no. 3 (2010): 8–35.

———. "H1N1 Is Not a Chinese Virus: The Racialization of People and Viruses in Post-SARS China." *Studies in Comparative International Development* 50, no. 4 (2015): 500–518.

———. *Infectious Change: Reinventing Chinese Public Health after an Epidemic.* Stanford, CA: Stanford University Press, 2016.

"The Medical Aftermath of the Conflict in Shanghai." *Chinese Medical Journal* 46 (1932): 329–32.

"Memorandum of the Members of Health and Finance Committee, March 28, 1939." Filed in SMA U1-4-212.

Meng Yuan 梦远, ed. *Zhongguo guanshang* 中国官商 (Officials and merchants in China). Beijing: Huanghe chubanshe, 1998.

———. "Zhongqing riyong huagong 'erxian' dingli kaituo xinpin diechu" 钟情日用化工'二仙'鼎力开拓新品迭出" ("Two Xians" who were committed to the daily chemical industry, and who consistently developed new items and sent them to market). In *Zhong-guo guanshang*, vol. 1, edited by Meng Yuan, 385–403. Beijing: Huanghe chubanshe, 1998.

Mengruo 夢若. "Tanyan: Weisheng yundong ying zhuyi de jidian" 談言: 衛生運動應注意的幾點 (Briefly noted: Some points that we should pay attention to regarding hygiene campaigns). *Shenbao benbu zengkan* 申報本埠增刊, June 6, 1934, 11.

Mine Kiyoshi 峯潔. "Shin koku Shanghai kenbun roku" 清国上海見聞録 (Travel experiences in Qing Shanghai). In *Taishō Chūgoku kenbun roku shūsei,* edited by Kojima Shinji, 24–35. Tokyo: Yumani shobō, 1997.

"Minguo sanshi niandu liuyuefen gongzuo baogao" 民國三十年度六月分工作報告 (Business report for June, 1941). Filed in SMA R50-299.

Mingyi yaolan bianshen weiyuanhui 名医摇篮编审委员会 (*Mingyi yaolan* editorial committee), ed. *Mingyi yaolan: Shanghai zhongyi yixueyuan* 名医摇篮: 上海中医医学院 (A cradle of prominent physicians: A history of Shanghai Chinese Medical School). Shanghai: Shanghai zhongyi daxue chubanshe, 1998.

Mizuno, Hiromi. *Science for the Empire: Scientific Nationalism in Modern Japan.* Stanford, CA: Stanford University Press, 2009.

Morris, Andrew. *Marrow of the Nation: A History of Sports and Physical Culture in Republican China.* Berkeley: University Of California Press, 2004.

Musgrove, Charles. "Cheering the Traitor: The Post-War Trial of Chen Bijun, April 1946." *Twentieth-Century China* 30, no. 2 (2005): 3–27.

Myers, Ramon, and Yeh-chien Wang. "Economic Developments, 1644–1800," In *The Ch'ing Empire to 1800*, volume 9 of *Cambridge History of China*, part one, edited by Willard Peterson, 563–645. Cambridge, UK: Cambridge University Press, 2008.

Nathan, Andrew. "Some Trends in the Historiography of Republican China." *Republican China* 17, no. 1 (1991): 117–31.

Nathan, Carl. *Plague Prevention and Politics in Manchuria, 1910–1931.* Cambridge, MA: East Asian Research Center, Harvard University, 1967.

Nedostup, Rebeccan. *Superstitious Regimes: Religion and the Politics of Chinese Modernity.* Cambridge, MA: Harvard University Asia Center, 2010.

Needham, Joseph. *Science and Civilisation in China.* Various volumes. Cambridge, UK: Cambridge University Press, 1954–.

North China Herald.

Ono Tokuichirō 小野得一郎, ed. *Zhonghua minguo yishi zonglan* 中華民國醫事綜覽 (A general guide to medical affairs of the Republic of China). Tokyo: Dōjinkai, 1935.

Pan Junxiang 潘君祥. *Jindai Zhongguo guohuo yundong yanjiu* 近代中国国货运动研究 (A study of the National Products Movement in modern China). Shanghai: Shanghai shehui kexueyuan chubanshe, 1998.

Pan, Tianshu. "Place Attachment, Communal Memory, and the Moral Underpinnings of Gentrification in Postreform Shanghai." In *Deep China: The Moral Life of the Person: What Anthropology and Psychiatry Tell Us about China Today*, edited by Arthur Kleinman, Yunxiang Yan, Jing Jun, Sing Lee, Everett Zhang, Pan Tianshu, Wu Fei, and Guo Jinhua, 152–76. Berkeley: University of California Press, 2011.

Pang Jingzhou 龐京周. *Shanghai jinshinianlai yiyao niaokan* 上海近十年來醫藥鳥瞰 (An overview of Shanghai's medicine in the last ten years). Shanghai: Zhongguo kexue gongsi, 1933.

Parker, Andrew, Mary Russo, Doris Sommers, and Patricia Yaeger, eds. *Nationalisms and Sexualities*. New York: Routledge, 1992.

Peng, Juanjuan. "Selling a Healthy Lifestyle in Late Qing Tianjin: Commercial Advertisements for Weisheng Products in the Dagong Bao, 1902–1911." *International Journal of Asian Studies* 9, no. 2 (2012): 211–30.

Peng Shanmin 彭善民. *Gonggong weisheng yu Shanghai dushi wenming, 1898–1949* 公共卫生与上海都市文明, 1898–1949 (Public health and urban civilization in Shanghai, 1898–1949). Shanghai: Shanghai renmin chubanshe, 2007.

Pernick, Martin. "Thomas Edison's Tuberculosis Films: Mass Media and Health Propaganda." *Hastings Center Report* 8, no. 3 (June 1978): 21–27.

Perry, Elizabeth J. *Anyuan: Mining China's Revolutionary Tradition*. Berkeley: University of California Press, 2014.

———. *Patrolling the Revolution: Worker Militias, Citizenship, and the Modern Chinese State*. Lanham, MD: Rowman and Littlefield, 2005.

———. *Shanghai on Strike: The Politics of Chinese Labor*. Stanford, CA: Stanford University Press, 1993.

Peter, W. W. "Popular Health Education in China; A Movement Adapted to the Psychology of the People." *American Journal of Public Health* 9, no. 10 (1919): 743–49. http://www.ncbi.nlm.nih.gov/pmc/articles/PMC1362607/.

Peterson, Willard, ed. *The Cambridge History of China, Volume 9, Part 1: The Ching Dynasty to 1800*. Cambridge, UK: Cambridge University Press, 2008.

Pickowicz, Paul G., Kuiyi Shen, and Yingjin Zhang, eds. *Liangyou, Kaleidoscopic Modernity and the Shanghai Global Metropolis, 1926–1945*. Leiden: Brill, 2013.

Poon, Shuk-wah. *Negotiating Religion in Modern China: State and Common People in Guangzhou, 1900–1937*. Hong Kong: Chinese University Press, 2011.

"Public Health Laboratory of the City Government of Greater Shanghai." *Chinese Medical Journal* 50 (1936): 864–66.

"Public Health Movement—Meeting of 'Order Maintenance' Section." Filed in SMA U1-16-298.

Qiao Shuming 譙枢铭, ed. *Shanghaishi yanjiu* 上海史研究 (A study of Shanghai history). Shanghai: Xuelin chubanshe, 1984.

Qin Lüzhi 秦绿枝. *Haipai shangren Huang Chujiu* 海派商人黄楚九 (Huang Chujiu, a Shanghai merchant). Shanghai: Shanghai shudian chubanshe, 1999.

Qingnian jinbu 青年進步 [Association Progress].

Quanguo zhengxie wenshi ziliao weiyuanhui 全国政协文史资料委员会, ed. *Wenshi ziliao xuanji* 文史资料选辑 (Accounts of culture and history, selected works), no. 119. Beijing: Zhongguo wenshi chubanshe, 1989.

Rankin, Mary Backus. *Elite Activism and Political Transformation in China: Zhejiang Province, 1865–1911*. Stanford, CA: Stanford University Press, 1986.

Rawski, Thomas. "SARS and China's Economy." In *SARS in China: Prelude to Pandemic?* edited by Arthur Kleinman and James L. Watson, 105–21. Stanford, CA: Stanford University Press, 2006.

Read, Benjamin L. *Roots of the State: Neighborhood Organization and Social Networks in Beijing and Taipei.* Stanford, CA: Stanford University Press, 2012.

Reardon-Anderson, James. *The Study of Change: Chemistry in China, 1840–1949.* Cambridge, UK: Cambridge University Press, 1991.

Reed, Christopher. *Gutenberg in Shanghai: Chinese Print Capitalism, 1876–1937.* Vancouver: University of British Columbia Press, 2004.

"Relationships between the Municipal Public Health Department and the Public Health Department of Greater Shanghai." Filed in SMA U1-16-319.

Renshaw, Michelle. *Accommodating the Chinese: The American Hospital in China, 1880–1920.* New York: Routledge, 2005.

Report of Annual Meeting of Subscribers Held on Tuesday 20 May 1934 at the Hospital Shantung Road. Filed in SMA U1-4-216.

Report of the International Plague Control Held at Mukden, April 1911. Manila: Bureau of Printing, 1912.

Rogaski, Ruth. *Hygienic Modernity: Meanings of Health and Disease in Treaty-Port China.* Berkeley: University of California Press, 2004.

———. "Nature, Annihilation, and Modernity: China's Korean War Germ-Warfare Experience Reconsidered." *Journal of Asian Studies* 61, no. 2 (2002): 381–415.

———. "Vampires in Plagueland: The Multiple Meanings of Weisheng in Manchuria." In *Health and Hygiene in Chinese East Asia,* edited by Angela Leung and Charlotte Furth, 132–59. Durham, NC: Duke University Press, 2010.

Rosenberg, Charles. *The Care of Strangers: The Rise of American Hospital System.* Baltimore, MD: Johns Hopkins University Press, 1995.

Ruan Renze 阮仁泽, and Gao Zhennong 高振农, eds. *Shanghai zongjiaoshi* 上海宗教史 (A history of religion in Shanghai). Shanghai: Shanghai renmin chubanshe, 1992.

Saich, Tony. "Is SARS China's Chernobyl or Much Ado about Nothing?" In *SARS in China: Prelude to Pandemic,* edited by Arthur Kleinman and James L. Watson, 71–104. Stanford, CA: Stanford University Press, 2006.

———. *Providing Public Goods in Transitional China.* New York: Palgrave Macmillan, 2008.

Sanshi nian fen Shanghai shiyi yiyuan baogaoshu 三十年份上海時疫醫院報告書 (Chinese Infectious Disease Hospital business report for 1941). Filed in SMA U1-4-220.

Scheid, Volker. *Currents of Tradition in Chinese Medicine, 1626–2006.* Seattle: Eastland Press, 2007.

———. "The People's Republic of China." In *Chinese Medicine and Healing: An Illustrated History,* edited by TJ Hinrichs and Linda L. Barnes, 239–83. Cambridge, MA: Belknap Press of Harvard University Press, 2013.

Scheid, Volker, and Sean Hsiang-Lin Lei. "The Institutionalization of Chinese Medicine." In *Medical Transitions in Twentieth-century China,* edited by Bridie Andrews and Mary Brown Bullock, 244–66. Bloomington: Indiana University Press, 2014.

Schneider, Helen M. *Keeping the Nation's House: Domestic Management and the Making of Modern China.* Vancouver: University of British Columbia Press, 2011.

Schneider, Laurence. *Biology and Revolution in Twentieth-Century China.* Lanham: Rowman and Littlefield, 2003.

Schoppa, Keith. "Patterns and Dynamics of Elite Collaboration in Occupied Shaoxing County." In *Chinese Collaboration with Japan, 1932–1945: The Limits of Accommodation,* edited by David P. Barrett and Larry N. Shyu, 156–79. Stanford, CA: Stanford University Press, 2001.

"The Second Health Campaign Mass Meeting Was Inaugurated Yesterday at the Nanshi Confucian Temple." Filed in SMA R1-12-388.

"Shanghai bōeki iinkai kitei" 上海防疫委員会規定 (Regulations of Shanghai Epidemic Control Committee). Filed in SMA R50-289.

"Shanghai Crematory." *Chinese Medical Journal* 51 (1936): 995–96.

"Shanghai Health Department." *Chinse Medical Journal* 41 (1927): 469–70.

Shanghai jilianhui 上海機聯會 (Organization of Shanghai machine manufacturers). *Gongshang shiliao* 工商史料 (Historical records of industry and commerce), vol. 1. Shanghai: Jiating gongyeshe, 1935. Filed in SMA Y9-1-101-114.

Shanghai jilianhui 上海機聯會. *Gongshang shiliao* 工商史料 (Historical records of industry and commerce), vol. 2. Shanghai: Jiating gongyeshe, 1935. Filed in SMA Y9-1-101-38.

Shanghai jilianhui 上海機聯會. "Jiating gongyeshe" 家庭工業社 (Household Industries Company). In vol. 1 of *Gongshang shiliao,* edited by Shanghai jilianhui, 113–18. Shanghai: Jiating gongyeshe, 1935.

Shanghai jilianhui 上海機聯會. "Zhongguo huaxue gongyeshe" 中國化學工業社 (China Chemical Industries Company). In vol. 2 of *Gongshang shiliao,* edited by Shanghai jilianhui, 37–44. Shanghai: Jiating gongyeshe, 1935.

Shanghai Municipal Council Public Health Department Annual Reports. Filed in SMA U1-16-4651.

Shanghai renmin chubanshe bianjibu 上海人民出版社編輯部 (Shanghai People's Press Editorial Department), ed. *Dali kaizhan yi chusihai wei zhongxin de aiguo weisheng yundong* 大力开展以除四害为中心的爱国卫生运动 (Give your best shot in the development of the patriotic hygiene campaign by eliminating four evils). Shanghai: Shanghai renmin chubanshe, 1958.

Shanghai riyong gongyepin shangyezhi bianzuan weiyuanhui ≪上海日用工业品商业志≫ 编纂委员会 (*Shanghai riyong gongyepin shangyezhi* editorial committee), ed. *Shanghai riyong gongyepin shangyezhi* 上海日用工业品商业志 (Records of the everyday-use industrial products business in Shanghai). Shanghai: Shanghai shehuikexueyuan chubanshe, 1999.

Shanghai shehui kexueyuan jingji yanjiusuo 上海社会科学院经济研究所 (Shanghai Academy of Social Sciences, Institute of Economics), ed. *Shanghai jindai xiyao hangyeshi* 上海近代西药行业史 (A history of modern Western pharmaceutical industries in Shanghai). Shanghai: Shanghai shehui kexueyuan chubanshe, 1988.

Shanghai shehui kexueyuan jingji yanjiusuo chengshi jingjizu 上海社会科学院经济研究所城市经济组 (Shanghai Academy of Social Sciences, Institute of Economics, Division of Urban Economy), ed. *Shanghai penghuqu de bianqian* 上海棚户区的变迁 (Transformation of Shanghai's shantytown areas). Shanghai: Shanghai renmin chubanshe, 1962.

Shanghai Shi dang'anguan 上海市档案馆 (Shanghai Municipal Archives).

Shanghai Shi dang'anguan 上海市档案馆, ed. *Shanghai Archives and Records Studies*, vol. 3. Shanghai: Shanghai sanlian shudian, 2007.

Shanghai Shi Ningbo jingji jianshe cujin xiehui 上海市宁波经济建设促进协会 (Shanghai Ningbo Economic Development Promotion Association), Shanghai Shi Ningbo tongxiang lianyihui 上海市宁波同乡联谊会 (Shanghai Ningbo Natives Friendship Association), and *Ningboren zai Shanghai* xilie congshu bianweihui 《宁波人在上海》系列丛书编委会 (*Ningboren zai Shanghai* series editorial committee), eds. *Chuangye Shanghaitan* 创业上海滩 (Creating Shanghai). Shanghai: Shanghai kexue jishu wenxian chubanshe, 2003.

Shanghai Shi shehuiju 上海市社會局 (Shanghai Social Affairs Bureau), ed. *Shanghai zhi jizhi gongye* 上海之機製工業 (Machine industries of Shanghai). Shanghai: Zhonghua shuju, 1933.

Shanghai Shi sinianlai weisheng gongzuo gaiyao 1932–1936 上海市四年來衛生工作概要 1932–1936 (An outline of public health works in Shanghai in the last four years, 1932–1936). Shanghai, n.d.

Shanghai Shi weishengju 上海市衛生局 (Shanghai Public Health Bureau). *A Brief Survey of Greater Shanghai Public Health Activities, 1927–1937*. Shanghai, n.d.

Shanghai Shi weishengju Gaoqiao weisheng shiwusuo 上海市衛生局高橋衛生事務所 (Shanghai Public Health Bureau Gaoqiao Health Station), ed. Shanghai Shi weishengju Gaoqiao weisheng shiwusuo ji guoli Shanghai yiyuan weishengke nianbao, minguo ershisan niandu 上海市衛生局高橋衛生事務所暨國立上海醫院衛生科年報,民國二十三年度 (Shanghai Public Health Bureau Gaoqiao Health Station and the Public Health Department of National Shanghai Medical School, annual report for 1934). Shanghai, 1935.

Shanghai Shi xinshenghuo yundong cujinhui 上海市新生活運動促進會 (The Shanghai New Life Movement Promotional Society). *Shanghai xinyun jiyao* 上海新運輯要 (A summary of the New Life Movement in Shanghai). Shanghai, 1937.

Shanghai shiyi yiyuan 上海時疫醫院 Chinese Infectious Disease Hospital, ed. *Shanghai shiyi yiyuan shiqi nian baogao jian zhengxinlu* 上海時疫醫院十七年報告兼徵信錄 (Chinese Infectious Disease Hospital business report and financial statement, 1928). n.p., 1929.

———, ed. *Shanghai shiyi yiyuan ershi nian baogao jian zhengxinlu* 上海時疫醫院二十年報告兼徵信錄 (Chinese Infectious Disease Hospital business report and financial statement, 1931). n.p., 1932.

Shanghai shiyi yiyuan zhangcheng 上海時疫醫院章程 (Chinese Infectious Disease Hospital charter). Filed in SMA U1-4-220.

Shanghai Shi zhengfu 上海市政府 (The Shanghai Municipal Government). *Shanghai Shi chengli shizhounian jinian gongye zhanlanhui tekan.* 上海市成立十週年紀念工業展覽會特刊 (Special issue about the industrial exhibition to commemorate the tenth anniversary of the opening of Shanghai Municipality). Shanghai, 1937. Filed in SMA Y9-1-37.

Shanghai Shi zhengfu shehuiju 上海市政府社會局 [Social Affairs Bureau, the City Government of Greater Shanghai]. *Shanghai Shi gongren shenghuo chengdu* 上海市工人生活程度 [Standard of Living of Shanghai Laborers]. Shanghai: Zhonghua shuju, 1934.

Shanghai Shi zhengxie wenshi ziliao weiyuanhui 上海市政协文史资料委员会 (Shanghai political consultation conference *wenshi ziliao* committee), ed. *Gongye shangye* 工業商業 (Industry and commerce). Vols. 6 and 7 of *Shanghai wenshi ziliao cungao huibian* 上海文史资料存稿汇编 (Accounts of Shanghai's culture and history, compiled records). Shanghai: Shanghai guji chubanshe, 2001.

Shanghai shizheng gaiyao 上海市政概要 (An outline of the Shanghai Municipal administration). Shanghai, 1934.

Shanghai tebieshi shehuiju 上海特別市社會局 (Social Affairs Bureau, Shanghai Special Municipality), *Shanghai zhi gongye* 上海之工業 (Industries in Shanghai). Shanghai: Zhonghua shuju, 1930.

Shanghai tebieshi weishengju 上海特別市衛生局 (Public Health Bureau, Shanghai Special Municipality). *Zhonghuo minguo sanshi niandu Shanghai tebieshi weishengju yewu baogao* 中華民國三十年度上海特別市衛生局業務報告 (Shanghai Special Municipality public health services, annual business report for 1941). Shanghai.

"Shanghai tebieshi weishengju gaikuang" 上海特別市衛生局概況 (Shanghai Special Municipality Public Health Bureau, an overview). Filed in SMA R50-1151.

Shanghai tongzhi bianzhuan weiyuanhui 上海通志編纂委員会 (*Shanghai tongzhi* editorial committee, ed. *Gongye* 工业 (Industry). Vol. 17 of *Shanghai tongzhi* 上海通志 (Historical accounts of Shanghai). Shanghai: Shanghai renmin chubanshe, Shanghai shehui kexueyuan chubanshe, 2005. http://www.shtong.gov.cn/node2/node22247/node4579/index.html.

Shanghai weisheng gongzuo congshu bianweihui <<上海卫生工作丛书>>编委会 (The editorial committee of "public health work in Shanghai" series), ed. *Shanghai weisheng* 上海卫生, *1949–1983* (Public health in Shanghai, 1949–1983). Shanghai: Shanghai kexue jishu chubanshe, 1986.

Shanghai weishengzhi bianzuan weiyuanhui <<上海卫生志>>编纂委员会 (*Shanghai weishengzhi* editorial committee), ed. *Shanghai weishengzhi* 上海卫生志 (Public health records in Shanghai). Shanghai: Shanghai shehui kexueyuan chubanshe, 1998.

Shanghai zhizaochang changzhi bianshen weiyuanhui <<上海制皂厂厂志>>编审委员会 (*Shanghai zhizaochang changzhi* editorial committee), ed. *Shanghai zhizaochang changzhi 1923–1990* 上海制皂厂厂志 (A history of Shanghai Soap Manufacturing Factory, 1923–1990). Shanghai: Shanghai shehuikexueyuan chubanshe, 1993.

Shanghaishi ziliao congkan: Shanghai gonggong zujie shigao 上海史资料丛刊：上海公共租界史稿 (Collections of materials about Shanghai history: A draft history of Shanghai's International Settlement). 1933; reprint, Shanghai: Shanghai renmin chubanshe, 1980.

Shapiro, Judith. *Mao's War against Nature: Politics and the Environment in Revolutionary China*. Cambridge, UK: Cambridge University Press, 2001.

Shen Yuwu 沈雨梧. "Fang Yexian yu Zhongguo huaxue gongyeshe" 方液仙与中国化学工业社 (Fang Yexian and China Chemical Industries Company). In *Jindai Zhongguo gongshang renwuzhi*, vol. 4, edited by Shou Chongyi, Shou Moliao, and Shou Leying, 1–8. Beijing: Zhongguo wenshi chubanshe, 1996.

Shenbao 申報.

Shenbao zengkan 申報增刊 (*Shenbao* special issues).

Shi Meijun 史美俊. "Shanghai dianye juxing Li Pingshu" 上海電業巨星李平書 (Li Pingshu, The great star of Shanghai's electric industries). In *Yangchang jushang, chuangye qicai*, edited by Zhao Yunsheng and Liu Mingtao, 319–487. Taipei: Wanwenshe, 1998.

Shibao 時報.

Shih, Shu-mei. *The Lure of the Modern: Writing Modernism in Semicolonial China, 1917–1937*. Berkeley: University of California Press, 2001.

Shimose Kentarō 下瀨謙太郎. "Shanghai no igaku oyobi byōin sankanki" 上海の医学及病院参観記 (A report on medicine and hospital observations in Shanghai). *Shanghai* 上海 875 (1931): 26–27.

Shou Chongyi 壽充一, Shou Moliao 壽墨聊, and Shou Leying 壽乐英, eds. *Jindai Zhongguo gongshang renwuzhi* 近代中國工商人物志 (Historical accounts of remarkable figures who were engaged in industry and commerce in modern China). Beijing: Zhongguo wenshi chubanshe, 1996.

Shouzi 痩子. "Wei benshi weisheng yundong yiyan" 爲本市衛生運動一言 (A few words about our city's hygiene campaign). *Shenbao benbu zengkan*, June 20, 1934, 1.

"Shōwa jūgo nendo Shanghai ni okeru korera ryūkō ni tuite" 昭和 15 年度上海における コレラ流行について (On the cholera outbreak in Shanghai in 1940). Filed in GK I-3-2-0-11, vol. 6.

Shue, Vivienne. "The Quality of Mercy: Confucian Charity and the Mixed Metaphors of Modernity in Tianjin." *Modern China* 32, no. 4: 411–52.

Shūhō 週報 (Weekly report) 13 (1941). Filed in GK I-3-2-0-11, vol. 6.

Shūhō 週報 (Weekly report) 23 (1939). Filed in GK I-3-2-0-8, vol. 3.

Shūhō 週報 (Weekly report) 26, 27, 29, 31 (1938). Filed in GK I-3-2-0-7, vol. 2.

Shūhō 週報 (Weekly report) 41 (1939). Filed in GK I-3-2-0-8, vol. 3.

Sidel, Victor W., and Ruth Sidel. *Serve the People: Observations on Medicine in the People's Republic of China*. New York: Josiah Macy, Jr. Foundation, 1973.

Sinn, Elizabeth. *Power and Charity: The Early History of the Tung Wah Hospital, Hong Kong*. Hong Kong: Oxford University Press, 1989.

Sivin, Nathan. *Science in Ancient China: Researches and Reflections*. Aldershot, UK: Variorum, 1995.

Sivulka, Juliann. *Stronger than Dirt: A Cultural History of Advertising Personal Hygiene in America, 1875 to 1940*. Amherst, NY: Humanity Books, 2001.

68th Annual Report of St. Luke's Hospital for Chinese for the Year Ending December 31, 1934. Filed in SMA U1-4-212.

Smith, S.A. *Like Cattle and Horses: Nationalism and Labor in Shanghai, 1895–1927*. Durham, NC: Duke University Press, 2002.

Song Guangbo 宋广波. *Ding Wenjiang tuzhuan* 丁文江图传 (A biography of Ding Wenjiang with photographs). Wuhan: Hubei renmin chubanshe, 2007.

Song Guobin 宋國賓. "Fakanci" 發刊詞 (Foreword). *Kangjian zazhi* 康健雜誌 1, no. 1 (1933): 1.

State Council Information Office of the People's Republic of China and Ministry of Health of the People's Republic of China. *Health Care in China*. Beijing: People's Medical Publishing House, 2012.

"Statement of Receipts and Disbursement for the Year of 1940." Filed in SMA U1-4-220.

"Statement of Receipts and Disbursement for the Year of 1941." Filed in SMA U1-4-220.

"Statement of Receipts and Disbursement for the Year of 1942." Filed in SMA U1-4-220.

Stepan, Nancy. *The Idea of Race in Science: Great Britain, 1800–1960.* Hamden, CT: Archon Books, 1982.

Stevens, Rosemary. *In Sickness and in Wealth: American Hospitals in the Twentieth Century.* New York: Basic Books, 1989.

Stop U.S. Germ Warfare: Protests, Statements, Appeals and Other Documents concerning the Criminal Use of Bacteriological Weapons against the People of Korea and China. Beijing: Chinese People's Committee for World Peace, 1952.

Strand, David. *"Civil Society" and "Public Sphere" in Modern China: A Perspective on Popular Movements in Beijing, 1919–1989.* Durham, NC: Asian/Pacific Studies Institute, Duke University Press, 1990.

———. *Rickshaw Beijing: City People and Politics in the 1920s.* Berkeley: University of California Press, 1993.

———. *An Unfinished Republic: Leading by Word and Deed in Modern China.* Berkeley: University of California Press, 2011.

Strauss, Julia C. *Strong Institutions in Weak Polities: State Building in Republican China, 1927–1940.* Oxford: Oxford University Press, 1998.

Sun Yat-sen 孙逸仙. "Sanmin zhuyi, minzu zhuyi, di-er jiang, 1924" 三民主义，民族主义，第二讲 (Three Principles of the People, nationalism, lecture 2). In Sun Yat-sen, *Sun Zhongsan quanji*, vol. 1, edited by Shang Mingxuan, 341–51. Beijing: Renmin chubanshe, 1989.

———. *Sun Zhongsan quanji* 孙中山全集 (Complete works of Sun Zhongshan), vol. 1. Edited by Shang Mingxuan 尚明轩. Beijing: Renmin chubanshe, 1989.

Sutphen, Mary P. "Not What, but Where: Bubonic Plague and the Reception of Germ Theories in Hong Kong and Calcutta, 1894–1897." *Journal of the History of Medicine* 52 (1997): 81–113.

Sutphen, Mary P., and Bridie Andrews. "Introduction." In *Medicine and Colonial Identity*., edited by Mary P. Sutphen and Bridie Andrews, 1–13. New York: Routledge, 2003.

Sutphen, Mary P., and Bridie Andrews, eds. *Medicine and Colonial Identity.* New York: Routledge, 2003.

Tan Yulin 谈玉林. "Huang Chujiu" 黄楚九. In *Zhongguo jindai qiye de kaituozhe*, vol. 2, edited by Kong Lingren and Li Dezheng, 427–37. Jinan: Shandong renmin chubanshe, 1991.

———. "Xiang Songmao, Xiang Shengwu" 项松茂，项绳武. In *Zhongguo jindai qiye de kaituozhe*, vol. 2, edited by Kong Lingren and Li Dezheng, 211–24. Jinan: Shandong renmin chubanshe, 1991.

Tang Zhenchang 唐振常, Shen Hengchun 沈恒春, and Qiao Shuming 樵枢铭. *Shanghai-shi* 上海史 (A history of Shanghai). Shanghai: Shanghai renmin chubanshe, 1989.

Tomes, Nancy. *The Gospel of Germs: Men, Women, and the Microbe in American Life.* Cambridge, MA: Harvard University Press, 1998.

Tsai, Weipin. *Reading Shenbao: Nationalism, Consumerism and Individuality in China 1919–37.* New York: Palgrave Macmillan, 2010.

Van de Ven, Hans J. *War and Nationalism in China, 1925–1926.* London: Routledge Curzon, 2003.

Vigarello, Georges. *Concepts of Cleanliness: Changing Attitudes in France since the Middle Ages.* Cambridge, UK: Cambridge University Press, 1988.

Wakeman, Frederic Jr. "The Civil Society and Public Sphere Debate: Western Reflections on Chinese Political Culture." *Modern China* 19, no. 2 (1993): 108–38.

———. *Policing Shanghai, 1927–1937.* Berkeley: University of California Press, 1995.

———. "A Revisionist View of the Nanjing Decade: Confucian Fascism." *China Quarterly* 150 (1997): 395–432.

———. *The Shanghai Badlands: Wartime Terrorism and Urban Crime, 1937–1941.* Cambridge, UK: Cambridge University Press, 1996.

Wakeman, Frederic Jr., and Richard Louis Edmonds, eds. *Reappraising Republican China.* Oxford: Oxford University Press, 2000.

Wang Daren 王达人. "Yingshang Zhongguo feizao gongsi zaihua jingying gaikuang" 英商中国肥皂公司在华经营概况 (The operation of China Soap Company, a British business, in China: An overview). In *Gongye shangye*, vol. 7, edited by Shanghai Shi zhengxie wenshi ziliao weiyuanhui, 192–201. Originally published in 1964. Shanghai: Shanghai guji chubanshe, 2001.

Wang, Di. *Street Culture in Chengdu: Public Space, Urban Commoners, and Local Politics, 1870–1930.* Stanford, CA: Stanford University Press, 2003.

Wang Ermin 王爾敏. *Jindai Shanghai keji xianqu zhi Renji yiyuan yu Gezhi shuyuan* 近代上海科技先驅之仁濟醫院與格致書院 (Renji Hospital and Polytechnic Institute, forerunners of science and technology in modern Shanghai). Taipei: Jidujiao yuzhou guang quanren guanhuai jigou, 2006.

Wang Shenmin 王慎敏, ed. *Riyong huaxuepin* 日用化学品 (Eveyday-use chemical products). Beijing: Huaxue gongye chubanshe, 2005.

Wang Shucheng 王书城, ed. *Zhongguo weisheng shiye fazhan* 中国卫生事业发展 (The development of public health services in China). Beijing: Zhongyi guji chubanshe, 2006.

Wang Shu-hwai. "Dispute over the Ownership of the Zhabei Electricity and Water Supply Works, 1920–1924." *Bulletin of the Institute of Modern History, Academia Sinica* 25 (1996): 167–209.

Wang Yansong 王延松 "Xu" 序 (Preface). In *Xiandai shiyejia*, 7–8.

Wang, Zuoyue. "Saving China through Science: The Science Society of China, Scientific Nationalism, and Civil Society in Republican China." *Osiris*, 2nd Series, vol. 17, *Science and Civil Society* (2002): 291–322

Wasserstrom, Jeffrey. *Student Protests in Twentieth Century China: The View from Shanghai.* Stanford, CA: Stanford University Press, 1991.

Wasserstrom, Jeffrey N., and Elizabeth J. Perry, eds. *Popular Protest and Political Culture in Modern China.* Boulder, CO: Westview Press, 1994.

Watt, John R. *Saving Lives in Wartime China: How Medical Reformers Built Modern Healthcare Systems amid War and Epidemics, 1928–1945.* Leiden: Brill, 2014.

"Wei benshi di-er jie xialing weisheng yundong gaoshiminshu" 爲本市第二屆夏令衛生運動告市民書 (Our city's second summer hygiene campaign: A notice to citizens). Filed in SMA R50-736.

"Wei benshi di-yi jie dongji weisheng yundong gaoshiminshu" 爲本市第一屆冬季衛生運動告市民書 (Our city's first winter hygiene campaign, a notice to citizens). Filed in SMA R50-731.

Weisheng gongbao 衛生公報 (Public health gazette). 1929.

Weisheng yuekan 衛生月刊 (Public health monthly). Various issues.

Weisheng yundong choubeihui 衛生運動籌備會 (Hygiene campaign preparation team). "Benshi di-shisi jie weisheng yundong baogaoshu" 本市第十四屆衛生運動報告書 (The fourteenth hygiene campaign report). *Weisheng yuekan* 5, no. 7 (1936): 375–87.

Weisheng yundong choubeihui 衛生運動籌備會 (Hygiene campaign preparation team). "Benshi di-shiwu jie weisheng yundong baogaoshu" 本市第十五屆衛生運動報告書 (The fifteenth hygiene campaign report). *Weisheng yuekan* 6, no. 7 (1936): 359–66.

Weisheng yundong choubeihui 衛生運動籌備會 (Hygiene campaign preparation team). "Benshi di-shiwu jie weisheng yundong baogaoshu (xu)" 本市第十五屆衛生運動報告書 (續) (The fifteenth hygiene campaign report, a sequel). *Weisheng yuekan* 6, no. 8 (1936): 392–402.

"Weisheng yundong choubei jingguo baogao" 衛生運動籌備經過報告 (Report of the hygiene campaign preparation process). *Weisheng yuekan* 4, no. 7: (1934): 282–84.

"Weisheng yundong kaimuji" 衛生運動開幕記 (A record of the opening of the hygiene campaign). *Weisheng yuekan* 4, no. 7 (1934): 295–97.

"Weisheng zhanlanhui kaimuji" 衛生展覽會開幕記 (A record of the opening of the health exhibition). *Weisheng yuekan* 4, no. 7 (1934): 297–99.

Winslow, Charles-Edward Amory. *The Evolution and Significance of the Modern Public Health Campaign*. New Haven, CT: Yale University Press, 1923.

Wong, Chimin, and Wu Lien-teh (Wu Liande). *History of Chinese Medicine*. Shanghai: National Quarantine Service, 1936.

Wright, David. *Translating Science: The Transmission of Western Chemistry into Late Imperial China, 1840–1900*. Leiden: Brill, 2000.

Wu Hanmin 吴汉民, ed. *Ershi shiji Shanghai wenshi ziliao wenku* 二十世纪上海文史资料文库 (A collection of accounts of twentieth-century Shanghai's culture and history). Shanghai: Shanghai shudian chubanshe, 1999.

Wu, Liande (Lien-teh Wu). *Plague Fighter: The Autobiography of a Modern Chinese Physician*. Cambridge, UK: Heffer, 1959.

Wu, Lien-teh, J. W. H. Chun, R. Pollitzer, and C. Y. Wu. *Cholera: A Manual for Medical Professions in China*. Shanghai, National Quarantine Services, 1934.

Xiandai shiyejia 現代實業家 (Contemporary businessmen). Shanghai: Shanghai shangbaoshe, 1935. Filed in SMA Y9-1-78.

Xiang Zenan 项泽楠. "Yingshang Zhongguo feizao gongsi jianshi" 英商中国肥皂公司简史 (A brief history of China Soap Company, a British business). In *Ershi shiji Shanghai wenshi ziliao wenku*, vol. 3, edited by Wu Hanmin, 27–39. Shanghai: Shanghai shudian chubanshe, 1999.

Xiao, Zhiwei. "Movie House Etiquette Reform in Early-Twentieth Century China." *Modern China* 32, no. 4 (2006): 513–36.

Xin Ping 忻平, Hu Zhenghao 胡正豪, and Li Xuechang 李学昌. *Minguo shehui daguan* 民国社会大观 (A panorama of the Republican society). Fuzhou: Fujian renmin chubanshe, 1991.

Xinkangwang 信康网, ed. *Zuixin Shanghai jiuyi zhinan* 最新上海就医指南 (The most up-to-date guidebook to finding a doctor in Shanghai). Shanghai: Zhongguo dabaike quanshu chubanshe, 2004.

Xinyun yuekan 新運月刊 (The New Life Movement monthly).

Xiong Yuezhi 熊月之, ed. *Shanghai tongshi* 上海通史 (A general history of Shanghai), vol. 3 *WanQing zhengzhi* 晚清政治 (Late Qing politics). Shanghai: Shanghai renmin chubanshe, 1999.

———, ed. *Shanghai tongshi*, vol. 5, *WanQing shehui* 晚清社会 (Late Qing society). Shanghai: Shanghai renmin chubanshe, 1999.

———, ed. *Shanghai tongshi*, vol. 7, *Minguo zhengzhi* 民国政治 (Republican politics). Shanghai: Shanghai renmin chubanshe, 1999.

———, ed. *Shanghai tongshi*, vol. 8, *Minguo jingji* 民国经济 (Republican economics). Shanghai: Shanghai renmin chubanshe, 1999.

———, ed. *Shanghai tongshi*, vol. 9, *Minguo shehui* 民国社会 (Republican society). Shanghai: Shanghai renmin chubanshe, 1999.

———, ed. *Shanghai tongshi*, vol. 10, *Minguo wenhua* 民国文化 (Republican culture). Shanghai: Shanghai renmin chubanshe, 1999

Xiong Yuezhi 熊月之, and Zhou Wu 周武, eds. *Sheng Yuehan daxueshi* 圣约翰大学史 (History of St. John's University). Shanghai: Shanghai renmin chubanshe, 2007.

Xu Gongsu 徐公肅, and Qiu Jinzhang 丘瑾璋. "Shanghai gonggong zujie zhidu" 上海公共租界制度 (The International Settlement of Shanghai). In *Shanghaishi ziliao congkan: Shanghai gonggong zujie shigao*, 1–297. 1933; reprint, Shanghai: Shanghai renmin chubanshe, 1980.

Xu Jinsheng 许金生. *Jindai Shanghai Rizi gongyeshi*, 1884–1937 近代上海日资工业史，1884–1937 (A history of Japanese-owned industries in Shanghai, 1884–1937). Shanghai: Xuelin chubanshe, 2009.

Xu Wancheng 許晚成. *Zhanhou Shanghai ji quanguo yiyaoye diaochalu* 戰後上海及全國醫藥業調查錄 (A survey of medical and pharmaceutical professions in post-war Shanghai and the nation). n.p., 1939.

Xu, Xiaoqun. *Chinese Professionals and the Republican State: The Rise of Professional Associations in Shanghai, 1912–1937*. Cambridge, UK: Cambridge University Press, 2003.

———. "'National Essence' vs. 'Science': Chinese Physicians' Fight for Legitimacy, 1912–37." *Modern Asian Studies* 31, no. 4 (1997): 847–77.

Xu Xinwu 徐新吾, and Huang Hanmin 黄汉民, eds. *Shanghai jindai gongyeshi* 上海近代工业史 (History of modern industries in Shanghai). Shanghai: Shanghai shehui kexueyuan chubanshe, 1998.

Xu, Yamin. "Policing Civility on the Streets: Encounters with Litterbugs, 'Nightsoil Lords,' and Street Corner Urinators in Republican Beijing." *Twentieth Century China* 30, no. 2 (2005): 28–71.

Xu Yi 徐逸. "Zuijin de jiaohui weisheng shiye" 最近的教會衛生事業 (Recent public health undertakings by the Church). *Zhonghua jidujiaohui nianjian* 中華基督教會年鑑 12 (1933): 155–58.

Xu Yihua 徐以骅, ed. *Shanghai Sheng Yuehan daxue* 上海圣约翰大学 (1879–1952) (Shanghai St. John's University, 1879–1952). Shanghai: Shanghai renmin chubanshe, 2009.

Xu Yihua 徐以骅, and Han Xinchang 韩信昌. *Haishang fanwangdu: Sheng yuehan daxue* 海上梵王渡：圣约翰大学 (Shanghai's St. John's University). Shijiazhuang: Hebei jiaoyu chubanshe, 2003.

Xue Li 雪犁. *Zhonghua minsu yuanliu jicheng, jieri suishi juan* 中华民俗源流集成 节日岁时卷 (A collection of origins of Chinese folk customs: Festivals in four seasons). Lanzhou: Gansu renmin chubanshe, 1994.

Xue Shunsheng 薛顺生, and Lei Chenghao 类承浩, eds. *Lao Shanghai de gongye jiuzhi* 老上海的工业旧址 (Former industrial sites in old Shanghai). Shanghai: Tongji daxue chubanshe, 2004.

Xue Ziren 薛子仁. "Xue Kunming yu Taipingyang feizaochang" 薛坤明与太平洋肥皂厂 (Xue Kunming and Pacific Soap Factory). In *Jindai Zhongguo gongshang renwuzhi*, edited by Shou Chongyi, Shou Moliao, and Shou Leying, 197–209. Beijing: Zhongguo wenshi chubanshe, 1996.

Yan Yiwei 颜宜葳, and Zhang Daqing 张大庆. "Jibingpu yu zhiliaoguan–zaoqi jiaohui yiyuan de anli fenxi" 疾病谱與治療觀—早期教會醫院的案例分析 (Records of diseases and an outlook on cure—an analysis of early medical cases from missionary hospitals). In *Qing yilai de jibing, yiliao he weisheng: yi shehui wenhuashi wei shijiao de tansuo*, edited by Yu Xinzhong, 109–25. Beijing: Shenghuo, dushu, xinzhi sanlian shudian, 2009.

Yan Zhiyuan 颜志渊. "Yixue jiaoyujia, gonggong weisheng xuejia Yan Fuqing" 医学教育家，公共卫生学家颜福庆 (Yan Fuqing: An expert on medical education and public health). In *Shanghai yike daxue qishi nian*, edited by Yao Tai, 339–51. Shanghai: Shanghai yike daxue chubanshe, 1997.

Yang Dajin 楊大金, ed. *Xiandai Zhongguo shiyezhi* 現代中國實業誌 (A survey of contemporary Chinese businesses). Shanghai: Shangwu yinshuguan, 1938.

Yang Dehui 楊德惠, and Dong Wenzhong 董文中. *Shanghai zhi gongshangye* 上海之工商業 (Industry and commerce of Shanghai). Shanghai: Zhongwai chubanshe, 1941.

Yang Ximeng 楊西孟. *Shanghai gongren shenghuo chengdu de yige yanjiu* 上海工人生活程度的一個研究 (A study of the living standard of Shanghai workers). Beiping: Shehui diaochasuo, 1930.

Yang Yun 楊筠. "Huaxia xiyao zongshi Huang Chujiu" 華夏西藥宗師黄楚九 (Huang Chujiu, a great master of Western drugs in China). In *Yangchang jushang, chuangye qicai*, edited by Zhao Yunsheng and Liu Mingtao, 143–316. Taipei: Wanwenshe, 1998.

Yang Zhiyi 楊志一. "Chi baoban weisheng yundong zhe 斥包辦衛生運動者" (Critical words for those who organize hygiene campaigns). *Yijie chunqiu* 醫界春秋 23 (1928): 1–2.

Yao Fei 姚霏. "Jindai Shanghai gonggong yushi yu shimin jieceng" 近代上海公共浴室与市民阶层 [Public Bathhouses and Civilian Estates in Modern Shanghai]. In *Shanghai Archives and Records Studies*, vol. 3, edited by Shanghai Shi dang'anguan, 82–92. Shanghai: Shanghai sanlian shudian, 2007.

Yao Tai 姚泰, ed. *Shanghai yike daxue qishi nian* 上海医科大学七十年 (Seventy years of the Shanghai Medical College). Shanghai: Shanghai yike daxue chubanshe, 1997.

Ye Juquan 葉桔泉. "Weisheng yundong yu jiufengsu" 衛生運動與舊風俗 (Hygiene campaigns and old customs). *Weisheng zazhi* 衛生雜誌 19 (1934): 28–29.

Yeh, Wen-hsin. *The Alienated Academy: Culture and Politics in Republican China, 1919–1937*. Cambridge, MA: Council on East Asian Studies, Harvard University Press, 1990.

———. *Provincial Passages: Culture, Space, and the Origins of Chinese Communism.* Berkeley: University of California Press, 1996.

———. "Shanghai Modernity: Commerce and Culture in a Republican City." In *Reappraising Republican China,* edited by Frederic Wakeman and Richard Louis Edmonds, 121–40. New York: Oxford University Press, 2000.

———. *Shanghai Splendor: Economic Sentiments and the Making of Modern China, 1843–1949.* Berkeley: University of California Press, 2007.

———, ed. *Wartime Shanghai.* New York: Routledge, 1998.

———, ed. *Becoming Chinese: Passages to Modernity and Beyond.* Berkeley: University of California Press, 2000

Yeh, Wen-hsin, and Christian Henriot, eds. *In the Shadow of the Rising Sun: Shanghai under the Japanese Occupation.* Cambridge, UK: Cambridge University Press, 2004.

Yi Bin 益斌, Liu Youming 柳又明, and Gan Zhenhu 甘振虎. *Lao Shanghai guanggao* 老上海广告 (Advertisements in old Shanghai). Shanghai: Shanghai huabao chubanshe, 1995.

Yin Wei 殷伟, and Ren Mei 任玫. *Zhongguo muyu wenhua* 中国沐浴文化 (China's bathing culture). Kunming: Yunnan renmin chubanshe, 2003.

Yip, Ka-che. *Health and National Reconstruction in Nationalist China: The Development of Modern Health Care Services, 1928–1937.* Ann Arbor, MI: Association for Asian Studies, 1995.

———. "Health and National Reconstruction: Rural Health in Nationalist China, 1928–1937." *Modern Asian Studies* 26, no. 2 (1992): 395–415.

———. "Health and Society in China: Public Health Education for the Community, 1917–1937." *Social Science and Medicine* 16 (1982): 1197–205.

Yoshida Jirōbē 吉田治郎兵衛. *Chūgoku shin iryō eisei taisei no keisei: ikōki no shijō to shakai* 中国新医療衛生体制の形成：移行期の市場と社会 (The formation of new medical-care systems in China: Market and society in transition). Tokyo: Tōhō Shoten, 2010.

You Qihua 尤其華. "Shenme jiaozuo weisheng yundong" 甚麼叫做衛生運動 (What is the hygiene campaign?). *Weisheng yuekan* 4, no. 3 (1934): 110–11.

Young, Ernest. "Introduction." In *Defining Modernity: Guomindang Rhetorics of a New China, 1920–1970,* edited by Terry Bodenhorn, 1–9. Ann Arbor, MI: Center for Chinese Studies, University of Michigan, 2002.

Yu, Xinzhong. "The Treatment of Night Soil and Waste in Modern China." In *Health and Hygiene in Chinese East Asia,* edited by Angela Ki Che Leung and Charlotte Furth, 51–72. Durham, NC: Duke University Press, 2010.

Yu Xinzhong 余新忠, ed. *Qing yilai de jibing, yiliao he weisheng: yi shehui wenhuashi wei shijiao de tansuo* 清以来的疾病，医疗和卫生：以社会文化史为视角的探索 (Disease, medicine, and hygiene since the Qing period: Exploration from the viewpoint of sociocultural history). Beijing: Shenghuo, dushu, xinzhi sanlian shudian, 2009.

Yuan Fu 元甫. "Tingle lutian zhenliaosuo yixiyu zhi hou" 聽了露天診療所一夕語之後 (After listening to a short conversation at an outdoor clinic). *Shehui yibao* 社會醫報 130 (1930): 1445–46.

Zeng Hongyan 曾宏燕. *Shanghai jushang Huang Chujiu* 上海巨商黄楚九 (Huang Chujiu, Shanghai's great merchant). Beijing: Renmin wenxue chubanshe, 2004.

Zhang Bingrui 張炳瑞. "Chengshi weisheng jiaoyu zhi sheshi" 城市衛生教育之設施 (The facilities of urban health education). *Weisheng yuekan* 4, no. 3 (1934): 105–9.

Zhang Huimin 張惠民. "Chen Diexian yu Jiating gongyeshe" 陈蝶仙与家庭工业社 (Chen Diexian and Household Industries Company). In *Jindai Zhongguo gongshang renwuzhi*, edited by Shou Chongyi, Shou Moliao, and Shou Leying, 179–187. Beijing: Zhongguo wenshi chubanshe, 1996.

———. "Chen Diexian" 陈蝶仙. In *Zhongguo jindai qiye de kaituozhe*, vol. 1, edited by Kong Lingren and Li Dezheng, 597–607. Jinan: Shandong renmin chubanshe, 1991.

Zhang Jishun 張济順. "Kindai ni ishoku sareta dentō: Nihon gunseika Shanghai no hokō seido" 近代に移植された伝統: 日本軍政下上海の保甲制度 (A tradition transplanted into modern times: The *Baojia* system in Shanghai under the Japanese occupation). Translated by Kohama Masako, *Chikaki ni arite* 近きにありて 28 (1996): 25–39.

Zhang Qifu 張圻福, and Wei Heng 韦恒. *Huochai dawang Liu Hongsheng* 火柴大王刘鸿生 (Liu Hongsheng, the majordomo of the match industry). Xinxiang: Henan renmin chubanshe, 1990.

Zhang, Yingjin, ed. *Cinema and Urban Culture in Shanghai, 1922–1943*. Stanford, CA: Stanford University Press, 1999.

Zhang, Zhen. *An Amorous History of the Silver Screen: Shanghai Cinema, 1896–1937*. Chicago: University of Chicago Press, 2005.

Zhang Zhikang 張智康. "Gonggong weisheng" 公共衛生 (Public health). In *Zhonghua minguo kaiguo wushinianshi lunji*, edited by Zhonghua minguo kaiguo wushinian shilunji bianzuan weiyuanhui, 198–219. Taipei: Guofang yanjiuyuan, 1962.

Zhao Yunsheng 趙雲聲, and Liu Mingtao 劉明濤, eds. *Yangchang jushang, chuangye qicai* 洋场巨商, 创业奇才 (Shanghai's great merchants, rare talents who have broken new ground), vol. 10 of *Zhongguo dazibenjia chuanqi* 中國大資本家傳奇 (Biographies of China's great capitalists). Taipei: Wangwenshe, 1998.

Zhao Zengjue 趙曾玨. *Shanghai zhi gongyong shiye* (Shanghai's public works) 上海之公用事業. Shanghai: Shangwu yingshuguan, 1949.

Zheng Zu'an 郑祖安. *Bainian Shanghaicheng* 百年上海城 (One hundred years of the city of Shanghai). Shanghai: Xuelin chubanshe, 1999.

Zhongguo Guomindang zhongyang zhixing weiyuanhui xuanchuanbu 中國國民黨中央執行委員會宣傳部 (Chinese Nationalist Party Central Executive Committee Propaganda Department), ed. *Weisheng yundong xuanchuan gangyao* 衛生運動宣傳綱要 (An outline of propaganda from hygiene campaigns). Nanjing: Zhongyang xuanchuanbu, 1929.

Zhongguo renmin zhengzhi xieshang huiyi Shanghai Shi weiyuanhui wenshi ziliao gongzuo weiyuanhui 中国人民政治协商会议上海市委员会文史资料工作委员会 (Shanghai committee of the Chinese people's political consultation conference, *wenshi ziliao* work committee), ed. *Haishang yilin* 海上医林 (Doctors in Shanghai), vol. 67 of *Shanghai wenshi ziliao xuanji* 上海文史资料选辑 (Accounts of Shanghai's culture and history, selected works). Shanghai: Shanghai renmin chubanshe, 1991.

Zhongguo renmin zhengzhi xieshang huiyi Shanghai Shi weiyuanhui wenshi ziliao gongzuo weiyuanhui 中国人民政治协商会议上海市委员会文史资料工作委员会, ed.

Shanghai renwu shiliao 上海人物史料 (Historical accounts of prominent figures in Shanghai), vol. 70 of *Shanghai wenshi ziliao xuanji* 上海文史资料选辑 (Accounts of Shanghai's culture and history, selected works). Shanghai: Shanghai zhengxie wenshi ziliao bianjibu, 1992.

Zhonghua minguo kaiguo wushinian lunji bianzuan weiyuanhui 中華民國開國五十年論集委員會 (*Zhonghuo minguo kaiguo wushinian lunji* Committee), ed. *Zhonghua minguo kaiguo wushinianshi lunji* 中華民國開國五十年論集 (A collection of studies on the fifty years of the Republic of China). Taipei: Guofang yanjiuyuan, 1962.

Zhou Xueliang 周学良, ed. *Riyong huaxuepin* 日用化学品 (Eveyday-use chemical products). Beijing: Huaxue gongye chubanshe, 2002.

Zhu Jianping 朱建平. *Zhongguo yixueshi yanjiu* 中国医学史研究 (A study of China's medical history). Beijing: Zhongguo guji chubanshe, 2003.

Zhu Mingde 朱明德, and Chen Pei 陈佩, eds. *Renji yiyuan yibai wushiwu nian* 仁济医院一百五十五年 (One hundred fifty-five years of Renji Hospital). Shanghai: Huadong ligong daxue chubanshe, 1999.

Zhu Peilian 朱沛莲. "Ding Wenjiang, Huang Fu yu da Shanghai" 丁文江, 黄郛与大上海 (Ding Wenjian, Huang Fu, and greater Shanghai). In *Ding Wenjiang yinxiang*, edited by Lei Qili, 136–45. Shanghai: Xuelin chubanshe, 1997.

Zurndorfer, Harriet T. "Imperialism, Globalization, and the Soap/Suds Industry in Republican China (1912–37): The Case of Unilever and the Chinese Consumer." Unpublished paper. 2006. http://www.lse.ac.uk/economicHistory/Research/GEHN/GEHNPDF/WorkingPaper19-Zurndorfer.pdf.

Index

Page numbers for figures are in italics.

Perry, Elizabeth, 4
personal hygiene items, 24, 184–86, 195, 196, 211–12, 225; in advertisements, 199, 201, 204, *205, 208,* 209; and chemistry, 190; and entrepreneurs, 194–95, 222–23; and hygiene campaigns, 135, 150; in mass movements, 198–99, 205; and *weisheng,* 223. *See also* soap; toothpaste; toothpowder
Peter, W. W., 141
pharmaceutical business, 73, 183, 230, 237–38; and SEH, 58–59
pharmacy, 27, 61
Plans and Ideas for the Health of Greater Shanghai, 139
police: and cholera control work, 119–20, 122–23; hygiene campaign, *161,* 171–73, 178; and injection, 108; and public health, 79, 89–90, 94–95, 98, 104, 110
printed materials. *See under* hygiene campaign
procession, 129, 168–70
promiscuous urination, 157, *160, 161*
public health bureau, 85. *See also* Shanghai Public Health Bureau (PHB)
Public Health Bureau of the Wusong-Shanghai Commercial Port. *See* Songhu Public Health Bureau
Public Health Department (International Settlement), 86–87, 90, 153, 154; on discussion about fine, 173–74
public health division, 85
Public Health Office, 23
public health sections, 112
public urination, 157. *See also* promiscuous urination
Public Utilities Bureau, 100
publishing companies (in Shanghai), 154
Pure and White brand toothpaste, 201, *203*

Qing: commerce, 194; exhibitions, 152; hygiene campaign, 130–31; medical policy, 79–80; medical syncretism, 65; reformers, 14, 141; science, 190, 192
Quaker Oatmeal, 7–8, *8*

radio broadcast, 54, 136, 162–63
Red Cross Society, 51, 56, 58, 235
red medical workers, 235
"Regulations on the Enforcement of Cholera Prevention," 118–19
"Regulations of the Wusong-Shanghai Public Health Bureau," 90
religious teaching: at Renji, 35–36; at Tongren, 42
Renji Hospital: community service, 36; donations, 37–38; finance, 37; grants from SMC, 38–39; history, 32–33, 36–37; patient fees, 39–40; religious activities, 35–36; scientific research, 46–47; soup kitchen, 36; Women's Auxiliary Department, 41
Renjij Yiguan (Renji Medical Office), 34
renshu jishi, 34
repertoire: of collective actions, 24, 132, 226; cultural, 232; of protest, 4
Republican period, 15–16, 130, 141; Chinese medicine, 66; medical market, 27; scholarship on, 16–17
residents' committees, 235–36, 243, 246
residents' committee health station, 235–36, 243
responsibility system, 237
rituals, 24, 170; of death, 56; of Duanwujie, 137; and hygiene campaign, 147, 164, 167–68
Rockefeller Foundation, 77, 81
Rockefeller, John D. Jr., 81
Roentgen, Wilhelm Konrad, 46
Rogaski, Ruth, 1, 19, 87, 114n138, 179, 206n62
Rosenberg, Charles, 46–47
Ruan Renze, 31

sanitary bureau, 79, 86
sanitation and hygiene campaign, 240–41
SARS, 244–48; and Chinese medicine, 248–49; and social life in Beijing, 246
Scheid, Volker, 66
scholar-physician, 60–61, 60n129
Schoppa, Keith, 126